Strategies for
Managing

Multisystem
Disorders

Strategies for *Managing*

Multisystem Disorders

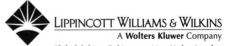

LIPPINCOTT WILLIAMS & WILKINS
A **Wolters Kluwer** Company

Philadelphia • Baltimore • New York • London
Buenos Aires • Hong Kong • Sydney • Tokyo

STAFF

Executive Publisher
Judith A. Schilling McCann, RN, MSN

Editorial Director
H. Nancy Holmes

Clinical Director
Joan M. Robinson, RN, MSN

Senior Art Director
Arlene Putterman

Editorial Project Manager
Jennifer P. Kowalak

Clinical Project Manager
Beverly Ann Tscheschlog, RN, BS

Design
Debra Moloshok (book design
and project manager)

Editor
Liz Schaeffer

Clinical Editors
Joanne M. Bartelmo, RN, MSN;
Maryann Foley, RN, BSN;
Collette Bishop Hendler, RN, BS, CCRN;
Tamara M. Kear, RN, MSN, CNN;
Kate McGovern, RN, MSN;
Jana Sciarra, RN, MSN, CRNP

Copy Editors
Kimberly Bilotta (supervisor), Heather Ditch,
Shana Harrington, Kelly Pavlovsky,
Pamela Wingrod

Digital Composition Services
Diane Paluba (manager), Joyce Rossi Biletz,
Donna S. Morris

Manufacturing
Patricia K. Dorshaw (director), Beth J. Welsh

Editorial Assistants
Megan L. Aldinger, Karen J. Kirk,
Linda K. Ruhf

Indexer
Barbara Hodgson

Library of Congress
Cataloging-in-Publication Data
Strategies for managing multisystem disorders
    p. ; cm.
  Includes bibliographical references and index.
  1. Catastrophic illness. 2. Internal medicine.
I. Lippincott Williams & Wilkins. [DNLM: 1. Diagnosis. 2. Therapeutics — methods. 3. Patient Care Team.]
  RC48.S77 2006
  616.07'5 — dc22
ISBN 1-58255-423-4 (alk. paper)   2005002803

Contents

Contributors and consultants

Beverly Anderson, RN, MSN
Associate Professor
Malcolm X College
Chicago

Peggy Bozarth, RN, MSN
Professor
Hopkinsville (Ky.) Community College

Deirdre Herr Byers, RN, BSN, CCRN
Staff Nurse
Southeast Georgia Health System
Brunswick

Merry Jahn Chandler, RN, MA, MSN
Assistant Professor, College of Nursing
McNeese State University
Lake Charles, La.

Margaret Davis, MSN, RN
Assistant Professor of Nursing
Central Florida Community College
Ocala

Louise M. Diehl-Oplinger, RN, MSN,
  APRN,BC, CCRN
Family Nurse Practitioner
Coventry Cardiology Associates
Phillipsburg, N.J.

Laurie Donaghy, RN, CEN
Staff Nurse
Frankford Hospital
Philadelphia

Shelba Durston, RN, MSN, CCRN
Nursing Instructor
San Joaquin Delta College
Stockton, Calif.
Staff Nurse
San Joaquin General Hospital
French Camp, Calif.

Carrin L. Dvorak, RN, MSN
Assistant Professor of Nursing
Cuyahoga Community College
Cleveland

Diane M. Ellis, RN, MSN, CCRN
Nursing Instructor
Villanova (Pa.) University
Service Excellence Consultant
Glen Mills, Pa.

Emilie M. Fedorov, RN, MSN, CS
Nurse Manager
Cleveland Clinic Foundation

Stephen Gilliam, FNP, PhD, APRN,BC
Assistant Professor
Medical College of Georgia
School of Nursing
Athens

Margaret M. Gingrich, RN, MSN
Associate Professor
Harrisburg (Pa.) Area Community College

Mary T. Kowalski, RN, BA, MSN
Director/Instructor Vocational Nursing &
  Health Career Programs
Cerro Coso Community College
Ridgecrest, Calif.

Grace G. Lewis, RN, MS, CNS, APRN,CS
Assistant Professor of Nursing
Georgia Baptist College of Nursing of Mercer
  University
Atlanta

Valerie Mignatti, RN, BSN
Clinical Cardiovascular Nurse
Hospital of the University of Pennsylvania
Philadelphia

Jolynne Myers, RNBC, MSN, MSEd, ANP
Employee Health & Worker's Compensation
  Coordinator
Baptist–Lutheran Medical Center
Kansas City, Mo.

Abby Plambeck, RN, BSN
Freelance Writer
Milwaukee

Cynthia A. Prows, RN, MSN, CNS
Clinical Nurse Specialist, Genetics
Children's Hospital Medical Center
Cincinnati

Donna Scemons, RN, MSN, FNP-C, CNS,
  CWOCN
Family Nurse Practitioner
Healthcare Systems, Inc.
Panorama City, Calif.

Colleen R. Walsh, RN, MSN, ONC, CS,
  ACNP-BC
Faculty, Graduate Nursing
University of Southern Indiana
  School of Nursing & Health Professions
Evansville

Foreword

It's a prevalent perception in the health care community that caring for patients in this millennium is challenging and, at times, complex, because of the high level of acuity of patients not only in hospitals but also in home-care agencies, long-term care facilities, and physicians' offices. Furthermore, the number of patients who have multiple diagnoses (with increasing severity) is on the rise. Health care professionals and students alike are required to have a broad knowledge base about these multisystem conditions, including their causes, assessment findings, and care management. Indeed, today's health care professional must see beyond the patient's primary diagnosis and be adept at uncovering coexisting disorders, anticipating complications, and determining how these problems interact and influence the progress and positive response of patients to treatment.

Strategies for Managing Multisystem Disorders covers more than 75 disorders and how each condition can interact and affect other diseases. One of the premier features of this book is its emphasis on the multidisciplinary team approach—a growing trend in today's health care arena regardless of the clinical setting. For example, the patient with myocardial infarction may also suffer from diabetes mellitus and thyroid disease, necessitating the counsel of an endocrinologist who can help adapt the treatment and care plan. The pregnant patient with asthma may need the services of a dietician to monitor weight gain during her pregnancy because excess weight gain may increase diaphragmatic elevation and decrease functional residual capacity.

Strategies for Managing Multisystem Disorders is organized A-to-Z for quick retrieval of information, when needed. Each multisystem disorder entry concisely covers overview, which includes description, incidence, risk factors, prognosis; etiology;

pathophysiology, including how multiple body systems are affected; assessment, which includes clinical findings and diagnostic test results; collaborative management; and treatment and care. The various charts, tables, and illustrations supplement and condense essential information throughout the text. Further, special icons highlight critical information including:

■ *Watchful eye*—describes what to look for and how to adapt care in patients with a multisystem disorder who may also have a coexisting disorder or who may develop complications.

■ *Red flag*—highlights emergency or life-threatening findings that signal immediate intervention.

■ *Up close*—diagrams the underlying pathophysiologic processes of the given multisystem disorder.

■ *Drug alert*—emphasizes possible complications of multisystem disorders related to drug therapy.

Helpful appendices include quick-reference guide to laboratory test results, blood factors and products, and Internet resources.

In summary, *Strategies for Managing Multisystem Disorders* addresses disorders that require comprehensive, coordinated, and integrated interventions. No doubt, it will help today's health care professional meet the challenge of providing the best possible care to patients with multisystem disorders.

Evelyn Yeaw, RN, PhD
Professor and Chairperson Nursing
    Education
Graduate Program
University of Rhode Island
South Kingston

Strategies for
Managing

Multisystem Disorders

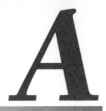

Abdominal trauma

Abdominal trauma may occur as a singular injury or, more commonly, as a part of combined multisystem and multiorgan trauma. Most patients with this type of injury are younger than age 50, and half are involved in motor vehicle accidents.

Morbidity and mortality of patients with abdominal trauma are directly affected by early diagnosis and prompt treatment. Early detection may prove challenging because about one-third of patients with abdominal injuries show no outward signs of trauma. Some patients develop delayed organ rupture or hemorrhage hours or days after the initial traumatic event.

ETIOLOGY

Abdominal trauma may be classified as blunt or penetrating. Blunt abdominal trauma involves the crushing, shearing, bursting, tearing, or compression of abdominal organs (especially the spleen, liver, pancreas, and intestines) and possibly secondary perforation from fracture fragments. Most commonly caused by motor vehicle accidents or falls, blunt abdominal trauma may also result from injuries sustained during assaults with blunt objects. Blunt abdominal trauma carries a higher mortality risk than penetrating trauma because patients can have severe internal damage with little external evidence of injury, resulting in delayed detection and treatment.

Penetrating trauma is most commonly caused by gunshot or stab wounds. Impalement by various objects can also cause this type of injury. The appearance of entrance and exit wounds doesn't determine the extent of internal injury. For example, bullets may fragment and change direction once inside the body.

Abdominal trauma may also occur in patients with associated spinal, thoracic, or pelvic injuries. Acceleration-deceleration injuries may produce spinal fractures and great vessel disruption, as well as abdominal injuries that may not be apparent for hours to days. Seat-belt restraints may produce pelvic disruption in addition to intraperitoneal or retroperitoneal injuries.

PATHOPHYSIOLOGY

Blunt and penetrating abdominal trauma may be associated with extensive damage to the abdominal organs, possibly resulting in massive blood loss. Generally, blunt trauma causes greater injury to solid organs (liver, spleen, pancreas, and kidneys), whereas penetrating trauma causes greater injury to hollow organs (stomach, small intestine, large intestine, and urinary bladder).

When a blunt object strikes a person's abdomen, it raises intra-abdominal pressure. Depending on the force of the blow, the trauma can lacerate the liver and spleen, rupture the stomach, bruise the duodenum, and even damage the kidneys.

Trauma to solid organs typically results in bleeding from lacerations or fractures; trauma to hollow organs results in rupture and release of organ contents into the abdominal cavity, which causes inflammation and infection. Regardless of whether the trauma is blunt or penetrating, the greater the speed or force behind the injury, the greater the degree of trauma sustained and the greater the risk of complications. (See *Disorders affecting management of abdominal trauma*, pages 2 to 5.)

Cardiovascular system
■ After abdominal trauma, massive fluid shifts can occur (for example, fluid shifts to the bowel wall or irritated peritoneum), resulting in decreased vascular volume.

(*Text continues on page 4.*)

WATCHFUL EYE

DISORDERS AFFECTING MANAGEMENT OF ABDOMINAL TRAUMA

This chart highlights disorders that affect the management of abdominal trauma.

DISORDER	SIGNS AND SYMPTOMS	DIAGNOSTIC TEST RESULTS
Disseminated intravascular coagulation (complication)	◆ Abnormal bleeding without a history of a hemorrhagic disorder ◆ Bleeding into the skin, such as cutaneous oozing, petechiae, ecchymoses, and hematomas ◆ Bleeding from surgical or invasive procedure sites, such as incisions or venipuncture sites ◆ Nausea and vomiting ◆ Severe muscle, back, and abdominal pain or chest pain ◆ Hemoptysis and epistaxis ◆ Seizures ◆ Oliguria ◆ Diminished peripheral pulses ◆ Hypotension ◆ Mental status changes, including confusion	◆ Platelet count is decreased. ◆ Fibrinogen level is less than 150 mg/dl. ◆ Prothrombin time is greater than 15 seconds. ◆ Partial thromboplastin time is greater than 60 seconds. ◆ Fibrin degradation products are increased, often greater than 45 mcg/ml. ◆ D-dimer test is positive at less than 1:8 dilution. ◆ Fibrin monomers are positive; levels of factors V and VIII are diminished with fragmentation of red blood cells (RBCs). ◆ Hemoglobin is less than 10 g/dl. ◆ Urine studies reveal blood urea nitrogen (BUN) greater than 25 mg/dl. ◆ Serum creatinine level is greater than 1.3 mg/dl.
Hypovolemic shock (complication)	*Minimal volume loss (10% to 15%)* ◆ Slight tachycardia ◆ Normal supine blood pressure ◆ Positive postural vital signs, including a decrease in systolic blood pressure that's greater than 10 mm Hg or an increase in pulse rate that's greater than 20 beats/minute ◆ Increased capillary refill time (longer than 3 seconds) ◆ Urine output more than 30 ml/hour ◆ Cool, pale skin on arms and legs ◆ Anxiety *Moderate volume loss (about 25%)* ◆ Rapid, thready pulse ◆ Supine hypotension ◆ Cool truncal skin ◆ Urine output of 10 to 30 ml/hour ◆ Severe thirst ◆ Restlessness, confusion, or irritability *Severe volume loss (40% or more)* ◆ Marked tachycardia ◆ Marked hypotension ◆ Weak or absent peripheral pulses ◆ Cold, mottled, or cyanotic skin ◆ Urine output less than 10 ml/hour ◆ Unconsciousness	◆ Complete blood count reveals low hematocrit and decreased hemoglobin level, RBC count, and platelet counts. ◆ Metabolic studies reveal elevated serum potassium, sodium, lactate dehydrogenase, creatinine, and BUN levels. ◆ Urine studies reveal increased urine specific gravity (greater than 1.020) and urine osmolality and urine sodium levels less than 50 mEq/L. ◆ Urine creatinine levels may be decreased. ◆ ABG analysis may reveal decreased pH and partial pressure of arterial oxygen and increased partial pressure of arterial carbon dioxide. ◆ Gastroscopy, X-rays, and aspiration of gastric contents through a nasogastric tube may reveal evidence of frank or occult bleeding. ◆ Coagulation studies may show evidence of coagulopathy.

TREATMENT AND CARE

◆ Ensure a patent airway, and assess breathing and circulation. Monitor vital signs and cardiac and respiratory status closely, at least every 30 minutes, or more frequently, depending on the patient's condition.

● Observe skin color and check peripheral circulation, including color, temperature, and capillary refill.

◆ Administer supplemental oxygen, and monitor oxygen saturation with continuous pulse oximetry and serial arterial blood gas (ABG) analysis; anticipate the need for endotracheal intubation and mechanical ventilation should the patient's respiratory status deteriorate.

◆ Assess neurologic status frequently – at least every hour, or more often as indicated – for changes.

● Assess the extent of blood loss, and begin fluid replacement. Obtain a blood type, and crossmatch for blood component therapy.

◆ If hypotension occurs, administer vasoactive drugs, such as amrinone (Inocor), dobutamine (Dobutrex), dopamine (Intropin), epinephrine, and nitroprusside (Nitropress).

◆ Assess hemodynamic parameters.

◆ Institute continuous cardiac monitoring to evaluate for possible arrhythmias, myocardial ischemia, or adverse effects of treatment.

◆ Administer heparin I.V. in low doses, antifibrinolytic agents cautiously, and vitamin K and folate (to correct deficiencies).

◆ Assess urine output hourly; check all stools and drainage for occult blood.

◆ Inspect skin and mucous membranes for signs of bleeding; assess all invasive insertion sites and dressings for evidence of frank bleeding or oozing. Weigh the dressings that are wet or saturated to aid in determining the extent of blood loss. Watch for bleeding from the GI and genitourinary tracts.

◆ Institute bleeding precautions. Limit all invasive procedures, such as venipunctures and I.M. injections, as much as possible. Apply pressure for 3 to 5 minutes over venous insertion sites and for 10 to 15 minutes over arterial sites.

◆ Institute safety precautions to minimize the risk of injury.

◆ Assess the extent of blood loss, and begin fluid replacement.

◆ Obtain a blood type, and crossmatch for blood component therapy.

◆ Assess airway, breathing, and circulation, and institute emergency resuscitative measures.

◆ Administer supplemental oxygen, and monitor oxygen saturation.

◆ Monitor vital signs and hemodynamic status continuously for changes. Observe skin color and check capillary refill.

◆ Institute continuous cardiac monitoring to evaluate for possible arrhythmias, myocardial ischemia, or adverse effects of treatment.

◆ Assess neurologic status frequently – about every 30 minutes until the patient stabilizes, and then every 2 to 4 hours.

◆ Monitor urine output at least hourly.

◆ Administer dopamine or norepinephrine (Levophed) I.V. to increase cardiac contractility and renal perfusion.

◆ During therapy, assess skin color and temperature, and note changes.

◆ Watch for signs of impending coagulopathy (such as petechiae, bruising, bleeding or oozing from gums or venipuncture sites).

◆ Prepare the patient for surgery (as appropriate).

(continued)

DISORDERS AFFECTING MANAGEMENT OF ABDOMINAL TRAUMA *(continued)*

DISORDER	SIGNS AND SYMPTOMS	DIAGNOSTIC TEST RESULTS
Peritonitis (complication)	◆ Vague or localized abdominal pain or diffuse pain over abdomen that becomes increasingly severe and unremitting; increases with movement and respirations; may be referred to the shoulder or the thoracic area ◆ Abdominal distention ◆ Anorexia, nausea, and vomiting ◆ Inability to pass feces and flatus ◆ Fever, tachycardia, and hypotension ◆ Lying still in bed with knees flexed to try to alleviate abdominal pain ◆ Shallow breathing ◆ Excessive sweating ◆ Cool, clammy skin ◆ Pallor ◆ Signs of dehydration ◆ Diminished to absent bowel sounds ◆ Abdominal rigidity and rebound tenderness	◆ White blood cell count shows leukocytosis (commonly more than 20,000/mm³). ◆ Serum electrolyte levels may be abnormal; albumin levels may be decreased, suggesting bacterial peritonitis. ◆ Abdominal X-rays show edematous and gaseous distention of the small and large bowel. With perforation of a visceral organ, the X-ray shows air in the abdominal cavity. ◆ Chest X-ray may reveal elevation of the diaphragm. ◆ Abdominal ultrasound may reveal fluid collections. ◆ Paracentesis discloses the nature of the exudate and permits bacterial culture so appropriate antibiotic therapy can be started.

■ Blood and fluid may be lost from an open penetrating abdominal wound, further decreasing vascular volume and increasing fluid loss.

■ Injury to the spleen or the abdominal aorta or inferior vena cava can lead to massive hemorrhage and fluid loss. If left untreated, hypovolemic shock can occur. If prolonged, hypovolemia can lead to organ ischemia and failure.

Gastrointestinal system

■ Rupture of the stomach, bowel, or liver can lead to spillage of organ contents and secretions into the normally sterile peritoneal cavity. This leakage initiates an inflammatory response.

■ The release of bacteria and intestinal contents into the peritoneum leads to peritonitis. If peritonitis progresses, sepsis may occur.

■ Electrolyte imbalances occur because of the disruption in the GI tract's integrity.

Hematologic system

■ Major abdominal trauma can result in the loss of massive amounts of blood and body fluid.

■ The body experiences systemic inflammation and metabolic changes secondary to the stress and the release of catecholamines that ultimately affect the vasculature.

■ Coagulation factors are mobilized in response to blood loss. These factors can become depleted, upsetting the delicate balance among the components needed for hemostasis.

■ If massive blood transfusions are necessary, hemostasis may be further disrupted. Subsequently, disseminated intravascular coagulation can occur.

ASSESSMENT

Abdominal trauma should be suspected in all patients who have experienced trauma, even if no signs of injury are apparent. Because deterioration in the patient's condition may occur rapidly (for example, because of

TREATMENT AND CARE

◆ Ensure a patent airway, and assess the patient's respiratory status at least every hour, or more frequently as indicated; auscultate lungs bilaterally for adventitious or diminished breath sounds.

◆ Assess oxygen saturation continuously with pulse oximetry or mixed venous oxygen saturation through a pulmonary artery catheter (if in place).

◆ Monitor serial ABG levels.

◆ If the patient's respiratory status deteriorates, assist with endotracheal intubation and mechanical ventilation.

◆ Place the patient in a comfortable position that maximizes air exchange.

◆ Closely monitor the patient's heart rate and blood pressure at least every hour, or more frequently as indicated; institute continuous cardiac monitoring, observe for arrhythmias, and prepare to treat.

◆ Monitor the patient's temperature every 1 to 2 hours; administer antipyretics, and use measures to reduce the patient's temperature, such as a hypothermia blanket and tepid sponge baths.

◆ Assess hemodynamic status closely – at least every hour, or more frequently as indicated.

◆ Insert or assist with intubation with a nasogastric or nasoenteric tube, if not already in place. Monitor tube drainage every 1 to 2 hours for color, amount, and characteristics.

◆ Assess the abdomen for evidence of bowel sounds and distention. Maintain nothing-by-mouth status until bowel function returns. Expect to administer histamine-2 receptor antagonists to reduce the risk of gastric ulcer formation.

◆ Administer I.V. fluid and electrolyte replacement; prepare to administer blood component therapy if hemorrhage occurs.

◆ Administer I.V. antimicrobial agents.

◆ Monitor intake and output closely; assess urine output hourly.

◆ Assess neurologic status for changes.

◆ Assess patient's complaints of pain and administer analgesics based on patient's degree of pain.

◆ Prepare the patient for surgery (as appropriate).

internal bleeding), accurate baseline data and astute assessment skills are essential for timely detection and treatment. During the initial history, the nurse should attempt to ascertain (if possible) the mechanism of injury, including:

■ if a fall, the height and point of impact

■ if a motor vehicle accident, the patient's placement in the car, use of a seat belt, speed and type of impact, and internal damage to the vehicle

■ if a gunshot wound, the caliber of gun and range of fire (as reported by the authorities)

■ if a stab wound, the length and type of object and the sex of the attacker (males are more likely to stab upward, whereas females tend to stab downward).

The history should also determine the location and quality of pain, any history of abdominal surgeries, and the presence of nausea and vomiting.

Clinical manifestations of abdominal trauma depend on the specific organs injured. Generally, signs and symptoms associated with abdominal trauma include obvious injury to the abdomen, hemodynamic instability, pain, nausea and vomiting, abdominal distention, and decreased or absent bowel sounds. (See *Assessing for abdominal organ injuries*, page 6.)

Assessment of the abdomen involves inspection, auscultation, percussion, and palpation — in that order. Auscultation must be done before percussion or palpation because those maneuvers may alter the frequency of bowel sounds. Additionally, painful or tender areas are always percussed and palpated last.

Clinical findings

■ Obvious signs of trauma (including on the back), such as stab, puncture, or gunshot wounds, bruising, or lacerations

■ Masses

■ Pulsations

■ Asymmetry

■ Discoloration

ASSESSING FOR ABDOMINAL ORGAN INJURIES

Specific organ injuries associated with abdominal trauma and their assessment findings are outlined below.

ORGAN	ASSESSMENT FINDINGS
Colon	◆ Possible rectal bleeding ◆ Peritoneal irritation due to perforation ◆ Signs of obstruction
Diaphragm	◆ Bowel sounds in chest ◆ Decreased breath sounds ◆ Chest pain
Duodenum	◆ Fever ◆ Jaundice ◆ Vomiting ◆ Pain ◆ Peritoneal signs
Esophagus	◆ Pain that radiates to the neck, chest, or shoulders ◆ Possible diffuse abdominal pain ◆ Dysphagia
Liver	◆ Tenderness of right upper quadrant with guarding ◆ Peritoneal irritation ◆ Right shoulder pain when lying flat or in Trendelenburg's position ◆ Positive Kehr's sign ◆ Positive Ballance's sign
Pancreas	◆ Positive Grey Turner's sign (ecchymosis in the flank area, suggesting retroperitoneal bleeding) ◆ Ileus ◆ Epigastric pain radiating to the back, or pain in the left upper quadrant ◆ Nausea and vomiting ◆ Positive Kehr's sign (pain in the left shoulder secondary to diaphragmatic irritation by blood)
Small intestine	◆ Ileus ◆ Peritoneal irritation ◆ Abdominal pain and tenderness ◆ Guarding ◆ Decreased or absent bowel sounds
Spleen	◆ Left-upper-quadrant pain radiating to the left shoulder ◆ Shock ◆ Positive Kehr's sign ◆ Positive Ballance's sign ◆ Peritoneal irritation ◆ Rigidity
Stomach	◆ Blood in nasogastric aspirate or hematemesis ◆ Epigastric pain and tenderness ◆ Signs of peritonitis due to release of acidic gastric contents ◆ Guarding ◆ Decreased or absent bowel sounds ◆ Shock

- Abdominal distention
- Decreased or absent bowel sounds (possibly caused by an irritant, such as blood or intestinal contents outside the bowel)
- Hyperactive bowel sounds (possibly the result of irritants inside the bowel)
- Bruits over the abdominal aorta, renal arteries, and femoral arteries

RED FLAG If bruits are auscultated, don't perform percussion or palpation because there's a risk of rupturing the aorta.

- Dullness on percussion, suggesting fluid
- Tympany, indicating air
- Rebound tenderness and guarding, indicating inflammation of the peritoneum
- Blood and possible anterior tenderness with peritoneal irritation on rectal palpation
- Possible coexisting injuries, such as head, thoracic, or orthopedic injuries, and their associated signs and symptoms

Diagnostic test results

- *Complete blood count* reveals an increase in the white blood cell (WBC) count. Early, mild elevation in the WBC count results from the neuroendocrine stress response; extreme elevation later on may indicate peritoneal inflammation. Hemoglobin and hematocrit levels are reduced with hemorrhage.
- *Serum amylase level* may be elevated with injuries to the duodenum or pancreas.
- *Serum bilirubin level* may be increased with duodenal or liver injuries.
- *Serum lipase level* may be increased with pancreatic injury.
- *Chest X-ray* may reveal lower rib fractures, raising the risk of injury to the liver or spleen. Abdominal contents in the chest cavity indicate a diaphragmatic tear. Right diaphragm elevation may be seen in injury to the liver.
- *Abdominal X-ray* may reveal foreign bodies or free air in the abdomen, which indicates perforation of abdominal organs.
- *Diagnostic peritoneal lavage* may be positive for blood, bile, or bacteria; WBC count is greater than 500/µl; red blood cell count is greater than 100,000/µl; amylase is greater than 175 U/dl.
- *Computed tomography* or *magnetic resonance imaging* may reveal bleeding, organ contusion, laceration, or rupture.

COLLABORATIVE MANAGEMENT

A patient experiencing abdominal trauma requires a multidisciplinary team approach, depending on the extent of his injuries. He may require the aid of neurologists, cardiologists, respiratory therapists, or surgeons. The patient and his family may also benefit from supportive and spiritual care as well as referral to community resources.

TREATMENT AND CARE

- The primary goals of treatment for the patient with abdominal trauma are to maintain hemodynamic stability, maintain organ function, and prevent major complications.

RED FLAG Perform emergency interventions, including maintaining airway, breathing, and circulation and a patent airway.

RED FLAG Never remove an object that has penetrated the abdomen. The object may provide a sealing effect to the surrounding tissues or organ; its removal could result in massive hemorrhage.

- Administer I.V. fluid replacement therapy and blood components to control hemorrhage and prevent hypovolemic shock. Monitor intake and output; report if urine output is less than 30 mL/hour.
- Monitor heart rate and rhythm, heart sounds, and blood pressure every hour for changes; use continuous cardiac monitoring to detect possible arrhythmias.
- Perform hemodynamic monitoring, including central venous pressure, pulmonary capillary wedge pressure, and cardiac output, as indicated, at least every 1 to 2 hours.
- Auscultate breath sounds at least every 2 hours, reporting a decrease in or absence of breath sounds or signs of congestion or fluid accumulation.
- Monitor oxygen saturation levels with serial arterial blood gas measurements. Administer supplemental oxygen at the ordered flow rate.
- Assist with endotracheal intubation and mechanical ventilation if the patient's respiratory status deteriorates or if the patient has difficulty maintaining a patent airway and adequate breathing.
- Assess dressings over penetrating trauma sites frequently, at least every 2 to 4 hours for the first 24 to 48 hours.

RED FLAG Report if dressings become saturated or require changing more

*than twice in 24 hours, or if drainage appears
bright red.*
■ Administer antiarrhythmics, inotropic
agents, or antibiotics.
■ Connect a nasogastric tube to intermittent suction to achieve gastric decompression.
■ Frequently monitor hemoglobin and
hematocrit levels for changes.
■ Assess the patient's pain and administer
analgesics.
■ Position the patient with the head of bed
elevated 30 to 45 degrees.
■ Perform pulmonary hygiene measures,
including coughing and deep breathing and
splinting the abdomen.
■ Provide frequent rest periods to decrease
oxygen demands.
■ Prepare for possible surgery when the patient is stabilized.

Acquired immunodeficiency syndrome

Acquired immunodeficiency syndrome
(AIDS) is marked by progressive failure of
the immune system. Although it's characterized by gradual destruction of cell-mediated
(T-cell) immunity, it also affects humoral immunity and autoimmunity because of the
central role of the CD4+ T lymphocyte in
immune reactions. The resultant immunodeficiency makes the patient susceptible to opportunistic infections, unusual cancers, and
other abnormalities.

The disease is disproportionately repre-
sented in:
■ homosexual and bisexual men
■ I.V. drug users
■ neonates of infected women
■ recipients of contaminated blood or
blood products
■ heterosexual partners of people in these
above groups.

Human immunodeficiency virus (HIV)
may enter the body through:
■ sexual contact with an infected person
(especially linked to the mucosal trauma of
rectal intercourse)

■ transfusion of contaminated blood or
blood products
■ sharing of contaminated injection needles
■ transplacental or postpartum transmission from an infected mother to her fetus
(by cervical or blood contact at delivery and
in breast milk).

ETIOLOGY
HIV, particularly the HIV-1 retrovirus, is the
primary cause of AIDS.

PATHOPHYSIOLOGY
HIV strikes helper T cells bearing the CD4+
antigen. Normally a receptor for major histocompatibility complex molecules, the antigen serves as a receptor for the retrovirus
and allows it to enter the cell. Viral binding
also requires the presence of a coreceptor
(believed to be the chemokine receptor
CCR5) on the cell surface. The virus also
may infect CD4+ antigen–bearing cells of the
GI tract, uterine cervix, and neuroglia.

Like other retroviruses, HIV copies its genetic material in a reverse manner compared
with other viruses and cells. Through the action of reverse transcriptase, HIV produces
deoxyribonucleic acid (DNA) from its viral
ribonucleic acid (RNA). Transcription is
usually poor, leading to mutations, some of
which make HIV resistant to antiviral drugs.

The viral DNA enters the nucleus of the
cell and is incorporated into the host cell's
DNA, where it's transcribed into more viral
RNA. If the host cell reproduces, it dupli-
cates the HIV DNA along with its own and
passes it on to the daughter cells. Thus, if
activated, the host cell carries this information and replicates the virus. Viral enzymes — proteases — arrange the structural
components and RNA into viral particles
that move to the periphery of the host cell,
where the virus buds and emerges. Thus, the
virus is now free to travel and infect other
cells. (See *How HIV replicates.*)

HIV replication may lead to cell death or
may become latent. HIV infection leads to
profound changes, either directly through
destruction of CD4+ cells or other immune
cells and neuroglial cells, or directly through
the secondary effects of CD4+ T-cell destruction and resulting immunosuppression. (See
Disorders affecting management of AIDS,
pages 10 to 13.)

(Text continues on page 14.)

How HIV replicates

This flowchart shows the steps in human immunodeficiency virus (HIV) cell replication.

HIV enters the bloodstream.

▼

HIV attaches to the surface of the CD4+ T lymphocyte.

▼

Proteins on the HIV cell surface bind to the protein receptors on the host cell's surface.

▼

HIV penetrates the host cell membrane and injects its protein coat into the host cell's cytoplasm.

▼

HIV's genetic information, ribonucleic acid (RNA), is released into the cell after its protective coat is partially dissolved.

▼

The single-stranded viral RNA, via the action of reverse transcriptase, is converted (transcribed) into double-stranded deoxyribonucleic acid (DNA).

▼

Viral DNA integrates itself into the host cell's nucleus.

▼

Integrase, an enzyme, inserts HIV's double-stranded DNA into the host cell's DNA.

▼

When the host cell is activated, the viral DNA takes over, telling the host cell to produce RNA (now viral RNA).

▼

Two strands of RNA are produced and transported out of the nucleus.

▼

One strand becomes the subunits of the HIV (that is, enzymes and structural proteins); the other becomes the genetic material for new viruses.

▼

Cleavage occurs (viral subunits are separated) through the action of protease, a viral enzyme.

▼

HIV subunits combine to make up new viral particles and begin to break down the host cell membrane.

▼

The genetic material in the new viral particles merges with the cell membrane that has been changed, forming a new viral envelope (outer covering).

▼

Viral budding occurs, in which the new HIV is released to enter the circulation.

DISORDERS AFFECTING
MANAGEMENT OF AIDS

This chart highlights disorders that affect the management of acquired immunodeficiency syndrome (AIDS).

DISORDER	SIGNS AND SYMPTOMS	DIAGNOSTIC TEST RESULTS
Cryptosporidiosis (complication)	◆ Frequent stools (6 to 26 per day) ◆ Fever ◆ Watery diarrhea ◆ Right-upper-quadrant pain and cramping ◆ Flatulence ◆ Nausea and vomiting ◆ Weight loss ◆ Malaise	◆ Stool testing is positive for ova and parasites.
Cytomegalovirus (CMV) (complication)	◆ Blind or dark spots in visual field (scotomas) ◆ Loss of peripheral vision ◆ Visual floaters ◆ Chorioretinitis ◆ Difficulty concentrating ◆ Sleepiness ◆ Mouth ulcerations ◆ Dysphagia ◆ Abdominal pain ◆ Bloody diarrhea ◆ Weight loss ◆ Rectal ulcers ◆ Persistent fever ◆ Fatigue ◆ Urine retention ◆ Incontinence	◆ Complement fixation studies and hemagglutination inhibition antibody tests isolate the virus. ◆ Chest X-ray reveals bilateral, diffuse, white infiltrates.
Kaposi's sarcoma (complication)	◆ Multicentric skin lesions that vary from brown to red to purple ◆ Swelling and pain in the lower extremities, penis, scrotum, or face	◆ With CNS involvement, lumbar puncture indicates increased pressure; cerebrospinal fluid analysis demonstrates increased protein levels and, possibly, pleocytosis. ◆ Tissue biopsy determines the lesion's type and stage. ◆ Computed tomography (CT) scan may show areas of metastasis.

TREATMENT AND CARE

◆ Closely monitor the patient's fluid and electrolyte balance.
◆ Encourage an adequate intake of fluids, especially those rich in electrolytes.
◆ Monitor the patient's intake and output, and weigh him daily to evaluate the need for fluid replacement. Watch him closely for signs of dehydration, and provide fluid replacement.
◆ Administer analgesics, antidiarrheal and antiperistaltic agents, and antibiotics. Observe the patient for signs of adverse reactions as well as therapeutic effects.
◆ Apply perirectal protective cream to prevent excoriation and skin breakdown.
◆ Encourage small, frequent meals to help prevent nausea.
◆ Administer amphotericin B with or without flucytosine (Ancobon), fluconazole (Diflucan), or itraconazole (Sporonox).

◆ Institute standard precautions before coming into contact with the patient's blood or other body fluids. Secretion precautions are especially important for infants.
◆ Administer medications to treat symptoms.
◆ Monitor intake and output. Offer nutritionally adequate meals. If the patient has diarrhea, replace fluids.
◆ Provide emotional support and counseling to the parents of a child with severe CMV infection. Help them find support systems, and coordinate referrals to other health care professionals.
◆ Monitor the patient with splenomegaly for signs of rupture, and protect him from excess activity and injury.
◆ For the patient with impaired vision, provide a safe environment and encourage independence. Make referrals to community resources.
◆ For the patient with respiratory involvement, frequently assess ventilation status and administer oxygen and assist ventilation as needed. Position the patient in semi-Fowler's or a sitting position to facilitate ventilation.
◆ Administer ganciclovir (Cytovene), foscarnet (Foscavir), or cidofovir (Vestide).

◆ Inspect the patient's skin every shift, looking for new lesions and skin breakdown.
◆ Administer pain medications.
◆ To help the patient adjust to changes in his appearance, urge him to share his feelings and give him encouragement.
◆ Plan meals around the patient's treatment. Supply the patient with high-calorie, high-protein meals. If he can't tolerate regular meals, provide frequent, smaller meals.
◆ If the patient can't take food by mouth, administer I.V. fluids.
◆ Give antiemetics and sedatives.
◆ Provide rest periods if the patient tires easily.
◆ Be alert for adverse effects of radiation therapy or chemotherapy — such as anorexia, nausea, vomiting, and diarrhea — and take steps to prevent or alleviate them.
◆ Systemic therapy may include vincristine (Oncovin), vinblastine (Velban), etoposide (VePesid), doxorubicin (Doxil), daunorubicin (Cerubidine), bleomycin (Blenoxane), and interferon alfa (Roferon-A) with or without an HIV-specific antiretroviral agent.

(continued)

DISORDERS AFFECTING
MANAGEMENT OF AIDS *(continued)*

DISORDER	SIGNS AND SYMPTOMS	DIAGNOSTIC TEST RESULTS
Mycobacterium avium–intracellular complex infection (complication)	◆ Weight loss ◆ Night sweats ◆ Persistent fever ◆ Weakness ◆ Diarrhea ◆ Anemia ◆ Fatigue ◆ Abdominal discomfort	◆ Sputum culture, bronchial wash, stool culture, acid-fast bacillus (AFB) blood culture, bone marrow aspiration, and tissue biopsy test positive for the bacteria.
Pneumocystis carinii pneumonia (complication)	◆ Low-grade, intermittent fever ◆ Increasing shortness of breath ◆ Nonproductive cough ◆ Tachypnea ◆ Dyspnea ◆ Accessory muscle use for breathing ◆ Cyanosis ◆ Dullness on percussion ◆ Crackles ◆ Decreased breath sounds	◆ Gallium scan reveals increased uptake over the lungs. ◆ Bronchoscopy and pleural washing show *P. carinii*. ◆ CD4+ T-cell count is less than 200 cells/µl. ◆ Sputum specimen is positive for *P. carinii*. ◆ Chest X-ray reveals slowly progressing, fluffy infiltrates; occasional nodular lesions; or spontaneous pneumothorax.
Toxoplasmosis (complication)	◆ Visual changes ◆ Constant dull headache ◆ Disorientation ◆ Seizures ◆ Asphasia ◆ Altered mental status ◆ Cranial nerve palsies ◆ Hemiparesis	◆ *Toxoplasma gondii* antibodies are detected in body fluid, blood, or tissue specimens.
Tuberculosis (complication)	◆ Night sweats ◆ Hemoptysis ◆ Fever ◆ Cough ◆ Shortness of breath ◆ Fatigue ◆ Headache ◆ Chills ◆ Nausea and vomiting ◆ Weight loss	◆ Purified protein derivative is positive. ◆ Chest X-ray reveals the penetrating lung parenchyma. ◆ Sputum smear and culture test positive for AFB.
Wasting syndrome (complication)	◆ Fever ◆ Nausea and vomiting ◆ Fatigue ◆ Abdominal pain ◆ Pain or discomfort while eating ◆ Diarrhea	◆ No specific diagnostic tests are used; diagnosis is based on evidence of underlying human immunodeficiency virus infection and assessment findings.

TREATMENT AND CARE

- Monitor WBC count and differential.
- Instruct the patient in ways to prevent infection.
- Teach the patient and his caregiver about the need to report possible infection.
- Monitor the patient for infection; fever, chills, and diaphoresis; cough; shortness of breath; oral pain or painful swallowing; creamy-white patches in the oral cavity; urinary frequency, urgency, or dysuria; redness, swelling, or drainage from wounds; and vesicular lesions on the face, lips, or perianal area.
- Administer combination therapy with two to five agents (clarithromycin [Biaxin], azithromycin [Zithromax], rifampin [Rifadin], rifabutin [Mycobutin], clofazimine [Lamprene], ethambutol [Myambutol], ciprofloxacin [Cipro], and amikacin [Amikin]).

- Use standard precautions.
- Give prescribed oral or I.V. TMP-SMZ (Bactrim, Septra) and oxygen.
- Encourage ambulation and use of incentive spirometry.
- Provide adequate rest periods.
- Encourage the patient to express his fears, feelings, or concerns.
- Provide emotional support.
- Assess for altered respiratory status, tachypnea, use of accessory muscles to breathe, cough, sputum color changes, abnormal breath sounds, dusky or cyanotic skin color, restlessness, confusion, or somnolence. Report abnormal findings.
- Monitor arterial blood gas values.
- Monitor fluid and electrolyte status.
- Provide pulmonary care (cough, deep breathing, postural drainage and percussion, and vibration) every 2 hours.

- Make sure the patient with fever, vomiting, and sore throat receives sufficient fluid intake.
- Provide nutritionally adequate foods and small, frequent feedings.
- Promote bed rest during the acute stage. Later, help the patient gradually increase his level of activity.
- Frequently assess respiratory status. Provide chest physiotherapy, administer oxygen, and assist with ventilation.
- Assess the patient for signs of neurologic involvement and increased intracranial pressure.
- Don't palpate the patient's abdomen vigorously; this could lead to a ruptured spleen.
- Modify the environment to protect a patient with neurologic manifestations or chorioretinitis.
- Administer pyrimethamine with sulfadiazine (Fansidar).
- Carefully monitor the patient's drug therapy.
- Because sulfonamides cause blood dyscrasias and pyrimethamine depresses bone marrow, closely monitor the patient's hematologic values.

- Initiate AFB isolation precautions immediately.
- Teach the infectious patient to cough and sneeze into tissues and to dispose of all secretions properly.
- Instruct the patient to wear a mask when outside of his room.
- Visitors and staff members should wear particulate respirators.
- Administer isoniazid (Nydrazid), rifampin, and (either) ethambutol or streptomycin.
- Remind the patient to get plenty of rest. Stress the importance of eating balanced meals. Record the patient's weight weekly.
- Be alert for adverse effects of medications. Because isoniazid sometimes leads to hepatitis or peripheral neuritis, monitor aspartate aminotransferase and alanine aminotransferase levels.
- To prevent or treat peripheral neuritis, give pyridoxine (vitamin B_6). If the patient receives ethambutol, watch for optic neuritis; if it develops, discontinue the drug. If he receives rifampin, watch for hepatitis and purpura. Observe the patient for other complications such as hemoptysis.

- Monitor weight; intake and output; and hematocrit, hemoglobin, and ferritin levels to evaluate nutritional status and fluid and electrolyte balance.
- Monitor for and report signs and symptoms of dehydration, such as extreme thirst and reduced skin turgor.

The HIV infectious process takes three forms:
■ immunodeficiency—causing opportunistic infections and unusual cancers
■ autoimmunity—causing lymphoid interstitial pneumonitis, arthritis, hypergammaglobulinemia, and the production of autoimmune antibodies
■ neurologic dysfunction—causing AIDS dementia complex, HIV encephalopathy, and peripheral neuropathies.

Immune system
■ As the immune system begins to compromise, opportunistic infections may develop.
■ The risk of cancer increases, most likely because HIV stimulates existing cancer cells or because the immune deficiency allows cancer-causing substances, such as viruses, to transform susceptible cells into cancer cells.

Gastrointestinal system
■ GI signs and symptoms may be related to the effect of HIV on the cells lining the intestine.
■ Oral candidiasis—a fungal infection—is a common manifestation in patients with AIDS.
■ Dehydration, altered skin integrity, and poor nutrition can also contribute to the development of candidiasis, which, in some patients, may spread to other body systems.
■ Involuntary weight loss, chronic diarrhea, and chronic fatigue may lead to a hypermetabolic state in which calories are burned at an excessively high rate and lean body mass is lost. This state can lead to organ failure.

Integumentary system
■ The overall effects of HIV infection, including weight loss, altered nutrition, weakness, and decreased mobility, predispose the patient to skin breakdown.
■ Skin breakdown along with the patient's immunodeficiency increases the risk of infection.

Neurologic system
■ Neurologic system dysfunction is directly related to the effect of HIV on nervous system tissue, opportunistic infections, primary or metastatic neoplasms, cerebrovascular

changes, metabolic encephalopathy, or complications secondary to therapy.
■ Central nervous system responses to HIV infection include atrophy, demyelination, inflammation, degeneration, and necrosis.

Respiratory system
■ Advanced and persistent immunosuppression allows opportunistic respiratory infections, such as *Pneumocystis carinii* pneumonia, to develop.
■ Tuberculosis may be a presenting illness in patients infected with HIV.

ASSESSMENT
The HIV-infected person usually experiences a mononucleosis-like syndrome, which may initially be attributed to influenza or another virus. The patient may then remain asymptomatic for years. In this latent stage, the only sign of HIV infection is laboratory evidence of antibody production.

Clinical findings
■ Persistent generalized adenopathy
■ Nonspecific signs and symptoms, such as weight loss, fatigue, night sweats, and fevers
■ Neurologic symptoms, such as confusion, disorientation, headache, ataxia, and cognitive impairments, resulting from HIV encephalopathy
■ Opportunistic infection causing signs and symptoms specific to the invading organism
■ Cancer

Diagnostic test results
■ *CD4+ T-cell count* is less than 200 cells/μl.
■ *Enzyme-linked immunosorbent assay* is positive.
■ *CD4+ and CD8+ T-lymphocyte subset ratios* are decreased.
■ *Erythrocyte sedimentation rate* varies but may be increased.
■ *Serum beta$_2$-microglobulin* shows increased protein levels with disease progression.
■ *p24 antigen studies* are positive for free viral protein.
■ *Neopterin levels* are increased as the disease progresses.
■ *Anergy testing* is positive.

ADVERSE EFFECTS OF COMMONLY USED HIV MEDICATIONS

This chart shows some of the adverse effects of commonly used human immunodeficiency virus (HIV) medications. These adverse effects may be confused with signs and symptoms of disease process complications or opportunistic infections.

MEDICATION	ASSESSMENT FINDINGS
Delavirdine (Rescriptor)	Rash, headache, fatigue, increased liver enzymes
Didanosine (ddI, Videx)	Upper abdominal pain, diarrhea, persistent nausea and vomiting, pain, tingling or numbness, difficulty breathing, mental confusion
Indinavir (Crixivan)	Nephrolithiasis, asymptomatic hyperbilirubinemia, hyperglycemia, anemia, elevated cholesterol and triglycerides
Lamivudine (3TC, Epivir)	Headache, fever, rash, severe abdominal pain, shortness of breath, fatigue, muscle pain, mania, psychosis, confusion, lactic acidosis, pancreatitis
Nevirapine (Viramune)	Thrombocytopenia, rash, fever, anemia, stomatitis
Ritonavir (Norvir)	Diarrhea, nausea, vomiting, anorexia, abdominal pain, body fat redistribution, hyperglycemia, hyperlipidemia
Saquinavir (Fortovase)	Diarrhea (if formulated with lactose), body fat redistribution, hyperglycemia
Stavudine (Zerit)	Numbness, pain or tingling of the extremities, neutropenia, thrombocytopenia
Zalcitabine (dideoxycytidine, ddC, Hivid)	Rashes, mouth sores, upper abdominal pain, itching, numbness or tingling, mental confusion, seizures, fever, hyperbilirubinemia
Zidovudine (AZT, Retrovir)	Headache, fever, rash, severe abdominal pain, shortness of breath, fatigue, muscle pain, anemia, leukopenia, cardiomyopathy, cholestatic jaundice

COLLABORATIVE MANAGEMENT

The patient requires the skill of an immunologist specializing in HIV infection. He may also need the assistance of pulmonary specialists, if his respiratory system is compromised, and nutritional therapy to optimize his condition. Supportive therapy (for pain relief and psychological support) promotes patient comfort. The patient (and his significant others) may also benefit from referrals to AIDS societies and support programs.

TREATMENT AND CARE

■ Primary therapy involves a combination of three types of antiretroviral agents to inhibit HIV replication. Current recommendations include using two nucleosides (to interfere with copying of viral RNA into DNA by reverse transcriptase) plus one protease inhibitor (to block replication of virus particles and reduce the number of new virus particles produced), or two nucleosides and one nonnucleoside (to interfere with reverse transcriptase) to inhibit production of resistant, mutant strains. (See *Adverse effects of commonly used HIV medications.*)

■ Immunomodulatory agents are used to boost the immune system.

■ Human granulocyte colony-stimulating growth factor is given to stimulate neutrophil production (retroviral therapy causes anemia, therefore patients may receive epoetin alfa).

■ Anti-infective and antineoplastic agents combat opportunistic infections and associated cancers (some are used prophylactically to help resist opportunistic infections).
■ Diligent practice of standard precautions prevents inadvertent transmission of AIDS and other infectious diseases.

Acute coronary syndrome

Acute coronary syndrome (ACS) is an all-inclusive term that describes the potential for three conditions: unstable angina, non–ST-segment elevation myocardial infarction (NSTEMI), and ST-segment elevation myocardial infarction (STEMI). The degree of occlusion defines the condition.

ACS involves the rupture or erosion of plaque — an unstable and lipid-rich substance. The rupture results in platelet adhesions, fibrin clot formation, and activation of thrombin. Symptoms are caused by myocardial ischemia, resulting from an imbalance between supply and demand for myocardial oxygen.

In cardiovascular disease — the leading cause of death in the United States and Western Europe — death usually results from cardiac damage after an MI. Each year, approximately 1 million people in the United States experience MI. Incidence is higher in males younger than age 70. (Females have the protective effects of estrogen.) Mortality is high when treatment is delayed, and almost one-half of sudden deaths caused by MI occur before hospitalization or within 1 hour of the onset of symptoms. The prognosis improves if vigorous treatment begins immediately.

ETIOLOGY

Atherosclerotic plaque disease is the predominant cause of ACS. Coronary artery vasospasm is a less common cause. Other causes of angina include ventricular hypertrophy resulting from hypertension, valvular disease, or cardiomyopathy; embolic occlusion of the coronary arteries; hypoxia from carbon monoxide poisoning or acute pulmonary disorders; cocaine and amphetamine use, which increases myocardial oxygen demand and may cause coronary vasospasm; underlying coronary artery disease, which may be found by severe anemia; and inflammation of epicardial arteries.

PATHOPHYSIOLOGY

ACS most commonly results when a thrombus progresses and occludes blood flow. The degree of blockage and the time that the affected vessel remains occluded determine the type of infarct that occurs. The underlying effect is an imbalance in myocardial oxygen supply and demand.

For patients with unstable angina, a thrombus full of platelets partially occludes a coronary vessel. The partially occluded vessel may have distal microthrombi that cause necrosis in some myocytes. The smaller vessels infarct, thus placing the patient at higher risk for a NSTEMI.

If a thrombus fully occludes the vessel for a prolonged time, it's classified as a STEMI. This type of MI involves a greater concentration of thrombin and fibrin.

Occlusion of a vessel progresses through three stages:
■ Ischemia occurs first, indicating that blood flow and oxygen demand are imbalanced. It can be resolved by improving flow or reduction of oxygen needs.
■ Injury occurs when the ischemia is prolonged enough to damage the heart area.
■ Infarct occurs when myocardial cells die.

Cardiovascular system
■ An area of viable ischemic tissue surrounds the zone of injury.
■ When the heart muscle is damaged, the integrity of the cell membrane is impaired.
■ Intracellular contents, including cardiac enzymes (such as creatine kinase, lactate dehydrogenase, and aspartate aminotransferase) and proteins (such as troponin T, troponin I, and myoglobin) are released. (See *Understanding CAD,* pages 18 and 19.)
■ Within 24 hours, the infarcted area becomes edematous and cyanotic.
■ During the next several days, leukocytes infiltrate the necrotic area and begin to remove necrotic cells, thinning the ventricular wall.
■ Scar formation begins by the third week after MI; by the 6th week, scar tissue is well established.

- The scar tissue that forms on the necrotic area inhibits contractility.
- Compensatory mechanisms (vascular constriction, increased heart rate, and renal retention of sodium and water) try to maintain cardiac output.
- Ventricular dilation may also occur in a process called remodeling.
- Functionally, MI may cause reduced contractility with abnormal wall motion, altered left ventricular compliance, reduced stroke volume, reduced ejection fraction, and elevated left ventricular end-diastolic pressure.
- Cardiogenic shock is caused by failure of the heart to perform as an effective pump and can result in low cardiac output, diminished peripheral perfusion, pulmonary congestion, and elevated systemic vascular resistance and pulmonary vascular pressures.
- Ineffective contractility of the heart leads to accumulation of blood in the venous circulation upstream to the failing ventricle.
- Arrhythmias can occur in the patient with acute MI as a result of autonomic nervous system imbalance, electrolyte disturbances, ischemia, and slowed conduction in zones of ischemic myocardium.

Neurologic system

- Hypoperfusion of the brain results in altered mental status, involving changes in levels of consciousness, restlessness, irritability, confusion, or disorientation.
- Stupor or coma may result if the decrease in cerebral perfusion continues.

Renal system

- Shock and hypoperfusion from MI cause the kidney to respond by conserving salt and water.
- Poor perfusion results in diminished renal blood flow, and increased afferent arteriolar resistance occurs, causing a decreased glomerular filtration rate.
- Increased amounts of antidiuretic hormone and aldosterone are released to help maintain perfusion. Urine formation, however, is reduced.
- Depletion of renal adenosine triphosphate stores results from prolonged renal hypoperfusion, causing impaired renal function.

Respiratory system

- Cardiogenic shock with left-sided heart failure results in increased fluid in the lungs. This process can overwhelm the capacity of the pulmonary lymphatics, resulting in interstitial and alveolar edema. (See *Disorders affecting management of ACS,* pages 20 and 21.)
- Lung edema occurs when pulmonary capillary pressure exceeds 18 mm Hg.
- Pulmonary alveolar edema develops when pressures exceed 24 mm Hg, impairing oxygen diffusion.
- Increased interstitial and intra-alveolar fluid causes progressive reduction in lung compliance, increasing the work of ventilation and increasing perfusion of poorly ventilated alveoli.

ASSESSMENT

Initial diagnosis of ACS is mostly based on the patient's history, risk factors, and electrocardiogram (ECG) findings.

Clinical findings

These findings are typical of angina:
- Burning, squeezing, and crushing tightness in the substernal or precordial chest that may radiate to the left arm, neck, jaw, or shoulder blade
- Pain (commonly following physical exertion but also possibly after emotional excitement, exposure to cold, or a large meal)

A patient with MI may present with these findings:
- Chest pain (uncomfortable pressure, squeezing, or fullness in the center of the chest, usually lasting longer than 15 minutes; pain may radiate to the shoulders, neck, arms, jaw, or back between the shoulder blades)
- Light-headedness, fainting, sweating, shortness of breath, palpitations, or a feeling of impending doom
- Fatigue, low body temperature, dyspnea, falls, tingling of the extremities, nausea, vomiting, weakness, syncope, or confusion without chest pain (in older adults, patients with diabetes, women, and those experiencing cocaine-induced MI; commonly called a *silent MI*)
- Jugular vein distention
- Reduced urine output (secondary to reduced renal perfusion and increased aldosterone and antidiuretic hormone)

(Text continues on page 22.)

UNDERSTANDING CAD

Coronary artery disease (CAD) results as atherosclerotic plaque fills the lumens of the coronary arteries and obstructs blood flow. The primary effect of CAD is a diminished supply of oxygen and nutrients to myocardial tissue.

Progression of CAD in atherosclerosis

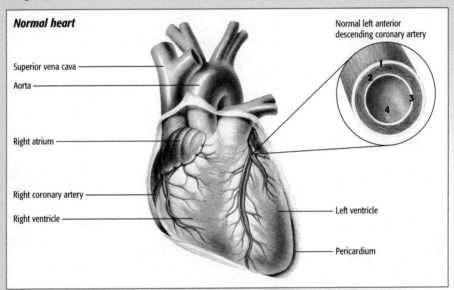

Normal heart

Normal left anterior descending coronary artery

Superior vena cava
Aorta
Right atrium
Right coronary artery
Right ventricle
Left ventricle
Pericardium

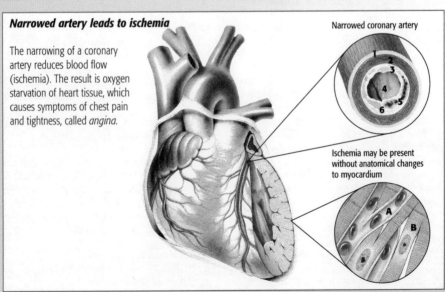

Narrowed artery leads to ischemia

Narrowed coronary artery

The narrowing of a coronary artery reduces blood flow (ischemia). The result is oxygen starvation of heart tissue, which causes symptoms of chest pain and tightness, called *angina*.

Ischemia may be present without anatomical changes to myocardium

Blocked artery leads to myocardial infarction (MI)

Sudden insufficient blood supply (ischemia) is commonly caused by ruptured plaque and thrombus formation that occludes the artery lumen. This produces an area of necrosis in heart muscle, which results in MI.

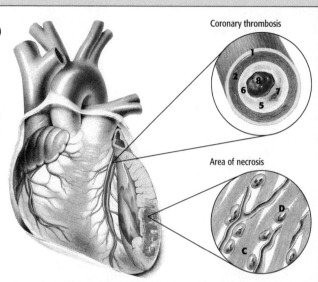

Coronary thrombosis

Area of necrosis

Recovery through collateral blood supply

Collateral (accessory) blood supply from adjacent vessels travels to the region affected by MI to provide fresh blood.

Collateral blood supply

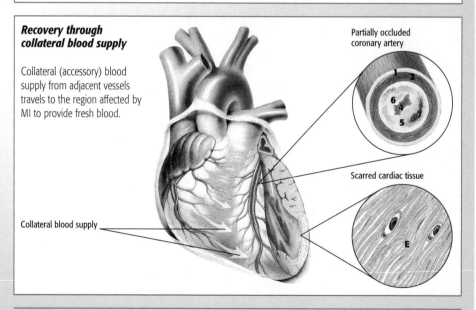

Partially occluded coronary artery

Scarred cardiac tissue

Key to circular insets

Coronary artery

1	Adventitia	5	Advanced plaque
2	Media	6	Fatty deposits
3	Intima	7	Hemorrhage
4	Lumen	8	Thrombus

Myocardium

A	Capillaries
B	Muscle fibers
C	Dead muscle fibers
D	Leukocytes
E	Scar tissue

DISORDERS AFFECTING MANAGEMENT OF ACS

This chart highlights disorders that affect the management of acute coronary syndrome (ACS).

DISORDER	SIGNS AND SYMPTOMS
Cardiogenic shock (complication)	*Compensatory stage* ◆ Tachycardia and bounding pulse caused by sympathetic stimulation ◆ Restlessness and irritability related to cerebral hypoxia ◆ Tachypnea to compensate for hypoxia ◆ Reduced urinary output secondary to vasoconstriction ◆ Cool, pale skin associated with vasoconstriction; warm, dry skin in septic shock resulting from vasodilation *Progressive stage* ◆ Hypotension as compensatory mechanisms begin to fail ◆ Narrowed pulse pressure associated with reduced stroke volume ◆ Weak, rapid, thready pulse caused by decreased cardiac output ◆ Shallow respirations as the patient weakens ◆ Reduced urinary output as poor renal perfusion continues ◆ Cold, clammy skin caused by vasoconstriction ◆ Cyanosis related to hypoxia *Irreversible (refractory) stage* ◆ Unconsciousness and absent reflexes caused by reduced cerebral perfusion, acid-base imbalance, or electrolyte abnormalities ◆ Rapidly falling blood pressure as decompensation occurs ◆ Weak pulse caused by reduced cardiac output ◆ Slow, shallow, or Cheyne-Stokes respirations secondary to respiratory center depression ◆ Anuria related to renal failure
Heart failure (complication)	◆ Cough that produces pink, frothy sputum ◆ Cyanosis of the lips and nail beds ◆ Pale, cool, clammy skin ◆ Diaphoresis ◆ Jugular vein distention ◆ Ascites ◆ Pulsus alternans ◆ Tachycardia ◆ Hepatomegaly ◆ Decreased pulse pressure ◆ Third and fourth heart sounds ◆ Moist, basilar crackles and rhonchi ◆ Expiratory wheezing ◆ Decreased pulse oximetry ◆ Peripheral edema ◆ Decreased urinary output

DIAGNOSTIC TEST RESULTS	TREATMENT AND CARE
◆ Arterial blood gas (ABG) analysis may show metabolic acidosis, respiratory acidosis, and hypoxia. ◆ Electrocardiography (ECG) shows possible evidence of acute myocardial infarction (MI), ischemia, or ventricular aneurysm. ◆ Thermodilution catheterization reveals a reduced cardiac index. ◆ Serum enzyme measurements display elevated levels of creatine kinase (CK), lactate dehydrogenase (LD), aspartate aminotransferase, and alanine aminotransferase, which indicate MI or ischemia and suggest heart failure or shock. ◆ CK-MB and LD isoenzyme levels may be elevated, confirming acute MI.	◆ Administer oxygen by face mask or artificial airway to ensure adequate oxygenation of tissues. ◆ Monitor and record blood pressure, pulse, respiratory rate, and peripheral pulses every 1 to 5 minutes until the patient stabilizes. ◆ Monitor cardiac rhythm continuously. ◆ Closely monitor pulmonary artery pressure (PAP), pulmonary artery wedge pressure (PAWP) and, if equipment is available, cardiac output. ◆ Record hemodynamic pressure readings every 15 minutes. ◆ Insert an indwelling urinary catheter, if needed, to measure hourly urine output. ◆ Administer dopamine (Intropin), amiodarone (Cordarone), dobutamine (Dobutrex), norepinephrine (Levophed), nitroglycerin (Tridil), and nitroprusside (Nitropress) as well as a vasopressor. ◆ Monitor ABG values, complete blood count, and electrolyte levels. Expect to administer sodium bicarbonate by I.V. push if the patient is acidotic. Administer electrolyte replacement therapy as indicated by laboratory results. ◆ During therapy, assess skin color and temperature and note changes. Cold, clammy skin may be a sign of continuing peripheral vascular constriction, indicating progressive shock. ◆ Move the patient with an intra-aortic balloon pump (IABP) as little as possible. Never flex the patient's ballooned leg at the hip because this may displace or fracture the catheter. ◆ Never place the patient on IABP in a sitting position while the balloon is inflated; the balloon will tear through the aorta and result in immediate death. ◆ During IABP use, assess pedal pulses and skin temperature and color to ensure adequate peripheral circulation. ◆ Check the dressing over the insertion site frequently for bleeding. Also check the site for hematoma or signs of infection; culture any drainage.
◆ B-type natriuretic peptide immunoassay may be elevated. ◆ Chest X-ray shows increased pulmonary vascular markings, interstitial edema, or pleural effusions and cardiomegaly. ◆ ECG reveals heart enlargement or ischemia, tachycardia, extrasystole, or atrial fibrillation. ◆ PAP, PAWP, and left ventricular end-diastolic pressure are elevated in the presence of left-sided heart failure; right atrial or central venous pressure is elevated in right-sided heart failure.	◆ Administer supplemental oxygen and mechanical ventilation. ◆ Place the patient in Fowler's position. ◆ Administer diuretics, inotropic drugs, vasodilators, angiotensin-converting enzyme inhibitors, angiotensin receptor blockers, cardiac glycosides, beta-adrenergic blockers, or electrolyte supplements. ◆ Initiate cardiac monitoring. ◆ Maintain adequate cardiac output, and monitor hemodynamic stability. ◆ Assess for deep vein thrombosis and apply antiembolism stockings.

- Systolic murmur (indicating papillary muscle dysfunction)
- Decrease in or abnormal heart sounds, such as third and fourth heart sounds (S_3 and S_4) or paradoxical splitting of the second heart sound (S_2)
- Hypotension or hypertension
- Pulmonary congestion, such as crackles and a productive cough

Diagnostic test results

- *12-lead ECG* may reveal characteristic changes, such as serial ST-segment depression in non–Q-wave MI and ST-segment elevation in Q-wave MI. The Q waves are considered abnormal when they appear greater than or equal to 0.4 second wide and their height is greater than 25% of the R-wave height in that lead. An ECG can also identify the location of MI, arrhythmias, hypertrophy, and pericarditis. The more combinations of leads affected with ECG changes, the more myocardial damage and the worse the prognosis.
- *Serial cardiac enzymes and proteins* may show a characteristic rise and fall of cardiac enzymes, specifically CK-MB, the proteins troponin T and I, and myoglobin.
- *Laboratory testing* may reveal elevated white blood cell count and erythrocyte sedimentation rate and changes in electrolytes.
- *Echocardiography* may show ventricular wall motion abnormalities and may detect septal or papillary muscle rupture or identify pericardial effusions.
- *Transesophageal echocardiography* may reveal areas of decreased heart muscle wall movement, indicating ischemia.
- *Chest X-rays* may show left-sided heart failure, cardiomegaly, or other noncardiac causes of dyspnea or chest pain.
- *Nuclear imaging scanning* using thallium 201 and technetium 99m can be used to identify areas of infarction and areas of viable muscle cells.
- *Multiple-gated acquisition scanning* is used to determine left ventricular function and identify aneurysms, problems with wall motion, and intracardiac shunting.
- *Cardiac catheterization* may be used to identify the involved coronary artery as well as to provide information on ventricular function and pressures and volumes within the heart.

COLLABORATIVE MANAGEMENT

A cardiologist is consulted for initial assessment and treatment. A cardiothoracic surgeon may also be consulted if the patient requires invasive therapy. Other specialists may be required after initial therapy and treatment, such as a physical therapist for cardiac rehabilitation and a nutritionist for dietary and lifestyle changes.

TREATMENT AND CARE

The goal of treatment for angina is to reduce myocardial oxygen demand or increase oxygen supply.

- Nitrates may be administered to reduce myocardial oxygen consumption.
- Beta-adrenergic blockers may be administered to reduce the workload and oxygen demands of the heart.
- Calcium channel blockers may be administered if angina is caused by coronary artery spasm.
- Antiplatelet drugs may be administered to minimize platelet aggregation and the danger of coronary occlusion.
- Antilipemics may be administered to reduce elevated serum cholesterol or triglyceride levels.
- Obstructive lesions may necessitate coronary artery bypass surgery or percutaneous transluminal coronary angioplasty (PTCA). Other alternatives include laser angioplasty, minimally invasive surgery, rotational atherectomy, or stent placement.

The goals of treatment for MI are to relieve pain, stabilize heart rhythm, revascularize the coronary artery, preserve myocardial tissue, and reduce cardiac workload. Here are some guidelines for treatment:

- Thrombolytic therapy (streptokinase [Streptase], alteplase [Activase], or reteplase [Retevase]) should be started within 3 hours of the onset of symptoms (unless contraindications exist).
- Oxygen is administered to increase oxygenation of the blood
- Nitroglycerin is administered sublingually to relieve chest pain (unless systolic blood pressure is less than 90 mm Hg or heart rate is less than 50 or greater than 100 beats/ minute)
- Morphine is administered for analgesia because pain stimulates the sympathetic nervous system, leading to an increase in heart rate and vasoconstriction.

■ Aspirin is administered to inhibit platelet aggregation

■ I.V. heparin is administered to patients who have received tissue plasminogen activator to increase the chances of patency in the affected coronary artery.

■ Lidocaine, transcutaneous pacing patches (or transvenous pacemaker), defibrillation, or epinephrine may be used if arrhythmias are present.

■ I.V. nitroglycerin is administered for 24 to 48 hours in patients without hypotension, bradycardia, or excessive tachycardia to reduce afterload and preload and relieve chest pain.

■ Glycoprotein IIb/IIIa inhibitors (such as abciximab [ReoPro]) are administered to patients with continued unstable angina or acute chest pain, or following invasive cardiac procedures to reduce platelet aggregation

■ I.V. beta-adrenergic blocker is administered early to those with an evolving acute MI (followed by oral therapy) to reduce heart rate, contractility, and myocardial oxygen requirements

■ ACE inhibitors are administered to those with an evolving MI, with ST-segment elevation or left bundle-branch block, to reduce afterload and preload and prevent remodeling

■ Lipid-lowering drugs are administered to patients with elevated low-density lipoprotein and cholesterol levels.

■ Laser angioplasty, atherectomy, PTCA, stent placement, or transmyocardial revascularization may also be initiated.

Acute GI bleeding

GI bleeding can occur anywhere in the GI tract and is classified as upper or lower. Upper GI bleeding occurs above the ligament of Treitz (where the duodenum meets the jejunum). Sites of upper GI bleeding include the esophagus, stomach, and duodenum. Lower GI bleeding occurs below the Treitz ligament. The most common site of lower GI bleeding is the colon.

Although GI bleeding stops spontaneously in most patients, *acute* GI bleeding accounts for significant morbidity and mortality. The incidence of upper GI bleeding is greater (100 patients per 100,000 adults) than that of lower GI bleeding (20 patients per 100,000 adults). On average, about 25% of patients who develop upper GI bleeding are already hospitalized with another condition, whereas only 5% of these patients develop lower GI bleeding.

ETIOLOGY

Common causes of upper GI bleeding include:

■ peptic ulcer disease (most common)
■ rupture of esophageal varices
■ esophagitis and esophageal ulcers
■ Mallory-Weiss syndrome
■ erosive gastritis
■ angiodysplasias
■ arteriovenous malformations.

Common causes of lower GI bleeding include:

■ diverticulitis
■ inflammatory bowel disease
■ polyps
■ neoplasms
■ arteriovenous malformation.

PATHOPHYSIOLOGY

With GI bleeding, the patient experiences a loss of circulating blood volume regardless of the underlying cause of bleeding. The extensive arterial blood supply near the stomach and esophagus can lead to a rapid loss of large amounts of blood, which may result in hypovolemia and shock. (See *Disorders affecting management of acute GI bleeding*, pages 24 and 25.)

Cardiovascular system

■ Loss of circulating blood volume leads to a decrease in venous return.
■ Cardiac output and blood pressure decrease, resulting in inadequate tissue perfusion.
■ Interstitial fluids shift to the intravascular space (in the body's attempt to compensate).
■ The sympathetic nervous system is stimulated, resulting in vasoconstriction and an increase in heart rate.

Renal system

■ The renin-angiotensin-aldosterone system is activated, causing increased secretion of antidiuretic hormone, thereby leading to

DISORDERS AFFECTING MANAGEMENT OF ACUTE GI BLEEDING

This chart highlights disorders that affect the management of acute GI bleeding.

DISORDER	SIGNS AND SYMPTOMS	DIAGNOSTIC TEST RESULTS
Hypovolemic shock (complication)	◆ Pale skin ◆ Decreased level of consciousness (LOC) ◆ Hypotension ◆ Tachycardia ◆ Urine output less than 25 ml/hour ◆ Cold, clammy skin	◆ Central venous pressure, right atrial pressure, pulmonary artery wedge pressure, and cardiac output are decreased. ◆ Hematocrit, hemoglobin, red blood cell count, and platelet count are low. ◆ Serum potassium, sodium, lactate dehydrogenase, blood urea nitrogen, and creatinine levels are elevated. ◆ Urine specific gravity is increased. ◆ Arterial blood gas analysis reveals respiratory acidosis.
Myocardial infarction (complication)	◆ Pressure, squeezing, pain, or fullness in the center of the chest lasting several minutes ◆ Pain radiating to the shoulders, neck, arms, or jaw ◆ Pain in the back between the shoulder blades ◆ Light-headedness ◆ Fainting ◆ Sweating ◆ Nausea ◆ Shortness of breath ◆ Palpitations ◆ Feeling of impending doom	◆ Serial electrocardiogram may reveal ST-segment depression or ST-segment elevatation. ◆ Serial cardiac enzymes (CK-MB) and proteins (troponin T and I) and myoglobin show a characteristic rise and fall. ◆ Nuclear imaging scanning may identify areas of infarction. ◆ Cardiac catheterization may show involved coronary and ventricular function. ◆ Chest X-rays may show left-sided heart failure or cardiomegaly. ◆ White blood cell count may be elevated. ◆ Echocardiography may show ventricular wall abnormalities.
Stroke (complication)	◆ Sudden onset of hemiparesis or hemiplegia ◆ Dizziness ◆ Seizures ◆ Aphasia ◆ Dysphagia ◆ Decreased LOC ◆ Hypertension	◆ Cardiac catheterization may identify the involved coronary artery. ◆ Computed tomography identifies ischemic stroke within 72 hours and hemorrhagic stroke immediately. ◆ Magnetic resonance imaging identifies the area of ischemia, infarction, or edema. ◆ Angiography reveals disruption of cerebral circulation.

fluid retention. These compensatory mechanisms lead to an increase in blood pressure.

■ If blood loss continues, the compensatory mechanisms ultimately fail; cardiac output continues to decrease, which leads to cellular hypoxia and a shift from aerobic to anaerobic metabolism (with the subsequent buildup of lactic acid), resulting in metabolic acidosis.

■ Eventually, all organs experience hypoperfusion and fail.

ASSESSMENT

Because GI bleeding can occur anywhere along the GI tract, assessment determines the amount of bleeding and its location.

Clinical findings

■ Asymptomatic, if total blood volume lost is 10% to 15% (500 to 750 ml)

■ Anxiety, agitation, confusion, tachycardia, hypotension, oliguria, diaphoresis, pallor, and cool, clammy skin, if total blood

TREATMENT AND CARE

- Assess extent of fluid loss.
- Immediately administer fluid and blood replacement.
- Administer supplemental oxygen.
- Monitor respiratory status and pulse oximetry.
- Monitor vital signs continuously for changes.
- Anticipate the need for intubation and mechanical ventilation
- Prepare the patient for surgery to control bleeding, if indicated.

- Percutaneous coronary intervention may be used; however, the patient with GI bleeding shouldn't receive heparin after the procedure.
- Administer morphine as prescribed to relieve chest pain.
- Administer oxygen as needed.
- Administer nitroglycerin cautiously to relieve chest pain and reduce blood pressure.
- Administer beta-adrenergic blockers to decrease the heart's workload.
- Fibrinolytics, anticoagulants, and antiplatelet drugs, such as aspirin, are contraindicated in patients with GI bleeding.

- Fibrinolytics, anticoagulants, and antiplatelet drugs, such as aspirin, are contraindicated in patients with GI bleeding.
- Percutaneous transluminal angioplasty or stent insertion may be used to open occluded vessels.
- Manage intracranial pressure with osmotic diuretics and corticosteroids.
- Administer anticonvulsants to treat or prevent seizures.
- Carotid endarterectomy may be indicated to open partially occluded carotid arteries.

volume lost is 35% to 50% (1,500 to 2,000 ml)

■ Bright red blood in nasogastric tube drainage or vomitus (hematemesis), indicating an upper GI source of bleeding

■ Drainage or vomitus that looks like coffee grounds (if blood has been held in the stomach)

■ Hematochezia (bright red blood from the rectum), typically indicating a lower GI source of bleeding, or possibly an upper GI source if the transit time through the bowel is rapid

■ Melena (black, tarry, sticky stools), usually indicating an upper GI bleeding source, or possible bleeding in the small bowel or proximal colon

■ Possible angina or even a myocardial infarction following an acute bleeding episode in patients with underlying cardiac disease

■ Aggravated heart failure or diabetes (with severe GI bleeding)

Diagnostic test results

■ *Upper GI endoscopy* reveals the source of bleeding, such as an ulcer, esophageal varice, or Mallory-Weiss tear.
■ *Colonoscopy* reveals the source of lower GI bleeding, such as polyps.
■ *Complete blood count* shows decreased hemoglobin level and hematocrit (usually 6 to 8 hours after the initial symptoms; hematocrit may be normal initially but can drop dramatically); increased reticulocyte and platelet levels; and a decrease in red blood cells.
■ *Arterial blood gas analysis* reveals low pH and bicarbonate levels, indicating lactic acidosis.
■ *12-lead electrocardiogram* may reveal evidence of cardiac ischemia secondary to hypoperfusion.
■ *Abdominal X-ray* may indicate air under the diaphragm, suggesting ulcer perforation.
■ *Angiography* may help visualize the site of bleeding if the bleeding is from an artery or large vein.
■ *Small-bowel follow-through* or a wireless capsule endoscope may help diagnose bleeding in the small bowel.

COLLABORATIVE MANAGEMENT

Medical and nursing care focuses on maintaining all body functions. Respiratory therapy may be necessary to ensure a patent airway and improve respiratory function. Nutritional support is indicated to ensure that the patient gets adequate nutrients for maximum tissue healing. Enteral or parenteral nutrition therapy may be necessary. Physical therapy can help minimize the risks associated with bed rest. Surgery may be necessary to repair the source of bleeding. Social services may be brought in to provide emotional support for the patient and his family.

TREATMENT AND CARE

Treatment focuses on stopping the bleeding and providing fluid resuscitation while maintaining the patient's vital functions. It includes:
■ fluid volume replacement with crystalloid solutions, initially, followed by colloids and blood component therapy

■ calcium supplementation (calcium binds to the citrate in the stored blood, thereby decreasing the body's free calcium levels)
■ respiratory support, including supplemental oxygen and, possibly, mechanical ventilation for the patient who experiences respiratory failure
■ gastric intubation with gastric lavage (unless the patient has esophageal varices) and gastric pH monitoring
■ histamine-2 receptor antagonists and other agents, such as misoprostol (Cytotec), and a proton pump inhibitor, such as omeprazole (Prilosec)
■ endoscopic or surgical repair of bleeding sites.

Acute pancreatitis

Acute pancreatitis (inflammation of the pancreas) is caused by an autodigestive process that produces swelling, hemorrhage, and vascular damage. In men, this disease is commonly associated with alcoholism, trauma, or peptic ulcer; in women, it's linked to biliary tract disease.

The incidence of acute pancreatitis varies with age. In the United States, it affects 270 out of every 100,000 people ages 15 to 44 and 540 out of every 100,000 people age 65 and older. Blacks have a higher incidence of acute pancreatitis than whites, and the disease affects men more commonly than women. In those with acquired immunodeficiency syndrome, acute pancreatitis affects 4 to 22 persons out of every 100. The disorder is uncommon in children.

The prognosis is good when acute pancreatitis follows biliary tract disease. However, when acute pancreatitis follows alcoholism, it's associated with necrosis and hemorrhage, and mortality rises as high as 60%.

ETIOLOGY

The most common causes of acute pancreatitis are biliary tract disease and alcoholism, but it can also result from trauma or the use of certain drugs, such as glucocorticoids, sulfonamides, chlorothiazide (Diuril), acetaminophen, and azathioprine (Imuran).

Acute pancreatitis may also develop as a complication of mumps. Less common causes include stenosis or obstruction of the sphincter of Oddi, hyperlipidemia, such metabolic endocrine disorders as hyperparathyroidism and hemochromatosis, vasculitis or vascular disease, viral infections, mycoplasmal pneumonia, renal failure, and such connective tissue disorders as systemic lupus erythematosus and sarcoidosis.

PATHOPHYSIOLOGY

Acute pancreatitis occurs in two forms:
■ edematous (interstitial), which causes fluid accumulation and swelling
■ necrotizing (hemorrhagic), which causes cell death and tissue damage.

Gastrointestinal system

■ Inflammation is caused by premature activation of enzymes (elastase and phospholipase A), which causes tissue damage. (See *Why enzymes activate prematurely.*) Enzymes back up and spill out into the pancreatic tissue, resulting in autodigestion of the pancreas.
■ Elastase is activated by trypsin. It digests the elastic tissue of the blood vessel walls, causing hemorrhage.
■ Phospholipase A may be activated by trypsin or bile acids. After it's activated, phospholipase A digests the phospholipids contained in the cell membranes.
■ Large amounts of fluid shift from the intravascular space to the peritoneal and interstitial spaces.
■ Additional fluid loss may occur because of vomiting, diarrhea, hemorrhage, and nasogastric suction.
■ Third-space fluid shifting may occur because of hypoalbuminemia.
■ Fluid losses eventually lead to hypovolemic shock.

Cardiovascular system

■ Trypsin activates kallikrein, which is thought to cause local damage and systemic hypotension. In turn, kallikrein causes vasodilation and increased vascular permeability, invasion of white blood cells, and pain.
■ Tachycardia occurs as a result of hypotension, pain, and fever.

WHY ENZYMES ACTIVATE PREMATURELY

Normally, the acini in the pancreas secrete enzymes in an inactive form. Sometimes, however, the enzymes are activated prematurely. Two theories attempt to explain why this occurs.

One theory suggests that a toxic agent, such as alcohol, alters the way the pancreas secretes enzymes. Increased pancreatic secretion then alters the metabolism of the acinar cells and encourages duct obstruction by causing pancreatic secretory proteins to precipitate.

Another theory suggests that reflux of duodenal contents containing activated enzymes enters the pancreatic duct, activating other enzymes and setting up a cycle for more pancreatic damage. This reflux may occur if atony and edema of the sphincter of Oddi occur, or if pancreatic duct obstruction or pancreatic ischemia is present.

Hematologic system

■ Pancreatic inflammation interferes with the absorption of vitamin K, resulting in vitamin K deficiency.
■ Vitamin K deficiency impairs clotting mechanisms, causing disseminated intravascular coagulation. (See *Disorders affecting management of acute pancreatitis*, pages 28 and 29.)

Immune system

■ The necrosed pancreatic tissue or the tissue surrounding the pancreas may become infected; leukocytosis and fever occur in response to the inflammatory process, if infection is present.
■ Secondary infections occur as microorganisms, typically from other body areas such as the colon, move to the necrosed pancreas.
■ As pancreatic enzymes cause tissue necrosis, purulent drainage collects within the pancreas. This material can erode through the retroperitoneum into the bowel, pleural space, mediastinum, or pelvis, subsequently leading to sepsis.

Respiratory system

■ Severe pain interferes with the patient's ability to breathe deeply and expand his

DISORDERS AFFECTING MANAGEMENT OF ACUTE PANCREATITIS

This chart highlights disorders that affect the management of acute pancreatitis.

DISORDER	SIGNS AND SYMPTOMS	DIAGNOSTIC TEST RESULTS
Acute respiratory distress syndrome (ARDS) (complication)	◆ Rapid, shallow breathing ◆ Tachycardia ◆ Cool, clammy skin ◆ Dyspnea ◆ Restlessness ◆ Agitation	◆ Initially, arterial blood gas (ABG) analysis shows respiratory alkalosis; as ARDS worsens, respiratory acidosis. ◆ Pulmonary artery wedge pressure (PAWP) is 12 mm Hg or less. ◆ Chest X-ray shows ground-glass appearance and, eventually, "whiteouts" of both lung fields.
Disseminated intravascular coagulation (complication)	◆ Bleeding from puncture sites ◆ Petechiae ◆ Ecchymoses ◆ Hematoma ◆ Nausea ◆ Vomiting ◆ Severe muscle, back, and abdominal pain ◆ Chest pain ◆ Hemoptysis	◆ Platelet count is decreased (less than 100,000/ml). ◆ Fibrinogen is less than 150 mg/dl. ◆ Prothrombin time (PT) is greater than 15 seconds. ◆ Fibrin degradation product level is greater than 45 mcg/ml. ◆ D-dimer is elevated. ◆ Blood urea nitrogen (BUN) and creatinine levels are elevated.
Hypovolemic shock (complication)	◆ Pale skin ◆ Decreased LOC ◆ Hypotension ◆ Tachycardia ◆ Urine output less than 25 ml/hour ◆ Cold, clammy skin	◆ Central venous pressure, right atrial pressure, PAWP, and cardiac output are decreased. ◆ Hematocrit, hemoglobin level, RBC count, and platelet counts are low. ◆ Serum potassium, sodium, lactate dehydrogenase, BUN, and creatinine levels are elevated. ◆ Urine specific gravity is increased. ◆ ABG analysis reveals respiratory acidosis.
Sepsis (complication)	◆ Agitation ◆ Anxiety ◆ Altered LOC ◆ Tachycardia ◆ Hypotension ◆ Rapid, shallow respirations ◆ Fever ◆ Urine output less than 25 ml/hour	◆ Blood cultures are positive for the infecting organism. ◆ Complete blood count reveals whether anemia, neutropenia, and thrombocytopenia are present. ◆ ABG studies show metabolic acidosis. ◆ BUN and creatinine levels are increased. ◆ Electrocardiogram shows ST-segment depression, inverted T waves, and arrhythmias.

lungs adequately, commonly resulting in pneumonia.

■ Pancreatic enzymes released into the circulation damage the pulmonary vessels, stimulate inflammation, and cause alveolo-capillary leakage, resulting in intrapul-monary shunting, hypoxemia and, possibly, pleural effusion.

ASSESSMENT

The severity of pancreatitis is predicted using Ranson's criteria. If the patient meets

TREATMENT AND CARE

- Assess respiratory status at least every 2 hours.
- Monitor pulse oximetry and ABG results.
- Monitor ventilator settings frequently.
- Suction only when necessary to maintain positive end-expiratory pressure.
- Administer neuromuscular blocking agents and sedation at regular intervals for maximum effect.
- Monitor heart rate and blood pressure hourly, or more frequently as indicated.
- Administer high-dose corticosteroids early in disease process.
- Administer diuretics to reduce interstitial and pulmonary edema.

- Treat underlying cause.
- Administer fresh frozen plasma, platelets, cryoprecipitate, and packed red blood cells (RBCs).
- Monitor vital signs at least every 30 minutes.
- Administer supplemental oxygen as indicated.
- Assess level of consciousness (LOC) hourly and when the patient's condition changes.
- Monitor serial hemoglobin and hematocrit, partial thromboplastin time, PT, fibrinogen levels, fibrinogen degradation products, and platelet counts.
- Administer low-dose heparin infusion.

- Administer vitamin K and folate.
- Institute safety precautions to minimize bleeding.
- Assess extent of fluid loss.
- Administer fluid and blood replacement immediately.
- Administer supplemental oxygen.
- Monitor respiratory status and pulse oximetry.
- Monitor vital signs continuously for changes.
- Anticipate the need for intubation and mechanical ventilation.
- Prepare the patient for surgery if indicated to control bleeding.

- Locate and treat the underlying cause of sepsis.
- Monitor vital signs frequently.
- Administer antibiotics.
- Administer I.V. fluids to replace intravascular volume.
- Administer vasopressors if fluid resuscitation doesn't maintain blood pressure.
- Assess respiratory status.
- Prepare for intubation and mechanical ventilation (if needed).

fewer than three of the criteria, the mortality rate is less than 1%. When three or four of the criteria are met, the mortality rate increases to 15% to 20%. When five or six criteria of the criteria are met, the mortality rate increases to 40%. (See *Ranson's criteria,* page 30.) The patient's history may reveal alcohol abuse, new or recent dietary changes, medications that are known to affect the pancreas, or cholelithiasis.

RANSON'S CRITERIA

Use Ranson's criteria – a set of 11 signs, 5 of which are measured on admission to the health care facility, and 6 in the first 48 hours after admission – to assess the severity of acute pancreatitis. The more criteria met by the patient, the more severe the episode of pancreatitis and, therefore, the greater the risk of mortality.

On admission
◆ Age older than 55
◆ White blood cell count greater than 16,000/mm³
◆ Serum glucose greater than 200 mg/dl
◆ Lactate dehydrogenase greater than 350 IU/L
◆ Aspartate aminotransferase greater than 250 U/L

After admission
◆ A 10% decrease in hematocrit
◆ Blood urea nitrogen increase greater than 5 mg/dl
◆ Serum calcium less than 8 mg/dl
◆ Base deficit greater than 4 mEq/L
◆ Partial pressure of arterial oxygen less than 60 mm Hg
◆ Estimated fluid sequestration greater than 6 L

Clinical findings
■ Steady epigastric pain centered close to the umbilicus, radiating between the 10th thoracic and 6th lumbar vertebrae (and unrelieved by vomiting) that's aggravated by fatty foods, alcohol, and lying in a recumbent position
■ In severe cases, extreme pain, persistent vomiting, abdominal rigidity, diminished bowel activity (suggesting peritonitis), crackles at lung bases, and left pleural effusion
■ Possible ileus caused by the proximity of the inflamed pancreas to the bowel
■ Diabetes mellitus (if pancreatitis damages the islets of Langerhans)
■ If onset is rapid, massive hemorrhage and total destruction of the pancreas, resulting in diabetic acidosis, shock, or coma
■ Mottled skin

■ Jaundice
■ Ascites
■ Tachycardia
■ Low-grade fever (100° F to 102° F [37.8° to 38.9° C])
■ Cold, sweaty extremities
■ Restlessness related to pain
■ Decreased pulmonary artery pressure (PAP) and cardiac output due to hemorrhage or dehydration
■ Elevated cardiac output and decreased systemic vascular resistance (if systemic inflammation or sepsis is present)

Diagnostic test results
■ *Serum amylase levels* are dramatically elevated – in many cases over 500 U/L.
■ *Urine and pleural fluid analysis amylase* is dramatically elevated in ascites.
■ *Serum lipase levels* are increased and rise slower than serum amylase.
■ *Serum calcium levels* are decreased because of fat necrosis and formation of calcium soaps.
■ *White blood cell counts* range from 8,000 to 20,000/mm³, with increased polymorphonuclear leukocytes.
■ *Glucose levels* are elevated – as high as 500 to 900 mg/dl.
■ *Abdominal X-rays* or *computed tomography (CT) scans* show dilation of the small or large bowel or calcification of the pancreas.
■ *Ultrasound* or *CT scan* reveals an increased pancreatic diameter.

COLLABORATIVE MANAGEMENT
Respiratory therapy may be included to ensure a patent airway and improve respiratory functioning. Nutritional support is indicated to assist with tissue healing and maintain a positive nitrogen balance. A pain management team may also be called upon to assist in that area. Additionally, social services may be involved to assist with emotional support for the patient and his family and with follow-up care.

TREATMENT AND CARE
■ The goal of therapy is to maintain circulation and fluid volume. Treatment measures must also relieve pain and decrease pancreatic secretions.
■ Monitor the patient's vital signs and PAP or central venous pressure closely. Give plasma or albumin to maintain blood pressure.

Record fluid intake and output (check urine output hourly), and monitor electrolyte levels. Assess for crackles, rhonchi, or decreased breath sounds.

■ For bowel decompression, maintain constant nasogastric suctioning and give nothing by mouth.

■ Watch for signs and symptoms of calcium deficiency — tetany, cramps, carpopedal spasm, and seizures. If you suspect hypocalcemia, keep airway and suction apparatus handy and pad side rails.

■ Administer analgesics to relieve the patient's pain and anxiety. Because anticholinergics reduce salivary and sweat gland secretions, warn the patient that he may experience dry mouth and facial flushing. Also note that atropine and its derivatives are contraindicated in patients with narrow-angle glaucoma.

■ Monitor glucose levels.

■ Emergency treatment of shock (the most common cause of death in early-stage pancreatitis) consists of vigorous I.V. replacement of electrolytes and proteins. Metabolic acidosis that develops secondary to hypovolemia and impaired cellular perfusion requires vigorous fluid volume replacement.

■ Drug treatment may include meperidine (Demeral) for pain; morphine (Duramorph) and codeine are usually avoided because of their effect on the sphincter of Oddi), diazepam (Valium) for restlessness and agitation, and antibiotics for bacterial infections.

■ If the patient has hypocalcemia, he needs an infusion of 10% calcium gluconate; if he has elevated serum glucose levels, he may require insulin therapy.

■ If the patient isn't ready to resume oral feedings after 5 to 7 days of I.V. therapy, total parenteral nutrition (TPN) may be necessary. Nonstimulating elemental gavage feedings may be safer because of the decreased risk of infection and overinfusion.

■ Watch for complications stemming from TPN, such as sepsis, hypokalemia, overhydration, and metabolic acidosis. Watch for fever, cardiac irregularities, changes in arterial blood gas measurements, and deep respirations. Use strict aseptic technique when caring for a central venous catheter insertion site.

■ In extreme cases, laparotomy to debride the pancreatic bed, partial pancreatectomy, or a combination of both plus a feeding jejunostomy may be needed.

Acute renal failure

Obstruction, reduced circulation (hypoperfusion), and renal parenchymatous disease can cause sudden interruption of kidney function, resulting in acute renal failure. Acute renal failure occurs in 5% of hospitalized patients and produces imbalances as the kidneys lose the ability to excrete water, electrolytes, metabolic wastes, and acid-base products in urine. Although acute renal failure is a critical illness, it's usually reversible with immediate medical treatment. If left untreated, however, it may progress to chronic renal failure, uremic syndrome and, ultimately, death.

ETIOLOGY
Acute renal failure can be classified as prerenal, intrarenal, or postrenal.

Prerenal failure is caused by decreased blood flow to the kidneys or decreased renal hypoperfusion. Conditions that cause decreased renal hypoperfusion include shock, embolism, blood loss, sepsis, ascites, burns, or such cardiac disorders as heart failure, arrhythmias, and cardiac tamponade. Other causes include disorders of the blood, such as idiopathic thrombocytopenia, purpura, transfusion reactions, malignant hypertension, and bleeding related to placental abruption or placenta previa. Autoimmune disorders, such as scleroderma, can also lead to prerenal failure.

Intrarenal failure occurs from damage to the kidneys, commonly from acute tubular necrosis. Damage may result from acute poststreptococcal glomerulonephritis, systemic lupus erythematosus, polyarteritis nodosa, vasculitis, sickle cell disease, bilateral renal vein thrombosis, nephrotoxin exposure, ischemia, renal myeloma, and acute pyelonephritis.

Postrenal failure results from bilateral obstruction of urine outflow. Possible causes include renal calculi, thrombus, papillae from papillary necrosis, tumors, benign prostatic hyperplasia, strictures, and urethral edema from catheterization.

PATHOPHYSIOLOGY

Acute renal failure usually occurs in three distinct phases: oliguric, diuretic, and recovery.

During the oliguric phase, which lasts a few days to several weeks, urine output drops below 400 ml/day. Intrarenal vasoconstriction; medullary hypoxia, causing cells to swell and neutrophils to adhere to capillaries and venules; and hypoperfusion lead to cellular injury and necrosis. Increasing ischemia and vasoconstriction further limit perfusion.

During the diuretic phase, which commonly lasts 10 days, urine output increases dramatically to approximately 150% of normal. However, waste products start to clear near the end of this phase.

The recovery, or final, phase may last 3 to 12 months or longer. During this phase, laboratory results return to normal levels, renal blood flow and oxygenation return to near normal levels, and the patient becomes asymptomatic.

Renal system

- Oliguria occurs as a result of decreased glomerular filtration rate (GFR).
- Hyperkalemia occurs as a result of decreased GFR and metabolic acidosis.
- Hyperphosphatemia and hypocalcemia occur because the kidney can't excrete phosphorus.
- Hypotension and dehydration may occur during the diuretic phase and lead to further ischemia of the kidneys.

Cardiovascular system

- Hypertension and edema occur with fluid accumulation and hypervolemia.
- Fluid overload may cause pulmonary and peripheral edema, possibly leading to heart failure because of how these conditions increase the heart's workload. (See *Disorders affecting management of acute renal failure*, pages 34 and 35.)
- Acute pulmonary edema and hypertensive crisis may result from nephron loss and decreased kidney size, causing decreased blood flow to the kidneys.
- Arrhythmias and cardiac arrest may result from hyperkalemia.

Endocrine and metabolic systems

- A hypermetabolic state caused by energy demands causes tissue catabolism and alterations in blood glucose levels.
- Metabolic acidosis occurs because the kidney can't excrete hydrogen ions and reabsorb sodium and bicarbonate.

Gastrointestinal system

- Nausea, vomiting, and anorexia occur with uremia.
- GI bleeding may occur with coagulation abnormalities and uremic gastric irritation.

Immune and hematologic systems

- Anemia occurs because of decreased erythropoiesis, glomerular filtration of erythrocytes, or bleeding associated with platelet dysfunction.
- Infection and sepsis may occur because of decreased white blood cell–mediated immunity.
- A hypercoagulable state results from anticoagulant abnormalities, which leads to bleeding and clotting difficulties.

Integumentary system

- Accumulation of uremic toxins leads to dryness, pruritus, pallor, purpura, and (rarely) the deposition of the uremic toxins on the skin (uremic frost).

Musculoskeletal system

- Muscle weakness may result from hyperkalemia.
- Pathological bone fractures may be caused by prolonged hypocalcemia.

Neurologic system

- Altered mental status and peripheral neuropathies are related to the effects of uremic toxins on the highly sensitive nerve cells.
- Headache, drowsiness, irritability, and seizures result from central nervous system involvement and, without treatment, may progress to coma.

Respiratory system

- Tachypnea and labored breathing result from anemia, causing tissue hypoxia. Respiratory rate and effort also increase to compensate for metabolic acidosis.

ASSESSMENT

A thorough assessment of the patient with acute renal failure is crucial because of the disorder's potential for affecting multiple body systems.

Clinical findings

■ Altered urinary elimination related to oliguria, anuria, or diuresis
■ Irritability, drowsiness, or confusion
■ Altered level of consciousness
■ Dry, pruritic skin
■ Infection related to an altered immune status
■ Hematuria, petechiae, and ecchymosis related to bleeding abnormalities
■ Fatigue, dyspnea, and malaise related to anemia
■ Anorexia, nausea, and vomiting
■ Edema related to fluid retention
■ Tachycardia and tachypnea
■ Bibasilar crackles
■ Uremic breath odor
■ Hypertension or hypotension (depending on the stage of acute renal failure)
■ Dry mucous membranes

Diagnostic test results

■ *Blood studies* show increased blood urea nitrogen, serum creatinine and potassium levels; serum phosphorus levels may be increased. Serum protein levels may be low.
■ *Laboratory studies* show a decrease in bicarbonate, hematocrit, hemoglobin, and acid pH levels.
■ *Urine studies* show casts, cellular debris, and decreased specific gravity. In glomerular disease, proteinuria and a urine osmolality close to the serum osmolality are present.
■ A *creatinine clearance test* will show a decreased number of functioning neurons and a decreased glomerular filtration rate.
■ *Electrocardiography* shows tall, peaked T waves; widening QRS complex; and disappearing P waves (if hyperkalemia is present).

COLLABORATIVE MANAGEMENT

A renal specialist or nephrologist can help evaluate, treat, and manage the patient's kidney function. Respiratory and cardiology specialists may be consulted depending on the patient's history and complications he may develop. Nutritional therapy may be involved to help institute necessary restrictions or supplementations. Physical and oc-cupational therapy may be necessary to help with energy conservation and rehabilitation depending on the patient's condition and length of stay. If a prolonged hospital stay is expected and the patient requires long-term or home care, social services may be consulted early on in the patient's care. The patient may also benefit from psychological or spiritual counseling if he's acutely ill or will require continued care even on discharge.

TREATMENT AND CARE

■ Monitor the patient's intake and output, daily weights, renal function studies, and vital signs.
■ Watch for multisystem effects of hypervolemia.
■ Monitor the dialysis access site, if applicable.
■ Place the patient on a high-calorie diet that's low in protein, sodium, phosphorous, and potassium to meet his metabolic needs.
■ Provide I.V. fluids to maintain fluid and electrolyte balance. Fluids may be restricted to minimize edema or may be increased during the diuretic phase.
■ Start diuretic therapy during the oliguric phase.

RED FLAG *Hyperkalemia is a medical emergency that must be promptly treated or it may lead to cardiac arrest.*

■ Dialytic therapies include hemodialysis, peritoneal dialysis, or continuous renal replacement therapy. These therapies are used to manage fluid, electrolyte, and acid-base imbalances. If the patient recovers renal function, long-term hemodialysis or peritoneal dialysis isn't necessary. If the patient doesn't recover renal function and progresses to chronic renal failure, long-term dialysis therapy or renal transplantation is required.
■ Monitor for signs of infection, and administer antibiotics as appropriate. Antibiotics shouldn't be administered immediately before hemodialysis because the process will remove the drug. Administer antibiotics and other medications after dialysis unless ordered otherwise.

RED FLAG *If the patient is prescribed an antihypertensive, avoid giving this drug immediately before hemodialysis to prevent the development of hypotension during treatment.*

(Text continues on page 36.)

DISORDERS AFFECTING
MANAGEMENT OF ACUTE RENAL FAILURE

This chart highlights disorders that affect the management of acute renal failure.

DISORDER	SIGNS AND SYMPTOMS	DIAGNOSTIC TEST RESULTS
Hyperkalemia (complication)	◆ Skeletal muscle weakness ◆ Flaccid paralysis ◆ Decreased heart rate ◆ Irregular pulse ◆ Decreased cardiac output ◆ Hypotension ◆ Cardiac arrest	◆ Electrocardiography (ECG) shows tall, tented T waves (characteristic); flattened P wave; and prolonged PR interval. ◆ Serum potassium levels are greater than 5 mEq/L; however, with severe hyperkalemia, levels are greater than 7mEq/L.
Hypertension (complication)	◆ Bounding pulse ◆ Fourth heart sound (S_4) ◆ Dizziness ◆ Fatigue ◆ Palpitations ◆ Chest pain ◆ Dyspnea ◆ Elevated blood pressure on at least two consecutive readings after initial screening	◆ Blood pressure is elevated (intermittent or sustained). ◆ Urinalysis may show protein, red blood cells, white blood cells, or glucose. ◆ Serum potassium levels are less than 3.5 mEq/L, possibly indicating adrenal dysfunction. ◆ Blood urea nitrogen (BUN) and creatinine levels are normal or elevated. ◆ ECG may reveal left ventricular hypertrophy. ◆ Arterial blood gas (ABG) analysis shows hypoxemia, hypercapnia, or acidosis. ◆ Chest X-ray shows diffuse haziness of the lung fields, cardiomegaly, and pleural effusion.
Pulmonary edema (complication)	◆ Restlessness and anxiety ◆ Rapid, labored breathing ◆ Intense, productive cough ◆ Frothy, bloody sputum ◆ Mental status changes ◆ Jugular vein distention ◆ Wheezing ◆ Crackles ◆ Third heart sound ◆ Tachycardia ◆ Hypotension ◆ Thready pulse ◆ Peripheral edema ◆ Hepatomegaly	◆ Pulse oximetry may reveal decreased oxygenation of the blood. ◆ Pulmonary artery catheterization may reveal increased pulmonary artery wedge pressures. ◆ ECG may show valvular disease and left ventricular hypokinesis or akinesis.

TREATMENT AND CARE

- Administer loop diuretics.
- Discontinue medications known to increase potassium, including antibiotics, angiotensin-converting enzymes, inhibitors, beta-adrenergic blockers, digoxin, heparin, nonsteroidal anti-inflammatory drugs, and potassium-sparing diuretics.
- Administer sodium polystyrene sulfonate (Kayexalate) (for mild hyperkalemia) or sorbitol. Watch for signs of heart failure when administering Kayexalate. Administer I.V. hypertonic glucose, insulin, and sodium bicarbonate (for severe hyperkalemia).
- Monitor serum potassium and other electrolytes frequently.
- Assess vital signs.
- Institute and maintain cardiac monitoring.
- Monitor intake and output, reporting an output of less than 30 ml/hour.
- Watch for signs of hypokalemia.
- Prepare the patient for dialysis if other treatments fail.

- Administer antihypertensives; adjust dosage to manage blood pressure.
- Monitor blood pressure.
- Monitor BUN and creatinine levels.
- Institute a sodium-restricted, low-fat diet.
- Encourage stress reduction, an exercise program, and behavior modification related to alcohol or tobacco use.
- Assess for bruits over the abdominal aorta and femoral arteries or the carotids.
- Assess for peripheral edema, bounding pulse, and respiratory distress related to hypervolemia.
- Assess for S_4.

- Identify and attempt to correct or manage the underlying disease.
- Closely monitor pulse oximetry and ABG results and hemodynamic values.
- Institute energy conservation strategies and space activities, as dictated by respiratory ability.
- Provide supplemental oxygen and mechanical ventilation.
- Restrict fluids and sodium.
- Closely monitor intake and output.
- Implement cardiac monitoring.
- Administer antiarrhythmics, diuretics, preload and afterload reducing agents, bronchodilators, or vasopressors.
- Maintain adequate cardiac output.
- Assess weight daily.

■ Provide emotional support and information on the disease process to the patient and his family members. Refer the patient to community resources if the disease progresses to chronic renal failure, thus requiring long-term dialysis.

Acute respiratory distress syndrome

Acute respiratory distress syndrome (ARDS) is a noncardiac form of pulmonary edema that can quickly lead to acute respiratory failure.

The prognosis for the patient with ARDS varies depending on the cause, the patient's age, and presence of comorbid conditions. Survival is high (over 90%) for patients who are young and relatively healthy before the event. If the patient is elderly or has a chronic disorder or multisystem organ dysfunction, the mortality rate ranges from 50% to 60%.

ETIOLOGY
Trauma is the most common cause of ARDS, possibly because trauma-related factors, such as fat emboli, sepsis, shock, pulmonary contusions, and multiple transfusions, increase the likelihood of microemboli developing.

Other common causes of ARDS include aspiration of gastric contents, diffuse pneumonia (especially viral), drug overdose (for example, heroin, aspirin, and ethchlorvynol), idiosyncratic drug reaction (to ampicillin and hydrochlorothiazide), blood transfusion reaction, inhalation of noxious gases (such as nitrous oxide, ammonia, and chlorine), near drowning, burn injury, and oxygen toxicity.

Less common causes of ARDS include coronary artery bypass grafting, hemodialysis, leukemia, acute miliary tuberculosis, pancreatitis, thrombotic thrombocytopenia purpura, uremia, and venous air embolism.

PATHOPHYSIOLOGY
In ARDS, the alveolar epithelium and the pulmonary capillary epithelium are injured by a specific agent or event, triggering a se-

ries of cellular and biochemical changes. (See *How ARDS develops*.)

Respiratory system
■ Damage to alveolar and pulmonary capillary epithelium triggers neutrophils, macrophages, monocytes, and lymphocytes to produce various cytokines that promote cellular activation, chemotaxis, and adhesion.
■ Damage can occur directly (by aspiration of gastric contents and inhalation of noxious gases) or indirectly (from chemical mediators released in response to systemic disease).
■ The activated cells produce inflammatory mediators, including oxidants, proteases, kinins, growth factors, and neuropeptides, which initiate the complement cascade, intravascular coagulation, and fibrinolysis.
■ Vascular permeability to proteins increases, ultimately affecting the hydrostatic pressure gradient of the capillary. Plasma and blood leak into the alveoli and interstitial space.
■ Fluid accumulates in the lung interstitium, the alveolar spaces, and the small airways, causing the lungs to stiffen and thus impairing ventilation and reducing oxygenation of the pulmonary capillary blood.
■ Pressure changes and decreased surfactant result in alveolar collapse and atelectasis.
■ Interstitial inflammation develops, and epithelial cells proliferate.
■ Fluid in the alveoli and alveolar cell damage reduce surfactant production. Without surfactant, surface tension in the alveoli increases.
■ Lung surface area is decreased as the lungs become less compliant and the alveoli collapse. (See *Disorders affecting management of ARDS*, pages 38 and 39.)
■ Gas exchange is impaired, and respirations increase to address hypoxia.
■ Initially, oxygenation is affected and carbon dioxide (CO_2) levels decrease because CO_2 is more easily diffused across the impaired alveolar-capillary membrane. As gas exchange worsens, hypercapnia develops.
■ Hyaline membranes form because of the lack of surfactant and the collection of tissue debris and white blood cells in the airway.
■ Inflammation leads to fibrosis, further impeding gas exchange. Fibrosis progres-

(*Text continues on page 40.*)

HOW ARDS DEVELOPS

These diagrams show the process and progress of acute respiratory distress syndrome (ARDS).

Phase 1. Injury reduces normal blood flow to the lungs. Platelets aggregate and release histamine (H), serotonin (S), and bradykinin (B).

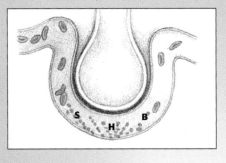

Phase 2. The released substances inflame and damage the alveolar capillary membrane, increasing capillary permeability. Fluids then shift into the interstitial space.

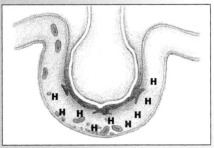

Phase 3. Capillary permeability increases and proteins and fluids leak out, increasing interstitial osmotic pressure and causing pulmonary edema.

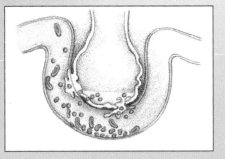

Phase 4. Decreased blood flow and fluids in the alveoli damage surfactant and impair the cell's ability to produce more. The alveoli then collapse, thus impairing gas exchange.

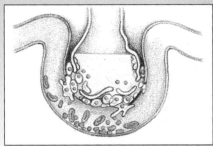

Phase 5. Oxygenation is impaired, but carbon dioxide (CO_2) easily crosses the alveolar capillary membrane and is expired. Blood oxygen (O_2) and CO_2 levels are low.

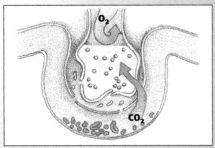

Phase 6. Pulmonary edema worsens, and inflammation leads to fibrosis. Gas exchange is further impeded.

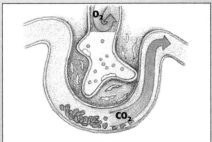

DISORDERS AFFECTING MANAGEMENT OF ARDS

This chart highlights disorders that affect the management of acute respiratory distress syndrome (ARDS).

DISORDER	SIGNS AND SYMPTOMS	DIAGNOSTIC TEST RESULTS
Metabolic acidosis (complication)	◆ Headache, lethargy progressing to drowsiness, central nervous system depression, Kussmaul's respirations, hypotension, stupor, and coma ◆ Anorexia, nausea, vomiting, diarrhea, and possibly dehydration ◆ Warm, flushed skin ◆ Fruity breath odor	◆ Arterial pH is below 7.35. ◆ Partial pressure of arterial carbon dioxide ($Paco_2$) may be normal or less than 34 mm Hg; bicarbonate level may be less than 22 mEq/L. ◆ Serum potassium level is greater than 5.5 mEq/L. ◆ Anion gap is greater than 14 mEq/L.
Multisystem organ dysfunction syndrome (complication)	◆ Hypotension ◆ Tachycardia ◆ Weak, thready peripheral pulses ◆ Decreased urine output ◆ Respiratory distress (tachypnea, accessory muscle use) ◆ Lung crackles on auscultation ◆ Peripheral edema ◆ Decreased LOC	◆ Complete blood count may reveal increased white blood cells and decreased hemoglobin. ◆ Serum studies show hyperglycemia in early stages, increased lactate levels, and electrolyte and enzyme abnormalities. ◆ Arterial blood gas (ABG) analysis shows metabolic acidosis with a pH less than 7.35 and a $Paco_2$ less than 32 mm Hg. ◆ Chest X-ray may show pulmonary edema.
Pneumonia (coexisting)	◆ Elevated temperature ◆ Cough with purulent, yellow, or bloody sputum ◆ Dyspnea ◆ Crackles ◆ Decreased breath sounds ◆ Pleuritic pain ◆ Chills ◆ Malaise ◆ Tachypnea	◆ Chest X-ray shows infiltrates. ◆ Sputum smear reveals acute inflammatory cells.
Pneumothorax (coexisting)	◆ Sudden, sharp pleuritic pain exacerbated by chest movement, breathing, and coughing ◆ Asymmetrical chest wall movement ◆ Shortness of breath ◆ Cyanosis and respiratory distress ◆ Absent breath sounds on the affected side ◆ Chest rigidity ◆ Tachycardia and hypotension ◆ Mediastinal shift and tracheal deviation	◆ Chest X-ray shows air in the pleural space and, possibly, mediastinal shift. ◆ ABG analysis may show hypoxemia, possibly with respiratory acidosis and hypercapnia.

TREATMENT AND CARE

- For severe cases, administer sodium bicarbonate I.V.
- Frequently monitor vital signs, laboratory results, and level of consciousness (LOC) because changes can occur rapidly.
- Evaluate and correct electrolyte imbalances.
- Correct the underlying cause.
- Because metabolic acidosis commonly causes vomiting, position the patient to prevent aspiration.
- Record intake and output carefully to monitor renal function.

- Monitor blood pressure, heart rate, and peripheral pulses continuously or every hour.
- Administer I.V. fluids, inotropic drugs, and vasodilators or vasopressors to maximize cardiac function.
- Watch the patient closely for signs of decreased cerebral perfusion (decreased LOC, restlessness) and decreased renal perfusion (urine output less than 0.5 ml/kg/hour, elevated serum blood urea nitrogen, creatinine, and potassium levels).
- Administer antibiotic therapy to treat underlying infection.
- Assess for interstitial edema, indicated by pretibial, sacral, ankle, and hand edema and lung crackles.
- Administer oxygen therapy as needed to increase oxygen available to tissues.
- Prepare for endotracheal intubation and mechanical ventilation if the patient exhibits impaired gas exchange.
- Maintain a patent airway by assisting with coughing or suctioning as needed.

- Administer antimicrobial therapy according to the causative organism.
- Provide humidified oxygen therapy for hypoxia and mechanical ventilation for respiratory failure.
- Administer an analgesic to relieve pleuritic chest pain.
- Provide a high-calorie diet, adequate fluid intake, and bed rest as needed.

- If the lung collapse is less than 30% and the patient shows no signs of dyspnea or other compromise, treatment includes bed rest, blood pressure monitoring, oxygen administration and, possibly, needle aspiration of the chest to remove air.
- If more than 30% of the lung is collapsed, treatment to reexpand the lung includes placing a thoracostomy tube and connecting it to an underwater seal or low-pressure suction.
- Watch for pallor, gasping respirations, and sudden chest pain.
- Carefully monitor vital signs at least every hour for indications of shock, increasing respiratory distress, or mediastinal shift.
- Ascultate for breath sounds over both lungs.
- Encourage the patient to cough and deep breathe at least once per hour to facilitate lung expansion after the chest tube is in place.
- Observe the chest tube site for leakage; change dressings around the chest tube insertion site as needed.
- Prevent potential barotraumas and pneumothorax by using the lowest pressures needed to reduce hypoxemia, or by ventilating with smaller volumes and permitting hypercapnia.

sively obliterates alveoli, respiratory bronchioles, and the interstitium. Functional residual capacity decreases, and shunting becomes more serious.
■ Increasing partial pressure of arterial carbon dioxide leads to respiratory acidosis.
■ Hypoxia further increases acidosis; pH decreases.
■ Hypoxia and acidosis result in mental changes.

Immune system
■ The lung injury causes an inflammatory response, which continues as ARDS progresses.
■ Platelets aggregate at the lung injury site and release substances — such as serotonin, bradykinin, and histamine — that attract and activate neutrophils. These substances inflame and damage the alveolar membrane and increase capillary permeability.
■ Additional chemotactic factors are released, including endotoxins (such as those present in septic states), tumor necrosis factor, and interleukin-1 (IL-1). The activated neutrophils also release several inflammatory mediators and platelet aggravating factors that damage the alveolar capillary membrane and increase capillary permeability.
■ Histamines and other inflammatory substances increase capillary permeability, allowing fluids to move into the interstitial space. As capillary permeability increases, proteins, blood cells, and more fluid leak out, increasing interstitial osmotic pressure and causing pulmonary edema.
■ Mediators released by neutrophils and macrophages cause varying degrees of pulmonary vasoconstriction, resulting in pulmonary hypertension and causing a ventilation-perfusion ($\dot{V}/\dot{Q}$) mismatch.
■ Systemically, neutrophils and inflammatory mediators cause generalized endothelial damage and increased capillary permeability throughout the body.
■ Multiple organ dysfunction syndrome (MODS) occurs as the cascade of mediators affects each body system.
■ Death may occur from the influence of ARDS and MODS.

ASSESSMENT
The patient's history will likely reveal one or more risk factors for ARDS, such as multiple trauma, severe pulmonary tissue injury, aspiration, pneumonia, or sepsis. Specific signs and symptoms will depend on the pathophysiologic processes contributing to the development of ARDS.

Clinical findings
■ Hypoxemia, which if uncorrected results in hypotension, decreasing urine output, respiratory and metabolic acidosis and, eventually, ventricular fibrillation or standstill
■ Rapid respirations
■ Dyspnea within hours to days of the initial injury (sometimes after the patient's condition appears to be stable)
■ Hypoxemia, causing an increased drive for ventilation
■ Intercostal and suprasternal retractions (because of the effort required to expand the stiff lung)
■ Crackles and rhonchi produced by fluid accumulation upon auscultation
■ Tachycardia, possibly with transient increased arterial blood pressure, as hypoxemia worsens
■ Restlessness, apprehension, mental sluggishness, confusion, and motor dysfunction as hypoxemia worsens

Diagnostic test results
■ *Arterial blood gas (ABG) analysis* (with the patient breathing room air) initially shows a partial pressure of arterial oxygen (Pao_2) less than 60 mm Hg and a $Paco_2$ less than 35 mm Hg. Blood pH usually reflects respiratory alkalosis. As ARDS worsens, ABG values show respiratory acidosis ($Paco_2$ more than 45 mm Hg) and metabolic acidosis (bicarbonate levels less than 22 mEq/L) and declining Pao_2 despite oxygen therapy.
■ *Pulmonary artery wedge pressure (PAWP)* values are 12 mm Hg or less.
■ *Serial chest X-rays* in early stages initially may be normal. In later stages, findings demonstrate lung fields with a ground-glass appearance and, eventually, "whiteouts" of both lung fields.
■ *Sputum analyses* (including Gram stain and culture and sensitivity tests), *blood cultures* (to identify infectious organisms), *toxicology tests* (to screen for drug ingestion), and *serum amylase tests* (to rule out pancreatitis) may reveal the causative factor.

COLLABORATIVE MANAGEMENT

A pulmonary specialist can help evaluate and treat the patient's respiratory system. If infectious agents are involved, an infectious disease specialist may be called in; if cardiac involvement is suspected, a cardiologist may be consulted. If the patient progresses through the later stages of ARDS and a prolonged course is expected, a nutritional consult for total parenteral nutrition may be needed as well as specialists in physical and occupational therapy to assist with rehabilitation. If this patient develops a prolonged dependency on ventilation, he may require an extended care facility that can accept ventilator-dependent patients (after he's stabilized). If a prolonged stay in the health care facility is expected and the patient requires long-term care, social services should be consulted. Alternatively, if ARDS is arrested in the initial stages, the patient may be discharged to home with instructions to follow up with his health care provider.

TREATMENT AND CARE

Therapy focuses on correcting the cause of the syndrome, if possible, and preventing the progression of life-threatening hypoxemia and respiratory acidosis. Supportive care may involve:

- administration of humidified oxygen by a tight-fitting mask, which facilitates the use of continuous positive airway pressure (if the patient's hypoxemia isn't corrected with this treatment, he may require intubation and mechanical ventilation with positive end-expiratory pressure; high-frequency jet ventilation may also be used)
- pressure-controlled inverse ratio ventilation to reverse the conventional inspiration-to-expiration ratio and minimize the risk of barotrauma (mechanical breaths are pressure-limited to prevent increased damage to the alveoli)
- permissive hypercapnia to limit peak inspiratory pressure
- suctioning, humidification, percussion, and vibration techniques to help clear secretions
- administration of sedatives, opioids, or neuromuscular blockers to patients who are mechanically ventilated to minimize restlessness, oxygen consumption, and carbon dioxide production and to facilitate ventilation

- sodium bicarbonate to reverse severe metabolic acidosis
- I.V. fluid administration to maintain blood pressure by treating hypovolemia
- vasopressors to maintain blood pressure
- antimicrobial drugs to treat nonviral infections
- diuretics to reduce interstitial and pulmonary edema
- correction of electrolyte and acid-base imbalances
- fluid restriction to prevent increased interstitial and alveolar edema
- positioning strategies to address $\dot{V}/\dot{Q}$ mismatch.

Acute respiratory failure

Acute respiratory failure results when the lungs can't adequately maintain arterial oxygenation or eliminate carbon dioxide (CO_2), leading to tissue hypoxia. In patients with normal lung tissue, respiratory failure is indicated by a partial pressure of arterial carbon dioxide ($Paco_2$) greater than 50 mm Hg and a partial pressure of arterial oxygen (Pao_2) less than 50 mm Hg.

Patients with chronic obstructive pulmonary disease (COPD), however, have a consistently high $Paco_2$ (hypercapnia) and a low Pao_2 (hypoxemia). Therefore, acute deterioration in arterial blood gas (ABG) values for these patients and corresponding clinical deterioration signify acute respiratory failure.

Depending on the age of the patient and the cause of respiratory failure, this disorder can progress rapidly, resulting in a poor outcome because the ongoing lack of oxygen and buildup of CO_2 eventually lead to hypoxia and cellular death. Therefore, rapid diagnosis and intervention is needed.

ETIOLOGY

Conditions that can result in alveolar hypoventilation, ventilation-perfusion ($\dot{V}/\dot{Q}$) mismatch, or right-to-left shunting can lead to respiratory failure. These include:
- COPD
- bronchitis

WATCHFUL EYE

DISORDERS AFFECTING MANAGEMENT OF ACUTE RESPIRATORY FAILURE

This chart highlights disorders that affect the management of acute respiratory failure.

DISORDER	SIGNS AND SYMPTOMS	DIAGNOSTIC TEST RESULTS
Myocardial infarction (MI) (complication)	◆ Persistent, crushing substernal chest pain that may radiate to the left arm, jaw, neck, or shoulder blades ◆ Cool extremities, perspiration, anxiety, and restlessness ◆ Blood pressure and pulse initially elevated ◆ Hypotension (if cardiac output is reduced) ◆ Bradycardia (associated with conduction disturbances) ◆ Fatigue and weakness ◆ Nausea and vomiting ◆ Shortness of breath ◆ Lung crackles on auscultation ◆ Jugular vein distension ◆ Reduced urine output	◆ Electrocardiography (ECG) shows ST-segment changes. ◆ Total creatine kinase (CK) and CK-MB isoenzyme levels are elevated over a 72-hour period. ◆ Myoglobin is elevated within 3 to 6 hours. ◆ Echocardiography shows ventricular-wall motion abnormalities. ◆ Multigated acquisition scan or radionuclide ventriculography identifies acutely damaged muscle. ◆ Homocysteine and C-reactive protein levels are elevated.
Respiratory acidosis (complication)	◆ Restlessness ◆ Confusion ◆ Apprehension ◆ Somnolence ◆ Fine or flapping tremor (asterixis) ◆ Coma ◆ Headaches ◆ Dyspnea and tachypnea ◆ Papilledema ◆ Depressed reflexes ◆ Hypoxemia (unless the patient is receiving oxygen) ◆ Tachycardia ◆ Hypertension ◆ Atrial and ventricular arrhythmias ◆ Hypotension with vasodilation ◆ Bounding pulses and warm periphery (in severe acidosis)	◆ Arterial blood gas (ABG) analysis shows partial pressure of carbon dioxide ($Paco_2$) greater than 45 mm Hg, pH less than 7.35, normal HCO_3^- (bicarbonate) in the acute stage, and elevated HCO_3^- in the chronic stage. ◆ Chest X-ray commonly shows such causes as heart failure, pneumonia, chronic obstructive pulmonary disease (COPD), and pneumothorax. ◆ Serum potassium level is greater than 5 mEq/L, and serum chloride is low. ◆ Urine pH is acidic.

TREATMENT AND CARE

◆ Be prepared to administer an antiarrhythmic, to possibly assist with pacemaker insertion and, rarely, to assist with cardioversion, to treat cardiac arrhythmias.

◆ Be prepared to administer thrombolytic therapy (streptokinase or recombinant tissue plasminogen) to preserve myocardial tissue.

◆ Percutaneous transluminal coronary angioplasty may be done to restore blood flow to the heart muscle.

◆ Be prepared to administer other drugs as needed, including antiplatelet drugs (aspirin) to inhibit platelet aggregation; sublingual or I.V. nitrates (nitroglycerin) to relieve pain, increase cardiac output, and reduce myocardial workload; morphine for pain and sedation; and angiotensin-converting enzyme inhibitors to improve survival rate in large anterior-wall MI.

◆ Administer oxygen at a modest flow rate for 3 to 6 hours.

◆ Assist with pulmonary artery catheterization, which is used to detect left- or right-sided heart failure and to monitor the patient's response to treatment.

◆ Assess and record the severity of chest pain.

◆ During episodes of chest pain, obtain ECG, blood pressure, and pulmonary artery catheter measurements for changes.

◆ Monitor vital signs frequently.

◆ Watch for signs and symptoms of fluid retention (crackles, cough, tachypnea, and edema).

◆ Carefully monitor daily weight, intake and output, and serum enzyme levels.

◆ The goal of treatment is to correct the underlying source of alveolar hypoventilation.

◆ Mechanical ventilation may be needed until the underlying condition can be treated. If so, maintain a patent airway and provide adequate humidification, perform tracheal suctioning regularly, and continuously monitor ventilator settings and respiratory status.

◆ Treatment for patients with COPD may include a bronchodilator, oxygen, a corticosteroid and, commonly, an antibiotic.

◆ Closely monitor the patient's ABG values.

◆ Watch for critical changes in the patient's respiratory, central nervous system, and cardiovascular functions.

◆ Maintain adequate hydration.

■ pneumonia
■ bronchospasm
■ ventilatory failure
■ pneumothorax
■ atelectasis
■ cor pulmonale
■ pulmonary edema
■ pulmonary emboli
■ central nervous system (CNS) disease
■ CNS depression caused by head trauma or injudicious use of sedatives, opioids, tranquilizers, or oxygen.

PATHOPHYSIOLOGY

Respiratory failure results from impaired gas exchange. Any condition associated with alveolar hypoventilation, $\dot{V}/\dot{Q}$ mismatch, and intrapulmonary shunting can cause acute respiratory failure if left untreated.

Respiratory system

■ Hypoxemia and hypercapnia stimulate strong compensatory responses by all of the body systems.

■ Decreased oxygen saturation may result from alveolar hypoventilation, in which chronic airway obstruction reduces alveolar minute ventilation. Pa_{O_2} levels fall and Pa_{CO_2} levels rise, resulting in hypoxemia. The most common cause of alveolar hypoventilation is airway obstruction, commonly seen with COPD (emphysema or bronchitis).

■ Most commonly, hypoxemia — $\dot{V}/\dot{Q}$ imbalance — occurs when such conditions as pulmonary embolism or acute respiratory distress syndrome interrupt normal gas exchange in a specific lung region. Too little ventilation with normal blood flow or too little blood flow with normal ventilation may cause the imbalance, resulting in decreased Pa_{O_2} levels and, thus, hypoxemia.

■ Although uncommon, a decreased fraction of inspired oxygen may lead to respiratory failure. Inspired air doesn't contain adequate oxygen to establish an adequate gradient for diffusion into the blood — for example, at high altitudes or in confined, enclosed spaces. As a result, hypoxemia occurs.

■ Tissue hypoxemia results in anaerobic metabolism and lactic acidosis. Respiratory acidosis occurs from hypercapnia. (See *Disorders affecting management of acute respiratory failure*.) Cyanosis occurs because of increased amounts of unoxygenated blood. As respiratory failure worsens, intercostal, supraclavicular, and suprasternal retractions may also occur.

Cardiovascular system
■ Untreated V̇/Q̇ imbalances can lead to right-to-left shunting, in which blood passes from the heart's right side to its left without being oxygenated. This results in unoxygenated blood reaching the arterial system to be distributed to the rest of the body.
■ Heart rate and stroke volume increases; heart failure may occur.
■ Hypoxemia deprives the myocardial tissue of oxygen and nutrients, possibly resulting in ischemia or myocardial infarction.

Neurologic system
■ In response to hypoxemia, the sympathetic nervous system triggers vasoconstriction, increases peripheral resistance, and increases the heart rate.
■ Hypoxemia or hypercapnia (or both) causes the brain's respiratory control center to increase respiratory depth (tidal volume) and then to increase the respiratory rate.

Hematologic system
■ Hypoxia of the kidneys results in release of erythropoietin from renal cells, causing the bone marrow to increase production of red blood cells — an attempt by the body to increase the blood's oxygen-carrying capacity.

ASSESSMENT
History may reveal an underlying respiratory condition or an acute process leading to respiratory failure (such as asphyxia, drug overdose, or trauma). However, because acute respiratory failure is life-threatening, time to conduct an in-depth patient interview is limited. Therefore, interviewing family members or reviewing the patient's medical records (at a later time) may help to determine the precipitating incident.

Clinical findings
■ Nasal flaring (secondary to hypoxia), ashen skin, and cyanosis of the oral mucosa, lips, and nail beds (due to hypoxemia)
■ Yawning
■ Use of accessory muscles to breathe

■ Restlessness, anxiety, depression, lethargy, agitation, or confusion (resulting from cerebral hypoxia)
■ Tachypnea (due to hypoxia), signaling impending respiratory failure
■ Cold, clammy skin (due to vasoconstriction)
■ Asymmetrical chest movement, suggesting pneumothorax
■ Tactile fremitus that typically decreases over obstructed bronchi or pleural effusion areas but increases over consolidated lung tissue
■ Hyperresonance upon percussion (especially in patients with COPD)
■ Dull or flat sound upon percussion (if acute respiratory failure results from atelectasis or pneumonia)
■ Diminished breath sounds upon auscultation, indicating areas of hypoventilation
■ Absent breath sounds (in patients with pneumothorax)
■ Adventitious breath sounds, such as wheezes (in asthma) and rhonchi (in bronchitis)
■ Possible crackles, suggesting pulmonary edema as the cause of respiratory failure

Diagnostic test results
■ *ABG analysis* reveals Pao_2 less than 50 mm Hg and $Paco_2$ greater than 50 mm Hg and a pH below 7.35.
■ *Chest X-ray* identifies emphysema, atelectasis, lesions, pneumothorax, infiltrates, and effusions.
■ *Electrocardiography* may reveal arrhythmias that are commonly found with cor pulmonale and myocardial hypoxia.
■ *Pulse oximetry* reveals a decreasing arterial oxygen saturation and a mixed venous oxygen saturation level of less than 50%.
■ *White blood cell count* may be increased if an underlying infection is the cause.
■ *Hemoglobin and hematocrit levels* are abnormally low.
■ *Electrolyte levels* may show imbalances resulting from hyperventilation, acidosis, or hypoxia.
■ *Blood cultures, sputum culture,* and *Gram stain* may identify pathogens.
■ *Pulmonary artery catheterization* helps to distinguish pulmonary and cardiovascular causes of acute respiratory failure and monitors hemodynamic pressures.

COLLABORATIVE MANAGEMENT

A pulmonary specialist can help evaluate and treat the patient's respiratory system. If infectious agents are involved, an infectious disease specialist may be called in; if cardiac involvement is suspected, a cardiologist may be consulted. The patient may require nutritional support to maintain and improve overall nutrition, strengthen the immune system, and meet metabolic needs. Initially, the patient may require total parenteral nutrition, depending on the severity of the condition and the patient's status. If the patient is able to eat, a registered dietitian can provide planning to meet the patient's needs. A respiratory therapy team member can assist with oxygen therapy and ventilatory support.

Physical and occupational therapy may be necessary to help with energy conservation and rehabilitation depending on the patient's condition and length of stay. If a prolonged hospital stay is expected and the patient requires long-term care, social services should be contacted early.

TREATMENT AND CARE

Treatment typically focuses on restoring adequate gas exchange to provide oxygen to the organs, tissues, and cells, and correcting the underlying causative condition. Treatment includes:

- oxygen therapy to promote oxygenation and raise PaO_2
- mechanical ventilation with an endotracheal or tracheostomy tube, if needed, to provide adequate oxygenation and to reverse acidosis
- opioid antagonists, such as naloxone (Narcan), if drug overdose is suspected
- antibiotics to treat infection
- bronchodilators to maintain patency of the airways
- corticosteroids to decrease inflammation
- fluid restrictions (in cor pulmonale) to reduce volume and cardiac workload
- positive inotropic agents to increase cardiac output
- vasopressors to maintain blood pressure
- diuretics to reduce edema and fluid overload
- deep breathing with pursed lips to prevent alveolar collapse if the patient isn't intubated and mechanically ventilated

- incentive spirometry to increase lung volume
- chest physiotherapy or nasotracheal suction to maintain airway clearance.

Acute tubular necrosis

Acute tubular necrosis (ATN) is the most common cause of acute renal failure in critically ill patients, accounting for about 75% of all cases of acute renal failure. ATN injures the tubular segment of the nephron, causing renal failure and uremic syndrome. Mortality rates range from 40% to 70%, depending on complications from the underlying diseases. Patients with nonoliguric forms of ATN have a better prognosis.

ETIOLOGY

ATN results from ischemic or nephrotoxic injury. Ischemic injury can result from:
- circulatory collapse
- severe hypotension (lasting longer than 30 minutes)
- trauma (crush injuries, myoglobin release)
- hemorrhage or cardiogenic, septic, or neurogenic shock
- dehydration
- major surgery
- transfusion reactions (red blood cell hemolysis, hemoglobin release).

Nephrotoxic injury commonly occurs in debilitated patients, such as the critically ill or those who have undergone extensive surgery. Nephrotoxic injury may result from exposure to specific chemical agents that are toxic to the kidneys, including:
- aminoglycosides
- antifungals
- chemotherapeutic agents
- contrast media
- heavy metals (mercury, arsenic)
- solvents.

PATHOPHYSIOLOGY

Sloughing of renal tubule epithelial cells and decreased glomerular filtration and waste clearance characterize ATN. One theory suggests that the resultant tubule obstruction

DISORDERS AFFECTING MANAGEMENT OF ATN

This chart highlights disorders that affect the management of acute tubular necrosis (ATN).

DISORDER	SIGNS AND SYMPTOMS	DIAGNOSTIC TEST RESULTS
GI hemorrhage (complication)	◆ Anxiety ◆ Agitation ◆ Confusion ◆ Tachycardia ◆ Hypotension ◆ Oliguria ◆ Diaphoresis ◆ Pallor ◆ Cool, clammy skin ◆ Bright red blood in nasogastric tube drainage or vomitus (hematemesis) ◆ Coffee-ground drainage or vomitus ◆ Hematochezia (bright red blood from the rectum) ◆ Melena (black, tarry, sticky stools)	◆ Complete blood count shows decreased hemoglobin level and hematocrit (usually 6 to 8 hours after the initial symptoms); increased reticulocyte and platelet levels; and a decrease in red blood cells. ◆ Arterial blood gas (ABG) analysis reveals low pH and bicarbonate levels ◆ 12-lead electrocardiogram (ECG) may reveal evidence of cardiac ischemia secondary to hypoperfusion. ◆ Abdominal X-ray may indicate air under the diaphragm, suggesting ulcer perforation. ◆ Angiography may help visualize the site of bleeding if the bleeding is from an artery or large vein.
Sepsis (complication)	◆ Agitation ◆ Anxiety ◆ Altered LOC ◆ Tachycardia ◆ Hypotension ◆ Rapid, shallow respirations ◆ Fever ◆ Urine output less than 25 ml/hour	◆ Blood cultures are positive for the infecting organism. ◆ Complete blood count reveals whether anemia, neutropenia, and thrombocytopenia are present. ◆ ABG studies show metabolic acidosis. ◆ Blood urea nitrogen and creatinine are increased. ◆ ECG shows ST-segment depression, inverted T waves, and arrhythmias.

leads to ischemia, damage to the basement membrane, tubule death, and renal failure.

Ischemic injury disrupts blood flow to the kidneys. Ischemic ATN can damage the epithelial and basement membranes and cause lesions in the renal interstitium.

Renal system

■ Oliguria occurs as a result of decreased glomerular filtration rate (GFR).

■ Hyperkalemia occurs as a result of decreased GFR and metabolic acidosis.

■ Hyperphosphatemia and hypocalcemia occur because the kidney can't excrete phosphorus.

■ Hypotension and dehydration may occur (during the diuretic phase), leading to further kidney ischemia.

Cardiovascular system

■ Hypotension may occur early, followed by hypervolemia as the disease progresses.

■ Hypertension and peripheral edema occur with hypervolemia.

■ Heart failure develops as hypervolemia and anemia increase the heart's workload, resulting in pulmonary edema (complication of heart failure).

■ Cardiac arrest and arrhythmias may result from hyperkalemia.

Endocrine and metabolic systems

■ A hypermetabolic state caused by the energy demands promotes tissue catabolism and altered glucose levels.

TREATMENT AND CARE

◆ Begin fluid resuscitation.
◆ Ensure a patent airway, and assess breathing and circulation.
◆ Monitor cardiac and respiratory status closely – at least every 15 minutes or more, depending on the patient's condition.
◆ Administer supplemental oxygen. Monitor oxygen saturation levels (via continuous pulse oximetry) or serial ABG levels for evidence of hypoxemia.
◆ Assist with the insertion of a central venous or pulmonary artery catheter to evaluate hemodynamic status.
◆ Assess level of consciousness (LOC) frequently – approximately every 30 minutes until the patient stabilizes, and then every 2 to 4 hours as indicated by the patient's status.
◆ Monitor intake and output closely.
◆ Assist with or insert a nasogastric tube, and perform lavage using room temperature saline to clear blood and clots from the stomach. Assess gastric pH every 2 to 4 hours or continuously if indicated; maintain gastric pH between 4.0 and 5.0. Administer pharmacologic agents to maintain pH.

◆ Locate and treat the underlying cause of sepsis.
◆ Monitor vital signs frequently.
◆ Administer antibiotics.
◆ Administer I.V. fluids to replace intravascular volume.
◆ Administer vasopressors if fluid resuscitation doesn't maintain blood pressure.
◆ Assess respiratory status.
◆ Prepare the patient for intubation and mechanical ventilation.

■ Metabolic acidosis occurs because the kidney can't excrete hydrogen ions and reabsorb sodium and bicarbonate.

Gastrointestinal system
■ Nausea, vomiting, and anorexia occur with uremia.
■ GI bleeding may occur in patients with coagulation abnormalities or uremic gastric irritation.

Immune and hematologic systems
■ Anemia may occur related to decreased renal production of erythropoietin, glomerular filtration of erythrocytes, or bleeding associated with platelet dysfunction.
■ Platelet dysfunction is related to uremia.

■ Infection and sepsis commonly occur because of decreased white blood cell–mediated immunity. (See *Disorders affecting management of ATN.*)
■ A hypercoagulable state results from anticoagulant abnormalities, resulting in bleeding and clotting difficulties.

Integumentary system
■ Dryness, pruritus, pallor, purpura, and uremic frost may occur because of the accumulation of uremic toxins.

Musculoskeletal system
■ Muscle weakness is related to hyperkalemia.

■ Osteoporosis and pathological bone fractures may occur related to hyperphosphatemia and resultant hypocalcemia.

Neurologic system
■ Altered mental status and peripheral neuropathies are related to the effects of uremic toxins on the highly sensitive nerve cells.
■ Headache, drowsiness, irritability, and seizures result from central nervous system involvement and may progress to coma without treatment.

Respiratory system
■ Anemia causes tissue hypoxia, which stimulates increased ventilation and work of breathing.
■ Increased respiratory effort and rate compensate for metabolic acidosis.

ASSESSMENT
ATN is usually difficult to recognize in its early stages because effects of the patient's primary disease may mask the initial symptoms. Diagnosis is usually delayed until the condition has progressed to an advanced stage.

Clinical findings
■ Altered urinary elimination (oliguria, anuria, diuresis)
■ Irritability, drowsiness, or confusion
■ Altered level of consciousness
■ Infection related to an altered immune status
■ Hematuria, petechiae, and ecchymosis related to bleeding abnormalities
■ Fatigue, dyspnea, and malaise related to anemia
■ Anorexia, nausea, and vomiting
■ Edema related to fluid retention
■ Tachycardia and tachypnea
■ Dry, pruritic skin
■ Bibasilar crackles
■ Uremic breath odor
■ Hypertension or hypotension (depending on whether necrosis has progressed to renal failure)
■ Dry mucous membranes

Diagnostic test results
■ *Urinalysis* reveals urinary sediment containing red blood cells and casts and dilute urine of a low specific gravity (1.010), low osmolality (less than 400 mOsm/kg), and high sodium level (40 to 60 mEq/L).
■ *Blood urea nitrogen* is increased.
■ *Serum creatinine level* is increased.
■ *Urine creatinine clearance* is decreased.
■ *Hemoglobin and hematocrit levels* are low.
■ *Red blood cell count* is decreased.
■ *Platelet count* is abnormal.
■ *Blood chemistry* shows hyperkalemia, hyperphosphatemia, and hypocalcemia.
■ *Arterial blood gas* (ABG) *analysis* shows metabolic acidosis.
■ *Electrocardiogram* (ECG) may show arrhythmias resulting from electrolyte imbalances.

RED FLAG Hyperkalemia is a medical emergency. ECG changes consistent with hyperkalemia include a widening QRS segment, disappearing P waves, and tall, peaked T waves. Rhythm changes are apparent in the apical pulse.

COLLABORATIVE MANAGEMENT
A renal specialist or nephrologist can help evaluate, treat, and manage the patient's kidney function. Respiratory and cardiology specialists may be consulted depending on the patient's history and complications he may develop. Nutritional therapy may be involved to help institute necessary restrictions or supplementations. Physical and occupational therapy may be necessary to help with energy conservation and rehabilitation depending on the patient's condition and length of stay. If a prolonged hospital stay is expected and the patient requires long-term or home care, social services may be consulted early in the patient's care. The patient may also benefit from psychological or spiritual counseling if he's acutely ill or will require continued care even after discharge.

TREATMENT AND CARE
■ Treatment of patients with ATN consists of vigorous supportive measures during the acute phase until normal kidney function resumes.
■ Initial treatment may include administering diuretics and infusing a high volume of fluids to flush tubules of cellular casts and debris and to replace fluid losses; however, administering a high volume of fluid carries the risk of hypervolemia and requires careful monitoring of the patient's fluid status.

■ Long-term fluid management includes replacing projected and calculated losses and includes insensible losses.

■ Nutritional management may include restricting potassium, sodium, phosphorus, and fluids. To achieve an anabolic state, the patient must receive adequate calories and essential amino acids. Protein is usually restricted to the average daily intake.

■ Monitor intake and output, vital signs, hemoglobin level, hematocrit, electrolyte balance, ABG values, and ECG changes.

■ Blood transfusions may be required for anemia. Note that blood transfusion reactions are also a cause for the onset of ATN.

■ Antibiotics may be ordered for infection.

■ Hyperkalemia requires immediate therapy with I.V. glucose, insulin, and sodium bicarbonate, or oral or rectal sodium polystyrene sulfonate (Kayexalate) to reduce extracellular potassium levels.

■ Hemodialysis, peritoneal dialysis, or continuous renal replacement therapy may be required for severe catabolism.

■ Provide emotional support and information on the disease process to the patient and his family.

Adrenal insufficiency

Adrenal insufficiency (also called *adrenal hypofunction*) has primary and secondary forms. Primary adrenal insufficiency (Addison's disease) originates within the adrenal gland and is characterized by decreased mineralocorticoid, glucocorticoid, and androgen secretion. Addison's disease is a rare disorder that occurs in people of all ages and both sexes.

Secondary adrenal insufficiency can occur because of a disorder outside of the adrenal gland (such as pituitary tumor with corticotropin deficiency), but aldosterone secretion may continue intact. With early diagnosis and adequate replacement therapy, the prognosis for both forms of adrenal insufficiency is good.

Acute adrenal crisis — also called *addisonian crisis* — is a *critical* deficiency of mineralocorticoids and glucocorticoids. Acute adrenal crisis is a medical emergency that re-

quires immediate, vigorous treatment. (See *How acute adrenal crisis develops*, page 50.)

ETIOLOGY

Addison's disease occurs when more than 90% of the adrenal gland is destroyed. Such massive destruction usually results from an autoimmune process in which circulating antibodies react specifically against the adrenal tissue.

Other causes of Addison's disease include tuberculosis, bilateral adrenalectomy, hemorrhage into the adrenal gland, neoplasms, and such infections as human immunodeficiency virus, histoplasmosis, meningococcal pneumonia, and cytomegalovirus. Rarely, a familial tendency toward autoimmune disease predisposes a patient to Addison's disease and to other endocrinopathies. Addison's disease has also been linked to congenital adrenal hyperplasia, enzyme inhibitors, and cytotoxic agents.

Secondary adrenal insufficiency that results in glucocorticoid deficiency can stem from hypopituitarism, which can cause decreased corticotropin secretion. It can also stem from abrupt withdrawal of long-term corticosteroid therapy, as when long-term exogenous corticosteroid stimulation suppresses pituitary corticotropin secretion and causes adrenal gland atrophy. In addition, secondary adrenal insufficiency can result from removal of a nonendocrine, corticotropin-secreting tumor.

Acute adrenal crisis occurs in a patient with adrenal insufficiency when trauma, surgery, or other severe physiologic stress completely exhausts the body's stores of glucocorticoids. (See *Disorders affecting management of adrenal insufficiency*, pages 52 and 53.)

PATHOPHYSIOLOGY

Addison's disease is a chronic condition that results from the partial or complete destruction of the adrenal cortex. It manifests as a clinical syndrome in which the symptoms are associated with deficient production of the adrenocortical hormones — cortisol, aldosterone, and androgens. High levels of corticotropin and corticotropin-releasing hormone accompany the low glucocorticoid levels.

HOW ACUTE ADRENAL CRISIS DEVELOPS

Acute adrenal crisis, the most serious complication of Addison's disease, involves a critical deficiency of glucocorticoids and mineralocorticoids. This life-threatening event requires prompt assessment and immediate treatment. The flowchart below highlights the underlying mechanisms responsible for the complication.

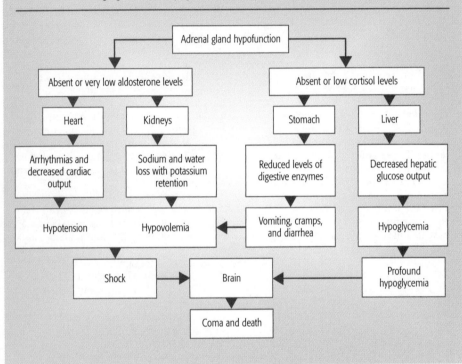

Corticotropin acts primarily to regulate the adrenal release of glucocorticoids (primarily cortisol); mineralocorticoids, including aldosterone; and androgens that supplement those produced by the gonads. Corticotropin secretion is controlled by corticotropin-releasing hormone from the hypothalamus and by negative feedback control by the glucocorticoids.

Addison's disease involves all zones of the cortex (although medullary involvement may occur, resulting in catecholamine deficiency), causing deficiencies of the adrenocortical secretions, glucocorticoids, androgens, and mineralocorticoids.

Renal system
■ Aldosterone deficiency causes increased renal sodium loss and enhances potassium reabsorption.
■ Sodium excretion causes a reduction in water volume that leads to hypotension.
■ Low plasma volume and arteriolar pressure stimulate renin release and a resulting increased production of angiotensin II.

Integumentary system
■ Androgen deficiency may decrease hair growth in axillary and pubic areas as well as on the extremities of women.

■ Abnormal bronze skin coloration results from decreased secretion of cortisol, which causes the pituitary gland to simultaneously secrete excessive amounts of melanocyte-stimulating hormone (MSH) and corticotropin.

ASSESSMENT

The history of a patient with adrenal insufficiency may reveal synthetic steroid use, adrenal surgery, or recent infection.

Clinical findings

■ Muscle weakness
■ Fatigue and syncope
■ Light-headedness when rising from a chair or bed
■ Weight loss
■ Cravings for salty food
■ Decreased tolerance for even minor stress
■ Various GI disturbances, such as nausea, vomiting, anorexia, and chronic diarrhea
■ Anxiety, irritability, and confusion
■ Reduced urine output and other symptoms of dehydration
■ In women, decreased libido resulting from reduced androgen production and amenorrhea
■ Poor coordination
■ Dry skin and mucous membranes
■ Decreased axillary and pubic hair in women
■ Bronze coloration of the skin that resembles a deep suntan, especially in the creases of the hands and over the metacarpophalangeal joints, elbows, and knees
■ Darkening of scars, areas of vitiligo (an absence of pigmentation), and increased pigmentation of the mucous membranes, especially the buccal mucosa
■ Weak, irregular pulse; tachycardia
■ Hypotension

Diagnostic test results

■ A *corticotropin stimulation test* demonstrates plasma cortisol response to corticotropin. In Addison's disease, plasma and urine cortisol levels fail to increase normally in response to corticotropin.
■ *Plasma cortisol levels* are decreased (less than 10 mcg/dl in the morning, with lower levels in the evening) in Addison's disease.

■ *Serum sodium levels* are reduced.
■ *Serum potassium, serum calcium,* and *blood urea nitrogen levels* are increased.
■ *Hematocrit, lymphocyte,* and *eosinophil counts* are elevated.
■ *X-rays* may show a small heart and adrenal calcification.

COLLABORATIVE MANAGEMENT

An endocrinologist may be involved in the management of the patient's adrenal function. As other organs become involved, however, the patient may need the assistance of a cardiologist and renal specialists. Respiratory therapists and nutritional consults may also be needed to assist the patient. Spiritual guidance may also be needed for the patient and his family.

TREATMENT AND CARE

■ Lifelong cortisone or hydrocortisone therapy is prescribed.

DRUG ALERT *Corticosteroids may cause cushingoid signs (such as fluid retention around the eyes and face) and gastric irritation. Signs of corticosteroid overdose include swelling and weight gain. Signs of underdose include lethargy or weakness.*

■ Administer oral fludrocortisone (Florinef), a synthetic mineralocorticoid, to prevent dangerous dehydration, hypotension, hyponatremia, and hyperkalemia.

DRUG ALERT *Mineralocorticoids may cause fluid and electrolyte imbalance, insomnia, and petechiae. Monitor the patient's weight and check his blood pressure to assess body fluid status.*

■ Administer I.V. bolus of hydrocortisone (initially for acute adrenal crisis), followed by hydrocortisone diluted with dextrose in I.V. saline solution to replace fluids, treat hyponatremia and hypoglycemia, and maintain blood pressure. With proper treatment, adrenal crisis usually subsides quickly; blood pressure stabilizes, and water and sodium levels return to normal. After crisis, give maintenance doses of hydrocortisone to preserve physiologic stability.
■ Administer vasopressors to treat hypotension uncorrected with initial treatment.

WATCHFUL EYE

DISORDERS AFFECTING MANAGEMENT OF ADRENAL INSUFFICIENCY

This chart highlights disorders that affect the management of adrenal insufficiency.

DISORDER	SIGNS AND SYMPTOMS	DIAGNOSTIC TEST RESULTS
Acute adrenal crisis (complication)	◆ Profound weakness ◆ Fatigue ◆ Nausea, vomiting, cramps, and diarrhea ◆ Hypotension ◆ Dehydration ◆ High fever followed by hypothermia (occasionally) ◆ Hypovolemia ◆ Shock ◆ Coma	◆ Plasma cortisol is less than 10 mcg/dl in the morning; less in the evening. ◆ Serum sodium and glucose levels are decreased. ◆ Serum potassium, blood urea nitrogen, and lymphocyte count are increased. ◆ Hematocrit is decreased. ◆ Eosinophil count is decreased. ◆ X-ray shows adrenal calcification if the cause is infection.
Diabetes mellitus (coexisting)	◆ Weight loss despite voracious hunger ◆ Weakness ◆ Vision changes ◆ Frequent skin and urinary tract infections ◆ Dry, itchy skin ◆ Poor skin turgor ◆ Dry mucous membranes ◆ Dehydration ◆ Decreased peripheral pulses ◆ Cool skin temperature ◆ Decreased reflexes ◆ Orthostatic hypotension ◆ Muscle wasting ◆ Loss of subcutaneous fat ◆ Fruity breath odor because of ketoacidosis	◆ At least two occasions of fasting plasma glucose level are ≥ 126 mg/dl, or a random blood glucose level is ≥ 200 mg/dl. ◆ Blood glucose level is ≥ 200 mg/dl 2 hours after ingestion of 75 grams oral dextrose. ◆ An ophthalmologic examination may show diabetic retinopathy.

Aortic aneurysm, abdominal

Abdominal aortic aneurysm (AAA) — an abnormal dilation in the arterial wall — generally occurs in the aorta between the renal arteries and iliac branches. Rupture — in which the aneurysm breaks open, resulting in profuse bleeding — is a common complication that occurs in larger aneurysms. Dissection occurs when the artery's lining tears and blood leaks into the walls. Up to 75% of aneurysms greater than 7 cm in diameter rupture within 5 years.

AAA is 7 times more common in men than in women and most prevalent in whites. Three-fourths of patients with AAA are older than age 60. Indeed, as the population ages, the incidence of AAA is expected to increase.

Patients with peripheral atherosclerotic vascular disease are at the greatest risk for developing an AAA. Patients with a first-degree relative with a history of AAA are also at increased risk. Smoking is another significant risk factor.

TREATMENT AND CARE

◆ Monitor vital signs closely.
◆ Watch for hypotension, volume depletion, decreased level of consciousness, reduced urine output, and other signs of shock.
◆ Monitor for hyperkalemia before treatment and for hypokalemia (from excessive mineralocorticoid effect) after treatment.
◆ Check for cardiac arrhythmias.
◆ Monitor blood pressure.
◆ Monitor sodium levels.
◆ Prepare prompt I.V. bolus administration of hydrocortisone. Doses are given I.M. or are diluted with dextrose in saline solution and given I.V. until the patient's condition stabilizes.
◆ Know that up to 300 mg/day of hydrocortisone and 3 to 5 L of I.V. saline solution may be required during the acute phase.

◆ Check blood glucose levels periodically because steroid replacement may require insulin dosage adjustment.
◆ Keep a late-morning snack available in case the patient becomes hypoglycemic.
◆ Keep accurate records of vital signs, weight, fluid intake, urine output, and calorie intake.
◆ Monitor serum glucose and urine acetone levels.
◆ Monitor for acute complications of diabetic therapy, especially hypoglycemia (vagueness, slow cerebration, dizziness, weakness, pallor, tachycardia, diaphoresis, seizures, and coma); immediately give carbohydrates in the form of fruit juice, hard candy, honey or, if the patient is unconscious, glucagon or I.V. dextrose.
◆ Be alert for signs of hyperosmolar coma (polyuria, thirst, neurologic abnormalities, and stupor). This hyperglycemic crisis requires I.V. fluids and insulin replacement.
◆ Monitor the patient for effects on the cardiovascular system, such as cerebrovascular, coronary artery, and peripheral vascular impairment.
◆ Monitor for effects on the peripheral and autonomic nervous systems.
◆ Provide meticulous skin care, especially to the feet and legs. Treat all injuries, cuts, and blisters.
◆ Observe for signs of urinary tract and vaginal infections.
◆ Encourage adequate fluid intake.

Ruptured AAA is the 13th-leading cause of death in the United States. Less than 50% of people with a ruptured AAA survive.

ETIOLOGY

AAA results from arteriosclerosis, hypertension, congenital weakening, cystic medial necrosis, trauma, syphilis, and other infections. In children, this disorder can result from blunt abdominal injury or Marfan's syndrome.

PATHOPHYSIOLOGY

Nearly 98% of all AAAs are located in the infrarenal aorta. They can be fusiform (spindle-shaped) or saccular (pouchlike) and generally develop slowly.

Cardiovascular system

■ A focal weakness in the muscular layer of the aorta (tunica media) allows the inner layer (tunica intima) and outer layer (tunica adventitia) to stretch outward.
■ Blood pressure within the aorta progressively weakens the vessel walls and enlarges the aneurysm.
■ The pressure of a large aneurysm causes damage to adjacent organs.
■ If dissection occurs, blood leaks into the space in between the vessel layers. The ves-

DISORDERS AFFECTING MANAGEMENT OF ABDOMINAL AORTIC ANEURYSM

This chart highlights disorders that affect the management of abdominal aortic aneurysm.

DISORDER	SIGNS AND SYMPTOMS	DIAGNOSTIC TEST RESULTS
Chronic obstructive pulmonary disease (coexisting)	◆ Dyspnea ◆ Abdominal discomfort ◆ Cyanosis	◆ Pulmonary function tests show increased residual volume, total lung capacity, and compliance. ◆ Chest X-ray shows hyperinflation. ◆ Arterial blood gas analysis shows decreased partial pressure of arterial oxygen (Pao_2) and normal or increased partial pressure of arterial carbon dioxide ($Paco_2$) (emphysema). ◆ Electrocardiogram (ECG) may show atrial arrhythmias and peaked P weaves in leads II, III, and aV_F (chronic bronchitis); tall, symmetrical P waves in leads II, III, and aV_F vertical QRS axis (emphysema).
Coronary artery disease (coexisting)	◆ Elevated blood pressure ◆ Chest pain that radiates to the left arm, neck, jaw, or shoulder ◆ Nausea and vomiting ◆ Fainting ◆ Cool extremities ◆ Decreased or absent peripheral pulses	◆ Stress echocardiography may show abnormal wall movement. ◆ Coronary angiography reveals the location and degree of coronary artery stenosis or obstruction. ◆ Exercise testing may detect ST-segment changes during exercise. ◆ ECG may show ischemic changes during exercise.
Hypertension (coexisting)	◆ Headache ◆ Dizziness ◆ Fatigue ◆ Bounding pulse ◆ Pulsating abdominal mass ◆ Elevated blood pressure ◆ Bruits over the abdominal aorta	◆ Urinalysis may show proteinuria, red blood cells, white blood cells, or glucose. ◆ Serum potassium levels are less than 3.5 mEq/L. ◆ Blood urea nitrogen is normal or elevated to more than 20 mg/dL. ◆ Serum creatinine levels normal or elevated to more than 1.5 mg/dL.

sels branching off the aorta become obstructed, causing decreased blood flow and tissue death.

■ Nearly all AAAs are fusiform, which causes the arterial walls to balloon on all sides. The resulting sac fills with necrotic debris and thrombi. Complications of this type of aneurysm include rupture, obstruction of blood flow to other organs, and embolization to a peripheral artery.

■ In the event of rupture, blood supply to vital organs is diminished and organ failure ensues.

■ Free intraperitoneal rupture leads to cardiovascular collapse.

Gastrointestinal system

■ If AAA ruptures into the duodenum, upper GI bleeding and hemorrhage occur.

■ Sigmoid colon ischemia may occur with loss of blood from the hypogastric artery during surgical repair of AAA.

Neurologic system

■ AAA rupture causes decreased blood flow to the brain, which alters mental status.

Renal system

■ Diminished perfusion of the kidneys may result from obstruction of the renal arteries, rupture of the aneurysm, or surgical repair.

accidentally through an X-ray or during a routine physical examination.

Clinical findings

- Possibly asymptomatic
- Symptoms that mimic renal calculi, lumbar disk disease, and duodenal compression (with a large aneurysm)
- Lumbar pain that radiates to the flank and groin from pressure on lumbar nerves (may signify enlargement and imminent rupture)
- Severe, persistent abdominal and back pain (signifies rupture)
- Signs of hemorrhage — such as weakness, sweating, tachycardia, and hypotension
- Pulsating mass in the periumbilical area
- Systolic bruit over the aorta
- Tenderness on deep palpation
- Diminished peripheral pulses or claudication (with embolization)
  With a ruptured AAA:
- Hypotension and cardiovascular collapse
- Constant severe pain
- Pulsating abdominal mass

Diagnostic test results

- *Abdominal ultrasonography* or *echocardiography* will determine the size, shape, and location of the aneurysm.
- *Anteroposterior* and *lateral X-rays* of the abdomen will detect aortic calcification, which outlines the mass, at least 75% of the time.
- *Computed tomography scan* will visualize the aneurysm's effect on nearby organs, particularly the position of the renal arteries in relation to the aneurysm.
- *Aortography* shows the condition of vessels proximal and distal to the aneurysm and the extent of the aneurysm.

COLLABORATIVE MANAGEMENT

A cardiologist may be brought in to treat potential coexisting disorders of hypertension, coronary artery disease, and atherosclerotic vascular disease. (See *Disorders affecting management of abdominal aortic aneurysm.*)

A vascular surgeon is consulted if the aneurysm exceeds 3 cm in diameter, if a segment of the aneurysm is one and one-half times bigger than the diameter of an adjacent segment, or if the patient is symptomatic of dissection or rupture. If the size of the aneurysm is smaller than 4 cm, a radiologist will monitor it biannually. A nephrolo-

---

TREATMENT AND CARE

- Help the patient adjust to lifestyle changes needed to decrease oxygen demands.
- Perform chest physiotherapy to maintain clear airways.
- Administer bronchodilators.
- Encourage daily activity to maximize lung capacity and promote psychological well being.
- Provide frequent rest periods to minimize oxygen demands.
- Provide a high-calorie, protein-rich diet.

- Monitor the patient for pain; have the patient grade the severity of his pain on a scale of 1 to 10.
- Observe for signs and symptoms that may signify worsening of condition or pain.
- Administer calcium channel blockers, beta-adrenergic blockers, or antilipemics.
- Advise the patient to follow the prescribed medication regimen to reduce the risk of cardiac disease.
- Help the patient identify risk factors and modify his lifestyle as appropriate.

- Monitor blood pressure for stability.
- Help the patient identify risk factors and modify his diet and lifestyle.
- Administer thiazide-type diuretics, angiotensin-converting enzyme inhibitors, angiotensin receptor blockers, beta-adrenergic blockers, or calcium channel blockers.
- Help the patient identify stress factors and establish effective coping mechanisms.

Ureteral stents may be placed during surgery as a precaution, causing decreased renal function.

- Retroperitoneal rupture causes a self-limiting hemorrhage to the retroperitoneal space, resulting in pain, hypotension, and flank ecchymosis.

Respiratory system

- Rupture of an AAA leads to impaired gas exchange, resulting in diminished perfusion of organs.

ASSESSMENT

Because abdominal aneurysms seldom produce symptoms, they're commonly detected

gist is needed if signs of renal failure occur after surgery. A pulmonologist may be consulted for ventilator management postoperatively and for such coexisting disorders as chronic obstructive pulmonary disease. A dietitian is needed for dietary management preoperatively and postoperatively if cardiac disease is present or if renal failure occurs. Physical therapy is used postoperatively to promote increased activity and prevent complications.

TREATMENT AND CARE

■ The patient should have regular physical examination and ultrasound checks to detect enlargement (which may signal rupture).

■ Risk factor modification, including control of hypocholesterolemia and hypertension and smoking cessation, helps prevent expansion and rupture.

■ Beta-adrenergic blockers are given to reduce the risk of aneurysm expansion and rupture.

■ Monitor for signs of acute blood loss (decreasing blood pressure; increasing pulse and respiratory rate; cool, clammy skin; restlessness; decreased sensorium) to detect signs of rupture.

■ Elective surgical procedures — including resection and placement of a Dacron graft, or a less invasive endovascular stent procedure — may be used to repair the aneurysm and prevent rupture.

■ If rupture occurs, immediate surgery may be necessary.

Asthma

Asthma — a chronic inflammatory airway disorder — is characterized by airflow obstruction and airway hyperresponsiveness to various stimuli. It's a type of chronic obstructive pulmonary disease (COPD), a long-term pulmonary disease characterized by increased airflow resistance.

Although asthma can strike at any age, about 50% of patients are younger than age 10, and twice as many boys as girls are affected in this age-group. One-third of patients develop asthma between ages 10 and 30; the incidence of asthma in this age-group affects each gender equally. About one-third of all patients share the disease with at least one immediate family member.

ETIOLOGY

Asthma may result from sensitivity to extrinsic (atopic) or intrinsic (nonatopic) allergens. Extrinsic allergens include pollen, animal dander, house dust or mold, kapok or feather pillows, food additives containing sulfites, and other sensitizing substances. Intrinsic allergens include irritants, emotional stress, fatigue, endocrine changes, temperature variations, humidity variations, exposure to noxious fumes, anxiety, coughing or laughing, or genetic factors.

Extrinsic asthma begins in childhood and is commonly accompanied by other hereditary allergies, such as eczema and allergic rhinitis. Typically, patients are sensitive to specific external allergens.

Patients with intrinsic asthma react to internal, nonallergenic factors; no extrinsic allergen can be implicated. Indeed, most episodes occur after a severe respiratory tract infection, especially in adults.

A significant number of adults acquire an allergic form of asthma or exacerbation of existing asthma from exposure to agents in the workplace. Such irritants as chemicals in flour, acid anhydrides, toluene diisocyanate, screw flies, river flies, and excreta of dust mites in carpets have been identified as agents that trigger asthma.

PATHOPHYSIOLOGY

In asthma, widespread but variable airflow obstruction is caused by bronchospasm, edema of the airway mucosa, and increased mucus production with plugging and airway remodeling.

Respiratory system

■ Bronchial linings overreact to various stimuli, causing episodic smooth muscle spasms that severely constrict the airways. (See *How asthma progresses*.)

■ Immunoglobulin (Ig) E antibodies, attached to histamine-containing mast cells and receptors on cell membranes, initiate intrinsic asthma attacks. When exposed to an antigen, such as pollen, the IgE antibody combines with the antigen.

■ During an attack, the narrowed bronchial lumen can still expand slightly on inhala-

HOW ASTHMA PROGRESSES

In asthma, hyperresponsiveness of the airways and bronchospasms occur. These illustrations show the progression of an asthma attack.

Histamine (H) attaches to receptor sites in larger bronchi, causing swelling of the smooth muscles.

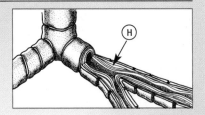

Leukotrienes (L) attach to receptor sites in the smaller bronchi and cause swelling of smooth muscle there. Leukotrienes also cause prostaglandins to travel through the bloodstream to the lungs, where they enhance the histamine's effects.

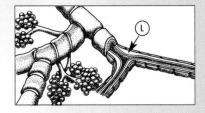

Histamine stimulates the mucous membranes to secrete excessive mucus, further narrowing the bronchial lumen. On inhalation, the narrowed bronchial lumen can still expand slightly; however, on exhalation, the increased intrathoracic pressure closes the bronchial lumen completely.

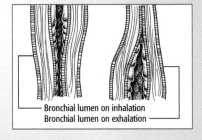

Bronchial lumen on inhalation
Bronchial lumen on exhalation

Mucus fills lung bases, inhibiting alveolar ventilation. Blood is shunted to alveoli in other parts of the lungs, but it still can't compensate for diminished ventilation.

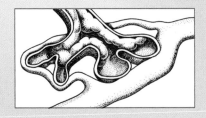

tion, allowing air to reach the alveoli. On exhalation, increased intrathoracic pressure closes the bronchial lumen completely. Air enters but can't escape. The patient develops a barrel chest and hyperresonance to percussion. (See *Disorders affecting management of asthma*, pages 58 and 59.)

■ Mucus fills the lung bases, inhibiting alveolar ventilation. Blood is shunted to alveoli in other lung parts but still can't compensate for diminished ventilation.
■ Hyperventilation is triggered by lung receptors to increase lung volume because of trapped air and obstructions.

(*Text continues on page 60.*)

DISORDERS AFFECTING MANAGEMENT OF ASTHMA

This chart highlights disorders that affect the management of asthma.

DISORDER	SIGNS AND SYMPTOMS	DIAGNOSTIC TEST RESULTS
Gastroesophageal reflux disease (complication)	◆ Regurgitation without associated nausea or belching ◆ Feeling of fluid accumulation in the throat without a sour or bitter taste ◆ Chronic pain radiating to neck, jaws, and arms	◆ Barium swallow shows evidence of recurrent reflux. ◆ Esophageal acidity test reveals degree of esophageal reflux. ◆ Gastroesophageal scintillation testing shows reflux. ◆ Acid perfusion (Bernstein) test results confirm esophagitis. ◆ Esophagoscopy and biopsy results confirm pathologic changes in the mucosa.
Infection (coexisting)	◆ Tachycardia ◆ Fever ◆ Crackles or rhonchi ◆ Rapid, shallow respirations ◆ Malaise	◆ Eosinophil count is increased. ◆ White blood cell (WBC) count and granulocyte count are increased.
Pregnancy (coexisting)	◆ Fatigue ◆ Tachypnea ◆ Bronchial wheezing ◆ Use of accessory muscles for breathing	◆ Pulmonary function tests reveal decreased vital capacity and increased total lung and residual capacities. ◆ Peak and expiratory flow rate measurements are less than 60% of baseline. ◆ Pulse oximetry shows arterial oxygen saturation (Sao_2) less than 90%. ◆ Chest X-ray reveals hyperinflation with areas of atelectasis. ◆ Electrocardiogram (ECG) may reveal sinus tachycardia during an attack. ◆ Sputum analysis may indicate increased mucus viscosity and the presence of mucus plugs. ◆ Eosinophil count is increased. ◆ WBC count and granulocyte count are increased (if infection is present).
Respiratory failure (complication)	◆ Nasal flaring ◆ Restlessness, anxiety, depression, lethargy, agitation, or confusion ◆ Cold, clammy skin ◆ Tachypnea ◆ Tactile fremitus ◆ Diminished breath sounds ◆ Crackles	◆ Chest X-ray shows atelectasis, infiltrates, and effusions. ◆ Arterial blood gas analysis shows decreased partial pressure of arterial oxygen and normal or increased partial pressure of arterial carbon dioxide. ◆ ECG may show arrhythmias. ◆ Pulse oximetry reveals a decreasing Sao_2 and a mixed venous oxygen saturation level of less than 50%. ◆ Electrolyte levels may reflect imbalances from hyperventilation, acidosis, or hypoxia.

TREATMENT AND CARE

- Assist with diet modifications to decrease reflux activity.
- Perform chest physiotherapy to maintain clear airways.
- Assist in identifying situations or activities that increase intra-abdominal pressure (such as tight clothing or certain exercises) in order to avoid reflux.
- Warn the patient to refrain from using substances that reduce sphincter control (such as alcohol).
- Advise the patient to remain in an upright position for at least 2 hours after eating.

- Monitor the patient's temperature, and treat elevations.
- Encourage increased fluid intake to avoid dehydration from increased metabolism and fever.
- Provide frequent rest periods to minimize oxygen demands.
- Monitor for complications such as worsening infection.
- Monitor WBC count and differential.
- Instruct the patient in ways to prevent infection.
- Teach the patient and his caregiver about the need to report possible infection.

- Advise the patient to follow her prepregnancy asthma therapy and to follow up with her obstetrician or nurse-midwife.
- Encourage frequent rest periods. Pregnancy increases oxygen demands and metabolism.
- Assist with dietary planning to monitor weight gain of pregnancy. Excess weight gain may increase diaphragmatic elevation and decrease functional residual capacity.
- Encourage prompt treatment of asthma attacks to decrease effects of hypoxic damage to the fetus.
- If the patient is taking beta-adrenergics to control her asthma, the dose will be tapered close to labor because these drugs have the potential to reduce labor contractions.
- Women who have been taking a corticosteroid during pregnancy may need parenteral administration of hydrocortisone during labor because of the added stress during this time.
- Advise the patient that corticosteroids should never be abruptly discontinued.

- Administer antibiotics (if infection is present).
- Help the patient adjust to lifestyle changes needed to decrease oxygen demands.
- Perform chest physiotherapy to maintain clear airways.
- Provide frequent rest periods to minimize oxygen demands.
- Provide a high-calorie, protein-rich diet.
- Administer diuretics, bronchodilators, vasopressors, positive inotropic agents, or corticosteroids.
- Perform incentive spirometry to increase lung volume.
- Administer oxygen therapy.
- Assist with endotracheal intubation and mechanical ventilation (if needed).

■ Intrapleural and alveolar gas pressures rise, causing a decreased perfusion of alveoli.
■ Increased alveolar gas pressure, decreased ventilation, and decreased perfusion result in uneven ventilation-perfusion ratios and mismatching within different lung segments.
■ As the airway obstruction increases in severity, more alveoli are affected. Ventilation and perfusion remain inadequate, and carbon dioxide retention develops, resulting in respiratory acidosis.
■ If status asthmaticus occurs (if the attack continues):
— hypoxemia worsens and expiratory flows and volumes continue to decrease
— obstructed airways impede gas exchange and increase airway resistance
— breathing becomes increasingly labored
— respiratory rate drops to normal (as the patient tires), partial pressure of carbon dioxide ($Paco_2$) levels rise, and the patient hypoventilates from exhaustion (as breathing and hypoxemia tire the patient).
— respiratory acidosis continues as partial pressure of arterial oxygen (Pao_2) levels drop and $Paco_2$ levels continue to rise
— the situation becomes life-threatening as no air becomes audible upon auscultation (a silent chest) and $Paco_2$ rises to over 70 mm Hg
— the patient experiences acute respiratory failure (without treatment).

Neurologic system
■ Hypoxia that occurs during an asthma attack triggers hyperventilation by respiratory center stimulation, which in turn decreases $Paco_2$ and increases pH, resulting in a respiratory alkalosis.

ASSESSMENT
An asthma attack may begin dramatically with simultaneous onset of severe, multiple symptoms, or insidiously with gradually increasing respiratory distress. Typically, the patient reports exposure to a particular allergen.

Clinical findings
■ Sudden dyspnea, wheezing, and tightness in the chest
■ Coughing that produces thick, clear, or yellow sputum
■ Tachypnea
■ Use of accessory respiratory muscles

■ Rapid pulse
■ Hyperresonant lung fields
■ Diminished breath sounds
■ Wheezing
If status asthmaticus develops:
■ Marked respiratory distress
■ Marked wheezing
■ Absent breath sounds
■ Pulsus paradoxus greater than 10 mm Hg
■ Chest wall contractions
■ Altered level of consciousness

Diagnostic test results
■ *Pulmonary function tests* reveal signs of airway obstructive disease, low-normal or decreased vital capacity, and increased total lung and residual capacities. Pulmonary function may be normal between attacks. Pao_2 and $Paco_2$ are usually decreased, except in severe asthma, when $Paco_2$ may be normal or increased, indicating severe bronchial obstruction.
■ *Serum IgE levels* may increase from an allergic reaction.
■ *Sputum analysis* may indicate the presence of Curschmann's spirals (casts of airways), Charcot-Leyden crystals, and eosinophils.
■ *Complete blood count with differential* reveals an increased eosinophil count.
■ *Chest X-rays* will diagnose or monitor the progress of asthma and may show hyperinflation with areas of atelectasis.
■ *Arterial blood gas analysis* detects hypoxemia (decreased Pao_2; decreased, normal, or increasing $Paco_2$) and guides treatment.
■ *Skin testing* may identify specific allergens. Results read in 1 or 2 days detect an early reaction; after 4 or 5 days, a late reaction.
■ *Bronchial challenge testing* evaluates the clinical significance of allergens identified by skin testing.
■ *Electrocardiography* shows sinus tachycardia during an attack; a severe attack may show signs of cor pulmonale (right axis deviation, peaked P wave) that resolve after the attack.

COLLABORATIVE MANAGEMENT
Managing asthma usually involves an allergy and asthma specialist or a pulmonologist to identify causative factors and prescribe therapy to help control attacks.

TREATMENT AND CARE

■ Pharmacologic therapy typically includes the use of bronchodilators, inhaled cortico-steroids, histamine antagonists, leukotriene antagonists, anticholinergic bronchodilators, and antibiotics.

■ In cases of acute asthma attack or status asthmaticus, emergency medical services will treat the patient before transporting him to the emergency department for more in-depth treatment.

■ The respiratory therapy team may be involved to deliver oxygen therapy and breathing treatments.

■ A nurse practitioner or clinical nurse specialist provides patient-specific education about how the patient should manage asthma in conjunction with his lifestyle or coexisting conditions.

B

Bronchiectasis

Bronchiectasis is a chronic obstructive pulmonary disease characterized by the abnormal dilation of and repeated damage (as a result of certain conditions) to the bronchial walls. It's usually associated with repeated cycles of impaired clearance of secretions and subsequent infection and inflammation, causing a breakdown of supporting tissue in the medium-sized bronchi.

Bronchiectasis may be congenital or acquired. This disorder is usually bilateral and involves segments of the lower lobes, although it can occur throughout the tracheobronchial tree. Bronchiectasis occurs in three forms: cylindrical, varicose, and saccular. (See *Forms of bronchiectasis.*)

ETIOLOGY

Bronchiectasis generally affects people of both sexes and all age-groups. However, although incidence has dramatically decreased over the past 20 years because of the availability of antibiotics to treat acute respiratory infections, the increase in the number of immunocompromised patients, such as those with human immunodeficiency virus and organ transplants, may cause a resurgence of the disease.

Individuals with cystic fibrosis are at particular risk for bronchiectasis.

Bronchiectasis may be caused by:
- mucoviscidosis
- immune disorders
- recurrent bacterial respiratory tract infections
- complications of measles, pneumonia, pertussis, or influenza
- obstruction with recurrent infection
- inhalation of corrosive gas
- repeated aspiration of gastric juices

- congenital anomalies (rare) such as bronchomalacia
- various rare disorders such as immotile cilia syndrome.

PATHOPHYSIOLOGY

Repeated damage to the bronchial walls and abnormal mucociliary clearance lead to a breakdown in the supporting tissue adjacent to the airways.

Respiratory system

- Hyperplastic squamous epithelium that's removed of its cilia replaces ulcerated columnar epithelia. This results in bronchial dilation and inflammatory changes in the walls of the airways.
- Cartilage, muscle, and elastic tissue are gradually destroyed and may be replaced by fibrous tissue.
- Abscess formation involving all layers of the bronchial walls occurs, which produces inflammatory cells and fibrous tissues, resulting in further dilation and narrowing of the airways.
- Sputum stagnates in the dilated bronchi and leads to secondary infection, characterized by inflammation and leukocytic accumulations. Additional debris collects in the bronchi and occludes them.
- Pressure from the retained secretions induces further mucosal injury.
- Inflammatory processes increase the vascularity of the bronchial wall. As vascularity increases, bronchial arteries enlarge and anastomoses form between the bronchial and pulmonary arterial circulations.
- Extensive vascular proliferation of bronchial circulation occurs, producing copious, foul-smelling secretions, commonly occurring with hemoptysis.
- As damage occurs to the bronchial and pulmonary beds, oxygenation is compromised and hypoxia results.

FORMS OF BRONCHIECTASIS

The three types of bronchiectasis are cylindrical, varicose, and saccular. In cylindrical bronchiectasis, bronchioles are usually symmetrically dilated, whereas in varicose bronchiectasis, bronchioles are deformed. In saccular bronchiectasis, large bronchi become enlarged and balloonlike.

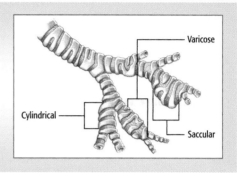

■ Airway obstruction can occur from bronchostenosis, impacted retained secretions, or compression by enlarged lymph nodes.

Cardiovascular system
■ Structural changes in the lungs can lead to increased pressure in the pulmonary arteries. This condition (called *pulmonary hypertension*) results in increased workload for the right ventricle, possibly leading to cor pulmonale and heart failure. (See *Disorders affecting management of bronchiectasis,* pages 64 and 65.)
■ Because the right side of the heart pumps blood through the lungs under much lower pressure, any condition that leads to prolonged pulmonary hypertension is poorly tolerated by the right ventricle.

Immune system
■ The host inflammatory response includes epithelial injury as a result of mediators released from neutrophils; thus protection against infection is compromised.
■ Dilated airways and retained secretions are more susceptible to colonization and growth of bacteria. This bacterial growth causes inflammation that produces airway damage, impairs clearance of secretions that harbor the microorganisms, and causes more infection, which then triggers more inflammation.

ASSESSMENT
Commonly, the patient's history reveals frequent bouts of pneumonia or a history of coughing up blood.

Clinical findings
■ Chronic cough that produces copious, foul-smelling, mucopurulent secretions, blood, or blood-tinged sputum
■ Dyspnea
■ Weight loss
■ Malaise
■ Sputum showing a cloudy top layer, a central layer of clear saliva, and a heavy, thick, purulent bottom layer
■ Clubbed fingers and toes
■ Cyanotic nail beds
■ Dullness over affected lung fields (if pneumonia or atelectasis is present)
■ Diminished breath sounds
■ Inspiratory crackles during inspiration over affected area
■ Occasional wheezes

Diagnostic test results
■ *Sputum culture* and *Gram stain* show predominant pathogens.
■ *Complete blood count* reveals anemia and leukocytosis.
■ *Computed tomography scan* shows inflammation, destruction, chronic inflammation, and increased mucus.
■ *Bronchography* shows location and extent of disease.
■ *Chest X-rays* show peribronchial thickening, atelectatic areas, and scattered cystic changes.
■ *Bronchoscopy* may show the source of secretions or, in cases of hemoptysis, the bleeding site.

DISORDERS AFFECTING
MANAGEMENT OF BRONCHIECTASIS

This chart highlights disorders that affect the management of bronchiectasis.

DISORDER	SIGNS AND SYMPTOMS	DIAGNOSTIC TEST RESULTS
Cor pulmonale (complication)	◆ Progressive dyspnea worsening on exertion ◆ Tachypnea and bounding pulse ◆ Orthopnea ◆ Dependent edema ◆ Weakness ◆ Distended neck veins ◆ Enlarged, tender liver ◆ Tachycardia ◆ Enlarged spleen	◆ Pulmonary artery pressure (PAP) shows increased right ventricular pressure. ◆ Echocardiography or angiography indicates right ventricular enlargement. ◆ Chest X-ray suggests right ventricular enlargement. ◆ Arterial blood gas (ABG) analysis shows decreased partial pressure of arterial oxygen (less than 70 mm Hg). ◆ Electrocardiography (ECG) may show various arrhythmias.
Heart failure (complication)	*Left-sided heart failure* ◆ Dyspnea ◆ Orthopnea ◆ Paroxysmal nocturnal dyspnea ◆ Fatigue ◆ Nonproductive cough ◆ Crackles ◆ Hemoptysis ◆ Tachycardia ◆ Third (S_3) and fourth (S_4) heart sounds ◆ Cool, pale skin ◆ Restlessness and confusion *Right-sided heart failure* ◆ Jugular vein distention ◆ Positive hepatojugular reflex ◆ Right-upper-quadrant pain ◆ Anorexia ◆ Nausea ◆ Nocturia ◆ Weight gain ◆ Edema ◆ Ascites or anasarca	◆ Chest X-rays may show pulmonary vascular markings, interstitial edema, or pleural effusion and cardiomegaly. ◆ ECG may indicate hypertrophy, ischemic changes, infarction, tachycardia, and extrasystoles. ◆ Liver function tests may be abnormal. ◆ Blood urea nitrogen (BUN) and creatinine levels may be elevated. ◆ Prothrombin time may be prolonged. ◆ Brain natriuretic peptide assay may be elevated. ◆ Echocardiography may reveal left ventricular hypertrophy, dilation, and abnormal contractility. ◆ PAP, pulmonary artery wedge pressure, and left ventricular end-diastolic pressure are elevated in the presence of left-sided heart failure; right atrial or central venous pressure is elevated in right-sided heart failure. ◆ Radionuclide ventriculography may reveal ejection fraction less than 40% in diastolic dysfunction.

■ *Pulmonary function tests* show hypoxemia and decreased vital capacity and expiratory flow.

■ A *sweat electrolyte test* may show cystic fibrosis as the underlying cause.

COLLABORATIVE MANAGEMENT

Respiratory therapists can assist with postural drainage, chest percussion, and administration of oxygen and bronchodilators. A pulmonary specialist or thoracic surgeon may be consulted if a bronchoscopy is needed to remove secretions. An infectious disease specialist may be needed to help identify the infectious organisms and recommend appropriate antibiotic therapy. If the patient is debilitated, nutritional therapy and physical therapy may help optimize the patient's outcome.

TREATMENT AND CARE

■ Administer antibiotic therapy (oral or I.V.) for 7 to 10 days, or until sputum production decreases (principal treatment).

■ If pulmonary function continues to be poor, segmental resection, bronchial artery emobilization, lobectomy, or surgical removal of the affected part of the lung may be required.

Burns

Burn injuries affect about 2 million people each year in the United States. Of this population, 300,000 are burned seriously, and more than 6,000 die, making burns this nation's third-leading cause of accidental death. About 60,000 people are hospitalized each year for burns. Most significant burns occur in the home, and home fires account for the highest burn fatality rate. In victims younger than age 4 and older than age 60, there's a higher incidence of complications, and thus a higher mortality.

A major burn is an injury that requires painful treatment and a long period of rehabilitation. It may be fatal or permanently disfiguring and emotionally and physically incapacitating. Immediate, aggressive burn treatment increases the patient's chance of survival. Supportive measures and strict sterile technique can help minimize infec

TREATMENT AND CARE

◆ Encourage bed rest to reduce myocardial oxygen demands.

◆ Administer digoxin, antibiotics, or pulmonary artery vasodilators, such as diazoxide, nitroprusside, hydralazine, angiotensin-converting enzyme inhibitors, calcium channel blockers, or prostaglandins to reduce pulmonary hypertension.

◆ Provide meticulous respiratory care, including low-dose oxygen therapy, suctioning, and deep-breathing and coughing exercises.

◆ Monitor ABG values, and look for signs of respiratory failure (change in pulse rate, deep labored respirations, and increased fatigue on exertion).

◆ Monitor fluid status carefully; limit fluid intake to 1,000 to 2,000 ml/day, and provide a low sodium diet.

◆ Monitor serum potassium levels if the patient is receiving diuretics; low serum potassium levels can potentiate arrhythmias.

◆ Place the patient in Fowler's position and give supplemental oxygen.

◆ Weigh the patient daily and check for peripheral edema. Monitor intake and output, vital signs, and mental status.

◆ Auscultate for S_3 and S_4 heart sounds and adventitious lung sounds, such as crackles or rhonchi.

◆ Monitor BUN, creatinine, and serum potassium, sodium, chloride, and magnesium levels.

◆ Institute continuous cardiac monitoring to promptly identify and treat arrhythmias.

◆ Administer diuretics, digoxin, beta-adrenergic blockers, inotropics, nesiritide, nitrates, or morphine.

◆ Administer supplemental oxygen.

◆ Encourage lifestyle modifications, such as weight loss, limited intake of sodium, smoking cessation, reduced alcohol consumption, and reduced intake of fat.

◆ Prepare the patient for coronary artery bypass grafting or heart transplantation (as appropriate).

DISORDERS AFFECTING MANAGEMENT OF BURNS

This chart highlights disorders that affect the management of burns.

DISORDER	SIGNS AND SYMPTOMS	DIAGNOSTIC TEST RESULTS
Burn shock (complication)	◆ Tachycardia ◆ Tachypnea ◆ Cyanosis ◆ Weak, rapid, thready pulse ◆ Cold, clammy skin ◆ Hypotension ◆ Reduced urinary output progressing to anuria ◆ Restlessness and irritability progressing to unconsciousness and absent reflexes ◆ Peripheral edema	◆ Potassium, serum lactate, and blood urea nitrogen levels are elevated. ◆ Urine specific gravity is greater than 1.020; urine osmolality is increased. ◆ Blood pH and partial pressure of arterial oxygen are decreased, and partial pressure of carbon dioxide is increased. ◆ Coagulation studies may detect disseminated intravascular coagulation (DIC).
Compartment syndrome (complication)	◆ Increased pain at the affected part ◆ Decreased touch sensation at the affected part ◆ Increased weakness of the affected part ◆ Increased swelling and pallor ◆ Decreased pulses and capillary refill	◆ Creatinine kinase levels are increased because of muscle tissue injury or necrosis. ◆ Intracompartmental tissue pressures are increased. ◆ Arteriograms or venograms show blocked vessels with embolus, thrombus, or other vascular injury. ◆ Transcutaneous Doppler venous flow studies show impaired venous flow.
Sepsis (complication)	◆ Labile temperature ◆ Tachycardia ◆ Tachypnea ◆ Hypotension ◆ Hyperglycemia ◆ Nausea and vomiting ◆ Lethargy and malaise	◆ Blood cultures as well as sputum, urine, and wound tissue cultures are done to isolate the organism. ◆ Platelet count is decreased and white blood cell count ranges from 15,000 to 30,000/mm³, suggesting leukocytosis.

tion. Survival and recovery from a major burn are more likely if the burn wound is reduced to less than 20% of the total body surface area.

ETIOLOGY

Burn injuries are classified based on their mechanism of injury. Thermal burns, the most common type, are caused by flame, flash, scald, or contact with hot objects. Factors that may cause thermal burns include residential fires, motor vehicle accidents, playing with matches, improperly stored

gasoline, use of a space heater, or electrical malfunctions. Other causes include improper handling of firecrackers, scalding accidents, and kitchen accidents (such as when a child climbs on top of a stove or grabs a hot iron). Burns in children are sometimes traced to parental abuse.

Chemical burns result from the contact, ingestion, inhalation, or injection of acids, alkalis, or vesicants that cause tissue injury and necrosis. Electrical burns result from coagulation necrosis caused by intense heat; they usually occur after contact with faulty

TREATMENT AND CARE

- Institute and monitor continuous cardiac monitoring.
- Administer analgesics and antiarrhythmics.
- Initiate and maintain I.V. fluid replacement therapy.
- Administer blood replacement therapy.
- Initiate prompt and adequate fluid volume replacement therapy to restore intravascular volume and raise blood pressure.
- Administer supplemental oxygen.
- Monitor vital signs, including central and peripheral pulses and capillary refill, approximately every 15 minutes.
- Monitor the patient for signs and symptoms of deficient fluid volume, such as tachycardia, hypotension, weak peripheral pulses, dry mucous membranes, and decreased urine output (less than 0.5 ml/kg/hour).
- Monitor the patient carefully for signs of neurological impairment, such as confusion, memory loss, insomnia, lethargy, and combativeness.
- Monitor the patient for signs of impaired peristalsis, such as vomiting or fecal impaction. To prevent Curling's ulcers, initiate early enteral feedings and maintain gastric pH greater than 5 by administering antacids and histamine-2 receptor antagonists.

- Assist with procedures to relieve the constricting forces. An emergency fasciotomy may be necessary.
- Apply ice and elevate the affected extremity to no more than 5″ (12.7 cm) above heart level.
- Provide pain relief. Opioids may be necessary.
- Monitor neurovascular status closely to detect developing or worsening compartment syndrome.
- Administer I.V. mannitol (Osmitrol), a systemic diuretic, to reduce intracompartmental pressures.

- Administer I.V. antibiotics to control the infection. Depending on the organism, a combination of antibiotics may be necessary.
- Monitor vital signs closely.
- Administer vasopressors.
- Monitor the patient closely for signs of septic shock and DIC.
- Monitor serum antibiotic levels.
- Provide meticulous burn wound and other care to prevent introducing microorganisms into the patient, who's typically immunocompromised.
- Apply topical antibiotics to the burn to prevent wound infection, which may develop into systemic sepsis depending on the patient's condition.

electrical wiring or high-voltage power lines, or when young children chew electric cords. Friction or abrasive burns happen when the skin is rubbed harshly against a coarse surface. Sunburn follows excessive exposure to sunlight.

PATHOPHYSIOLOGY

Many changes occur as a result of a burn injury. The injuring agent denatures cellular proteins. Some cells die because of traumatic or ischemic necrosis. Loss of collagen cross-linking also occurs with denaturation, creating abnormal osmotic and hydrostatic pressure gradients, which cause the movement of intravascular fluid into interstitial spaces. Cellular injury triggers the release of mediators of inflammation, contributing to local and, in the case of major burns, systemic increases in capillary permeability. Specific pathophysiologic events depend upon the severity of the burn. (See *Disorders affecting management of burns.*)

Cardiovascular system

■ Burns may cause fluid shifts or directly injure the heart and blood vessels, leading to impaired circulation.

■ The inflammatory response increases capillary permeability. As a result, intravascular fluid shifts to the interstitial spaces, leading to edema, decreased circulating fluid volume, and increased blood viscosity. This hemoconcentration places the patient at risk for thrombus formation.

Gastrointestinal system

■ As blood is shunted away from the abdominal area and GI tract, peristalsis is slowed or absent altogether.

■ Gastric dilation and vomiting may occur, possibly increasing the risk of aspiration.

■ Curling's ulcers may result (stomach and intestinal ulcerations and hemorrhage).

Integumentary system

■ Impaired skin integrity increases the risk of infection and causes hypothermia and rapid fluid losses.

■ Contractures and impaired range-of-motion in extremities may result from hypertrophic scar formation.

■ Edema associated with circumferential burns constricts underlying blood vessels, tissue, and muscle, impairing circulation to the affected area or extremity.

Immune and hematologic systems

■ One theory suggests burn cells release a toxin that interferes with the immune system's ability to function properly. Subsequently, major burns may result in immunosuppression.

■ Generalized sepsis is a common and serious complication; the larger the wound, the greater the risk of infection.

■ More severe burn states may result in the development of disseminated intravascular coagulation.

Renal system

■ Hemoconcentration and decreased intravascular volumes cause decreased renal perfusion and decreased urinary output.

■ Prolonged decreased renal perfusion leads to acute tubular necrosis and renal failure.

Respiratory system

■ Neck burns or swelling from heat and smoke exposure or chemical injury to the mucosa of the respiratory tract can lead to respiratory distress.

■ Restricted respiratory expansion from chest burns or eschar formation can lead to respiratory distress.

■ Smoke inhalation or inhalation of other caustic substances results in pulmonary injury, such as bronchitis or respiratory distress.

■ Hypoxia may result from a decreased amount of oxygen circulating through the blood that may be caused by inhalation of carbon monoxide, a by-product of combustion that displaces oxygen from hemoglobin molecules.

ASSESSMENT

Assessment of the patient with a burn injury should begin with a thorough history. A description of events surrounding the burn injury should include the cause and the duration the agent was in contact with the skin. The history also consists of how and when the injury occurred, treatment of the burn already administered, and history of previous burns. When performing the initial assessment of a patient with burn injury, remember to cover the ABCDEFs (Airway, Breathing, Circulation, Disability or neurologic deficits, Exposure and evaluation, and Fluid resuscitation).

Traditionally, burn depth is gauged by degrees, although most burns are a combination of different degrees and thicknesses. With a first-degree burn, also called a *superficial burn,* damage is limited to the epidermis, causing erythema and pain. A second-degree burn, also known as a *deep partial-thickness burn,* affects the epidermis and part of the dermis, producing blisters and mild to moderate edema and pain. With a third-degree burn, or full-thickness burn, the epidermis and the dermis are damaged. No blisters appear, but white, brown, or black leathery tissue and thrombosed vessels are visible. A fourth-degree burn (also considered a full-thickness burn) extends through deeply charred subcutaneous tissue to muscle and bone. (See *Classifications of burns.*)

CLASSIFICATIONS OF BURNS

The depth of skin and tissue damage determines burn classification. This illustration shows the four degrees of burn classifications.

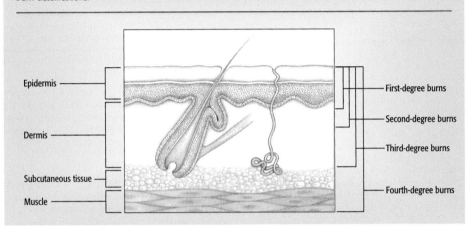

Epidermis — First-degree burns

— Second-degree burns

Dermis — Third-degree burns

Subcutaneous tissue — Fourth-degree burns

Muscle

Because the proportion of body surface area (BSA) varies with growth, burn severity may also determined by an individual's age:

■ *Rule of Nines chart* determines percentage of BSA covered by the burn in adults.

■ *Lund-Browder classification* (also known as the *Berkow method*) determines the extent of an infant's or child's burn.

Correlating the burn's depth and size allows for determination of the burn's severity. Minor burns are classified as:

■ third-degree burns over less than 2% of BSA

■ second-degree burns over less than 15% of adult BSA (10% in children).

Moderate burns are classified as:

■ third-degree burns over 2% to 10% of BSA

■ second-degree burns over 15% to 25% of adult BSA (10% to 20% in children).

Major burns are classified as:

■ third-degree burns over more than 10% of BSA

■ second-degree burns over more than 25% of adult BSA (over 20% in children)

■ burns of the hands, face, feet, or genitalia

■ burns complicated by fractures or respiratory damage

■ electrical burns

■ all burns in poor-risk patients.

Clinical findings

■ Localized pain and erythema, usually without blisters in the first 24 hours (first-degree burn)

■ Chills, headache, localized edema, and nausea and vomiting (more severe first-degree burn)

■ Thin-walled, fluid-filled blisters appearing within minutes of the injury, with mild to moderate edema and pain (second-degree burn)

■ White, waxy appearance to damaged area (more severe second-degree burn)

■ White, brown, or black leathery tissue and visible thrombosed vessels due to destruction of skin elasticity, without blisters (third- or fourth-degree burn)

■ Silver-colored, raised area, usually at the site of electrical contact (electrical burn)

■ Singed nasal hairs, mucosal burns, voice changes, coughing, wheezing, soot in mouth or nose, and darkened sputum (with smoke inhalation and pulmonary damage)

Diagnostic test results

■ *Complete blood count* may reveal a decreased hemoglobin (due to hemolysis), increased hematocrit (secondary to hemoconcentration), and leukocytosis (resulting from a systemic inflammatory response).

FLUID REPLACEMENT: THE FIRST 24 HOURS AFTER A BURN

Use the Parkland formula as a general guideline for the amount of fluid replacement. Administer 4 ml/kg of crystalloid × % total burn surface area; give half of the solution over the first 8 hours (calculated from time of injury) and the balance over the next 16 hours. Vary the specific infusions according to the patient's response, especially his urine output.

■ *Urinalysis* may reveal myoglobinuria and hemoglobinuria.
■ *Chest X-ray* will reveal alveolar damage.
■ *Arterial blood gas analysis* may be normal early on but may reveal hypoxia and metabolic later.
■ *Fiber-optic bronchoscopy* will reveal tracheal and bronchial burn damage.
■ *Carboxyhemoglobin level* may reveal the extent of smoke inhalation (because of the presence of carbon monoxide).

COLLABORATIVE MANAGEMENT

Management of minor burns can usually take place in a hospital or the health care provider's office. However, if the burn involves a large BSA or critical body parts (as in moderate and major burns), it usually requires treatment at a specialized burn center. Additionally, surgeons may be needed to perform escharotomy and fasciotomy to remove burn tissue. Wound care specialists may be needed to prevent wound infections and complications (such as contractures) and promote wound healing. Respiratory therapy is needed to maximize respiratory function in cases of inhalation injury.

As the patient improves, physical therapy is necessary to maintain or improve range of motion and prevent contractures. Nutritional therapists can prescribe an optimal diet to promote wound healing. Referral to a therapist and a support group may help the patient deal with psychological effects of the traumatic injury. Similar referrals are needed if severe scarring or disfigurement is anticipated.

TREATMENT AND CARE

Burn treatments are based on the type of burn and may include:
■ immersing the burned area in cool water (55° F [12.8° C]) or applying cool compresses (minor burns)
■ administering pain medication or anti-inflammatory medications as needed
■ covering the area with an antimicrobial agent and a nonstick bulky dressing (after debridement)
■ administering a prophylactic tetanus injection as needed
■ preventing hypoxia by maintaining an open airway; assessing ABCDEFs; checking for smoke inhalation immediately on receipt of the patient; assisting with endotracheal intubation; and giving 100% oxygen (first immediate treatment for moderate and major burns)
■ controlling active bleeding
■ covering partial-thickness burns over 30% of BSA or full-thickness burns over 5% of BSA with a clean, dry, sterile bed sheet (because of drastic reduction in body temperature, don't cover large burns with saline-soaked dressings)
■ removing smoldering clothing (first soaking it in saline solution if clothing is stuck to the patient's skin), jewelry (such as rings), and other constricting items
■ immediate I.V. therapy to prevent hypovolemic shock and maintain cardiac output (lactated Ringer's solution or a fluid replacement formula; additional I.V. lines may be needed) (see *Fluid replacement: The first 24 hours after a burn*)
■ antimicrobial therapy (all patients with major burns)
■ closely monitoring intake and output, frequently checking vital signs, and possibly inserting an indwelling urinary catheter
■ nasogastric tube to decompress the stomach and avoid aspiration of stomach contents
■ irrigating the wound with copious amounts of normal saline solution (chemical burns)
■ surgical intervention, including skin grafts and more thorough surgical cleaning (major burns)
■ nutritional therapy to ensure increased caloric intake because of increased metabolic rate and to promote healing and recovery.

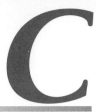

Cardiac tamponade

Cardiac tamponade is a rapid, unchecked rise in intrapericardial pressure that compresses the heart, impairs diastolic filling, and reduces cardiac output. The increase in pressure usually results from blood or fluid accumulation in the pericardial sac.

In children, cardiac tamponade is twice as common in males as in females. In adults, males have only a slightly higher incidence than females.

Without prompt diagnosis and treatment, cardiac tamponade is fatal.

ETIOLOGY

Cardiac tamponade may be idiopathic (Dressler's syndrome) or may result from:
- effusion (in cancer, bacterial infections, tuberculosis and, rarely, acute rheumatic fever)
- hemorrhage from trauma (gunshot or stab wounds of the chest, perforation by catheter during cardiac or central venous catheterization, or after cardiac surgery)
- hemorrhage from nontraumatic causes (rupture of the heart or great vessels or anticoagulant therapy in a patient with pericarditis)
- viral, postirradiation, or idiopathic pericarditis
- acute myocardial infarction
- chronic renal failure during dialysis
- connective tissue disorders (rheumatoid arthritis, systemic lupus erythematosus, rheumatic fever, vasculitis, and scleroderma).

PATHOPHYSIOLOGY

Typically, a patient has a coexisting disorder that prompts fluid accumulation. If it accumulates *rapidly* around the heart, as little as 50 ml of fluid can create an emergency situa-tion. Pericardial effusion associated with cancer may not produce immediate signs and symptoms because the fibrous wall of the pericardial sac can *gradually* stretch to accommodate as much as 1 to 2 L of fluid. (See *Understanding cardiac tamponade*, page 72.)

Cardiovascular system
- Pressure resulting from fluid accumulation in the pericardium decreases ventricular filling and cardiac output, resulting in cardiogenic shock and death if left untreated.

RED FLAG Cardiac tamponade may cause a cardiac condition called pulseless electrical activity (PEA). In PEA, isolated electrical activity occurs sporadically without evidence of myocardial contraction. Unless the underlying cardiac tamponade is identified and treated quickly, PEA will result in death.

Gastrointestinal system
- Cardiac tamponade alters systemic venous return secondary to increased compression of the right atrium. This results in increased volume in the right ventricle. Blood then accumulates in the venous circulation, causing hepatomegaly.

Immune system
- Exudative fluid accumulation may occur secondary to the inflammatory process that occurs in certain autoimmune disorders such as systemic lupus erythematosus; infections such as human immunodeficiency virus (HIV); or malignancy such as cancer.

Respiratory system
- Large pleural effusions have been associated with cardiac tamponade. These effusions cause increased intrapleural pressure, which transmits to the pericardial space and impairs ventricular filling, causing the same physiologic outcome as cardiac tamponade.

UNDERSTANDING CARDIAC TAMPONADE

The pericardial sac, which surrounds and protects the heart, is composed of several layers. The fibrous pericardium is the tough outermost membrane; the inner membrane, called the serous membrane, consists of the visceral and parietal layers. The visceral layer clings to the heart and is also known as the epicardial layer. The parietal layer lies between the visceral layer and the fibrous pericardium. The pericardial space—between the visceral and parietal layers—contains 10 to 30 ml of pericardial fluid. This fluid lubricates the layers and minimizes friction when the heart contracts.

In cardiac tamponade, blood or fluid fills the pericardial space, compressing the heart chambers, increasing intracardiac pressure, and obstructing venous return. As blood flow into the ventricles falls, so does cardiac output. Without prompt treatment, low cardiac output can be fatal.

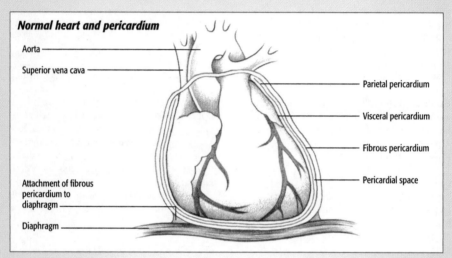

Normal heart and pericardium

Aorta

Superior vena cava

Parietal pericardium

Visceral pericardium

Fibrous pericardium

Pericardial space

Attachment of fibrous pericardium to diaphragm

Diaphragm

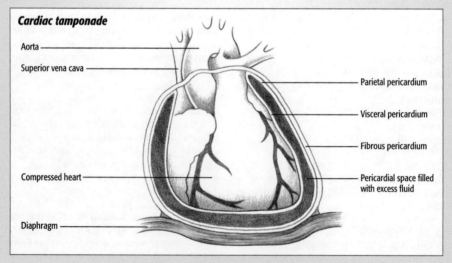

Cardiac tamponade

Aorta

Superior vena cava

Parietal pericardium

Visceral pericardium

Fibrous pericardium

Compressed heart

Pericardial space filled with excess fluid

Diaphragm

ASSESSMENT

The patient's history may reveal an underlying disorder that can lead to cardiac tamponade.

Clinical findings

- Acute chest pain
- Dyspnea
- Orthopnea
- Diaphoresis
- Anxiety
- Restlessness
- Pallor
- Cyanosis
- Beck's triad (jugular vein distention, hypotension, and muffled heart sounds)
- Rapid, weak peripheral pulses
- Widening area of flatness across the anterior chest wall on percussion
- Hepatomegaly
- Pulsus paradoxus (an abnormal inspiratory drop in systemic blood pressure greater than 15 mm Hg) and narrow pulse pressure
- Cardiac arrhythmia
- Possible sinus or atrial tachyarrhythmias or atrial fibrillation

Diagnostic test results

- *Chest X-rays* show slightly widened mediastinum, enlargement of the cardiac silhouette and, possibly, left pleural effusion.
- *Electrocardiography (ECG)* reveals that the QRS amplitude may be reduced and that electrical alternans of the P wave, QRS complex, and T wave may be present. Generalized ST-segment elevation is noted in all leads except aV_R and V_1.
- *Pulmonary artery pressure monitoring* detects increased right atrial pressure, right ventricular diastolic pressure, and central venous pressure.
- *Echocardiography* records pericardial effusion with signs of right ventricular and atrial compression.

COLLABORATIVE MANAGEMENT

If fluid accumulation is slow or chronic, a cardiothoracic surgeon will remove the fluid by direct needle aspiration (pericardiocentesis), pericardiotomy (sclerosing the pericardium), pericardio-peritoneum shunt, pericardiectomy, or by creating an opening called a pericardial window. Other members of the health care team may include a trauma health care provider (if secondary to trauma), an infectious disease specialist (if caused by infection, such as HIV or tuberculosis), or a nephrologist (for patients with renal disease). (See *Disorders affecting management of cardiac tamponade,* pages 74 and 75.)

TREATMENT AND CARE

- The goal of treatment is to relieve intrapericardial pressure and cardiac compression by removing accumulated blood or fluid.
- Supplemental oxygen is administered to improve oxygenation.
- Continuous ECG and hemodynamic monitoring are instituted (in an intensive care unit) to monitor for complications and effects of therapy.
- Pericardiocentesis (needle aspiration of the pericardial cavity) may be performed to reduce fluid in the pericardial sac and improve systemic arterial pressure and cardiac output. (A catheter may be left in the pericardial space attached to a drainage container to allow for continuous fluid drainage.)
- If pericardiocentesis fails, a pericardial window may be created to remove accumulated fluid from the pericardial sac.
- Pericardiectomy (resection of a portion or all of the pericardium) may be performed if repeated pericardiocentesis fails to prevent recurrence of cardiac tamponade.
- Trial volume loading with crystalloids, such as I.V. normal saline solution, may be administered to maintain systolic blood pressure.
- Inotropic drugs, such as isoproterenol (Isuprel) or dopamine (Inotropn), may be administered to improve myocardial contractility until fluid in the pericardial sac can be removed.
- Blood transfusion or a thoracotomy may be implemented to drain any reaccumulation of fluid or to repair bleeding sites in cases of traumatic injury.
- The heparin antagonist protamine sulfate may be administered to stop bleeding (in heparin-induced tamponade).
- Vitamin K may be administered to stop bleeding (in warfarin-induced tamponade).

(Text continues on page 76.)

DISORDERS AFFECTING
MANAGEMENT OF CARDIAC TAMPONADE

This chart highlights disorders that affect the management of cardiac tamponade..

DISORDER	SIGNS AND SYMPTOMS	DIAGNOSTIC TEST RESULTS
End-stage renal disease (coexisting)	◆ Reduced urine output ◆ Hypotension or hypertension ◆ Pleural friction rub ◆ Altered level of consciousness	◆ Blood urea nitrogen (BUN) is elevated. ◆ Creatinine clearance and potassium levels are increased. ◆ Urine specific gravity, blood pH, bicarbonate level, hemoglobin, and hematocrit are decreased.
Lung cancer (coexisting)	◆ Dyspnea ◆ Pleural friction rub ◆ Wheezing ◆ Decreased breath sounds ◆ Dilated chest and abdominal veins ◆ Pain	◆ Cytologic sputum analysis shows dense pulmonary malignancy. ◆ Liver function tests are abnormal, especially with metastasis. ◆ Chest X-ray shows advanced lesions. ◆ Contrast studies of the bronchial tree demonstrate the size and location as well as spread of the lesion. ◆ Computed tomography scan of the chest can detect malignant pleural effusion.
Myocardial infarction (MI) (coexisting)	◆ Severe, persistent chest pain ◆ Feeling of impending doom ◆ Fatigue ◆ Nausea and vomiting ◆ Shortness of breath ◆ Anxiety ◆ Muffled heart sounds ◆ Hypotension or hypertension	◆ Electrocardiogram (ECG) reveals ST-segment changes. ◆ Total creatine kinase (CK) and CK-MB isoenzyme levels are elevated over a 72-hour period. ◆ Myoglobin is elevated within 3 to 6 hours. ◆ Echocardiography shows ventricular-wall motion abnormalities. ◆ Multigated acquisition scan or radionuclide ventriculography identifies acutely damaged muscle. ◆ Homocysteine and C-reactive protein levels are elevated.

TREATMENT AND CARE

- Monitor intake and output; check weight daily.
- Monitor vital signs for signs of decreased cardiac output.
- Assess lungs for changes in breath sounds.
- Watch for signs of infection.
- Monitor serum laboratory results, including BUN, creatinine, and electrolyte levels.

- Monitor respiratory status for dyspnea and changes in breath sounds.
- Administer oxygen.
- Assess the patient's pain level, and administer medications.
- Monitor chest X-ray for development of pleural effusion.
- Provide support for patients undergoing testing for metastatic disease.
- Check for pulsus paradoxus.

- Assess the patient for specific type of pain, and monitor him for changes.
- Note cardiac rhythm and check peripheral pulses.
- Assess heart sounds for muffled tones, and auscultate for pericardial friction rub.
- Check for pulsus paradoxus.
- Assess for jugular vein distention.
- Be alert for signs of decreased cardiac output, such as decreased blood pressure and dyspnea.
- Be prepared to administer an antiarrhythmic, to possibly assist with pacemaker insertion and, rarely, to assist with cardioversion to treat cardiac arrhythmias.
- Be prepared to administer thrombolytic therapy (streptokinase or recombinant tissue plasminogen) to preserve myocardial tissue.
- Percutaneous transluminal coronary angioplasty may be performed to restore blood flow to the heart muscle.
- Be prepared to administer other drugs, including antiplatelet drugs (such as aspirin) to inhibit platelet aggregation; sublingual or I.V. nitrates (such as nitroglycerin) to relieve pain, increase cardiac output, and reduce myocardial workload; morphine for pain and sedation; and angiotensin-converting enzyme inhibitors to improve survival rate in large anterior-wall MI.
- Administer oxygen at 2 to 4 L/minute or at a flow rate to maintain oxygen saturation higher than 90%.
- Assist with pulmonary artery catheterization, used to detect left- or right-sided heart failure and to monitor the patient's response to treatment.
- Assess and record the severity of chest pain.
- During episodes of chest pain, monitor ECG, blood pressure, and pulmonary artery catheter measurements for changes.
- Monitor vital signs frequently.
- Watch for signs and symptoms of fluid retention (crackles, cough, tachypnea, and edema).
- Carefully monitor daily weight, intake and output, and serum enzyme levels.

Cardiomyopathy

Cardiomyopathy involves disease of the heart muscle fibers. It occurs in three main forms: dilated, hypertrophic, and restrictive (extremely rare). Cardiomyopathy is the second most common direct cause of sudden death. About 5 to 8 Americans out of 100,000 have *dilated cardiomyopathy,* the most common type. At greatest risk for dilated cardiomyopathy are men and blacks; other risk factors include coronary artery disease, hypertension, pregnancy, viral infections, and alcohol or illegal drug use. Because dilated cardiomyopathy usually isn't diagnosed until its advanced stages, the prognosis is usually poor.

There are two types of *hypertrophic cardiomyopathy:* nonobstructive hypertrophic cardiomyopathy and hypertrophic obstructive cardiomyopathy (HOCM). Almost 50% of all sudden deaths in competitive athletes age 35 or younger are caused by HOCM.

If severe, *restrictive cardiomyopathy* is irreversible.

ETIOLOGY
Most patients with dilated cardiomyopathy have idiopathic (or primary) disease; however, in some cases, dilated cardiomyopathy is caused by another condition. (See *Comparing cardiomyopathies,* pages 78 and 79.)

The course of hypertrophic cardiomyopathy is variable. The more common form — nonobstructive hypertrophic cardiomyopathy — is caused by pressure overload hypertension or aortic valve stenosis. The second form, HOCM, is almost always inherited as a non-sex-linked autosomal dominant trait. Some patients progressively deteriorate, whereas others remain stable for years. Restrictive cardiomyopathy results from cardiac muscle fibrosis secondary to infiltration.

PATHOPHYSIOLOGY
Dilated cardiomyopathy results from extensively damaged myocardial muscle fibers. Consequently, contractility in the left ventricle is reduced. As systolic function declines, stroke volume, ejection fraction, and cardiac output fall. As end-diastolic volumes rise, pulmonary congestion may occur. The elevated end-diastolic volume is a compensatory response to preserve stroke volume despite a reduced ejection fraction. The sympathetic nervous system is also stimulated to increase heart rate and contractility.

Cardiovascular system
Dilated cardiomyopathy
■ When the renin-angiotensin system, which has been stimulated to regulate cardiac output, can no longer do its job, the heart begins to fail. Left ventricular dilation occurs as venous return and systemic vascular resistance rise.
■ Eventually, the atria dilate as more work is required to pump blood into the full ventricles. Cardiomegaly occurs as a consequence of dilation of the atria and ventricles.
■ Blood pooling in the ventricles increases the risk of emboli. (See *Disorders affecting management of cardiomyopathy,* pages 80 to 83.)

Nonobstructive hypertrophic cardiomyopathy
■ Unlike dilated cardiomyopathy, which affects systolic function, hypertrophic cardiomyopathy primarily affects diastolic function.
■ The hypertrophied ventricle becomes stiff, noncompliant, and unable to relax during ventricular filling.
■ Ventricular filling is reduced and left ventricular filling pressure rises, causing a rise in left atrial and pulmonary venous pressures and leading to venous congestion and dyspnea. Ventricular filling time is further reduced as a compensatory response to tachycardia, leading to low cardiac output.
■ If papillary muscles (attached to the atrioventricular valves) become hypertrophied and don't close completely during contraction, mitral insufficiency occurs.

Hypertrophic obstructive cardiomyopathy
■ The features of HOCM include asymmetrical left ventricular hypertrophy; hypertrophy of the intraventricular septum; rapid, forceful contractions of the left ventricle; impaired relaxation; and obstruction to left ventricular outflow.
■ The forceful ejection of blood draws the anterior leaflet of the mitral valve to the intraventricular septum, which causes early

COMPARING DIAGNOSTIC TESTS IN CARDIOMYOPATHY

DIAGNOSTIC TEST	DILATED CARDIOMYOPATHY	HYPERTROPHIC CARDIOMYOPATHY	RESTRICTIVE CARDIOMYOPATHY
Electrocardiography	Biventricular hypertrophy, sinus tachycardia, atrial enlargement, atrial and ventricular arrhythmias, bundle-branch block, and ST-segment and T-wave abnormalities	Left ventricular hypertrophy, ST-segment and T-wave abnormalities, left anterior hemiblock, Q waves in precordial and inferior leads, ventricular arrhythmias and, possibly, atrial fibrillation	Low voltage, hypertrophy, atrioventricular conduction defects, and left-axis deviation
Echocardiography	Left ventricular thrombi, global hypokinesia, enlarged atria, left ventricular dilation and, possibly, valvular abnormalities, decreased ejection fraction, and possible pericardial effusion	Asymmetrical thickening of the left ventricular wall and intraventricular septum and left atrial dilation	Increased left ventricular muscle mass, normal or reduced left ventricular cavity size, and decreased systolic function; rules out constrictive pericarditis
Chest X-ray	Cardiomegaly, pulmonary congestion, pulmonary venous hypertension, and pleural or pericardial effusions	Cardiomegaly	Cardiomegaly, pericardial effusion, and pulmonary congestion
Cardiac catheterization	Elevated left atrial and left ventricular end-diastolic pressures, left ventricular enlargement, and mitral and tricuspid incompetence; may identify coronary artery disease as a cause	Elevated ventricular end-diastolic pressure and, possibly, mitral insufficiency, hyperdynamic systolic function, and aortic valve pressure gradient (if aortic valve is stenotic)	Reduced systolic function and myocardial infiltration; increased left ventricular end-diastolic pressure; rules out constrictive pericarditis
Radionuclide studies	Left ventricular dilation and hypokinesis, and reduced ejection fraction	Reduced left ventricular volume, increased muscle mass, and ischemia	Left ventricular hypertrophy with restricted ventricular filling and reduced ejection fraction

closure of the outflow tract, decreasing ejection fraction.
■ Intramural coronary arteries are abnormally small and may not be sufficient to supply the hypertrophied muscle with enough blood and oxygen to meet the increased needs of the hyperdynamic muscle.

Restrictive cardiomyopathy
■ Stiffness of the ventricle is caused by left ventricular hypertrophy and endocardial fibrosis and thickening, which reduce the ability of the ventricle to relax and fill during diastole.
■ The rigid myocardium fails to contract completely during systole, resulting in decreased cardiac output.

Renal system
■ The kidneys are stimulated to retain sodium and water to maintain cardiac output, resulting in vasoconstriction.

COMPARING CARDIOMYOPATHIES

Cardiomyopathies include various structural or functional abnormalities of the ventricles. They're grouped into three main pathophysiologic types – dilated, hypertrophic, and restrictive. These conditions may lead to heart failure by impairing myocardial structure and function.

NORMAL HEART	DILATED CARDIOMYOPATHY
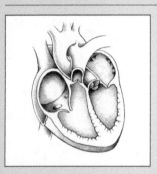	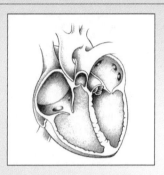
Ventricles	◆ Greatly increased chamber size ◆ Thinning of left ventricular muscle
Atrial chamber size	◆ Increased
Myocardial mass	◆ Increased
Ventricular inflow resistance	◆ Normal
Contractility	◆ Decreased
Possible causes	◆ Viral or bacterial infection ◆ Hypertension ◆ Peripartum syndrome related to toxemia ◆ Ischemic heart disease ◆ Valvular disease ◆ Drug hypersensitivity ◆ Chemotherapy ◆ Cardiotoxic effects of drugs or alcohol ◆ Adverse effects of chemotherapy

ASSESSMENT

Onset of dilated or restrictive cardiomyopathy is generally insidious. As the disease progresses, exacerbations and hospitalizations occur frequently — regardless of the cardiomyopathy type. For patients with dilated cardiomyopathy, findings may be overlooked until left-sided heart failure occurs.

In such cases, the patient's current condition must be compared with his condition over the past 6 to 12 months.

Clinical findings

Findings associated with *dilated cardiomyopathy* may include:

■ shortness of breath

HYPERTROPHIC CARDIOMYOPATHY	RESTRICTIVE CARDIOMYOPATHY

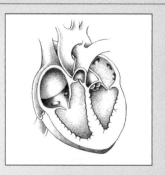

◆ Normal right and decreased left chamber size	◆ Decreased ventricular chamber size
◆ Left ventricular hypertrophy	◆ Left ventricular hypertrophy
◆ Thickened interventricular septum (hypertrophic obstructive cardiomyopathy [HOCM])	
◆ Increased on left	◆ Increased
◆ Increased	◆ Normal
◆ Increased	◆ Increased
◆ Increased or decreased	◆ Decreased
◆ Autosomal dominant trait (HOCM)	◆ Amyloidosis
◆ Hypertension	◆ Sarcoidosis
◆ Obstructive valvular disease	◆ Hemochromatosis
◆ Thyroid disease	◆ Infiltrative neoplastic disease
	◆ Collagen-vascular diseases
	◆ Tumors

- tachypnea
- orthopnea
- dyspnea on exertion
- paroxysmal nocturnal dyspnea
- fatigue
- dry cough at night caused by left-sided heart failure
- peripheral edema

- hepatomegaly
- right-upper-quadrant pain (secondary to hepatic engorgement)
- jugular vein distention
- weight gain caused by right-sided heart failure
- peripheral cyanosis associated with a low cardiac output

(Text continues on page 82.)

DISORDERS AFFECTING
MANAGEMENT OF CARDIOMYOPATHY

This chart highlights disorders that affect the management of cardiomyopathy.

DISORDER	SIGNS AND SYMPTOMS	DIAGNOSTIC TEST RESULTS
Arrhythmias (complication)	◆ Irregularly irregular pulse rhythm with normal or abnormal heart rate ◆ Radial pulse rate slower than apical pulse rate ◆ Palpable peripheral pulse with stronger contractions ◆ Evidence of decreased cardiac output, such as hypotension and light-headedness, with new-onset atrial fibrillation and a rapid ventricular rate	◆ Electrocardiography (ECG) shows atrial fibrillation (no clear P waves, irregularly irregular ventricular response, uneven baseline fibrillatory waves, and a wide variation in R-R intervals resulting in loss of atrial kick). Atrial fibrillation may be preceded by premature atrial contractions.
Heart failure (complication)	◆ Cough that produces pink, frothy sputum ◆ Cyanosis of the lips and nail beds ◆ Pale, cool, clammy skin ◆ Diaphoresis ◆ Jugular vein distention ◆ Ascites ◆ Pulsus alternans ◆ Tachycardia ◆ Hepatomegaly ◆ Decreased pulse pressure ◆ Third (S_3) and fourth (S_4) heart sounds ◆ Moist, basilar crackles ◆ Rhonchi ◆ Expiratory wheezing ◆ Decreased pulse oximetry ◆ Peripheral edema ◆ Decreased urinary output	◆ B-type natriuretic peptide immunoassay is elevated. ◆ Chest X-ray shows increased pulmonary vascular markings, interstitial edema, or pleural effusions and cardiomegaly. ◆ ECG reveals heart enlargement, ischemia, tachycardia, extrasystole, or atrial fibrillation. ◆ Pulmonary artery pressure, pulmonary artery wedge pressure, and left ventricular end-diastolic pressure are elevated in the presence of left-sided heart failure; right atrial or central venous pressure is elevated in right-sided heart failure.
Systemic or pulmonary embolization (complication)	◆ Dyspnea, which may be accompanied by anginal or pleuritic chest pain ◆ Tachycardia ◆ Productive cough ◆ Blood-tinged sputum ◆ Low-grade fever ◆ Pleural effusion ◆ Massive hemoptysis ◆ Chest splinting ◆ Leg edema ◆ Pleural friction rub ◆ Signs of circulatory collapse (weak, rapid pulse and hypotension) ◆ Signs of hypoxia (restlessness and anxiety)	◆ Chest X-ray helps to rule out other pulmonary diseases; areas of atelectasis, elevated diaphragm and pleural effusion, prominent pulmonary artery and, occasionally, the characteristic wedge-shaped infiltrate suggesting pulmonary infarction or focal oligemia of blood vessels are apparent. ◆ Lung scan shows perfusion defects in areas beyond occluded vessels; however, it doesn't rule out microemboli. ◆ Pulmonary angiography (the most definitive test) reveals evidence of emboli.

TREATMENT AND CARE

◆ Interventions aim to reduce the ventricular response rate to less than 100 beats/minute, establish anticoagulation, and restore and maintain a sinus rhythm.
◆ Treatment typically includes drug therapy to control the ventricular response or a combination of electrical cardioversion and drug therapy.
◆ If the patient is hemodynamically unstable, synchronized electrical cardioversion should be performed immediately.
◆ A transesophageal echocardiogram may be obtained before cardioversion to rule out the presence of thrombi in the atria.
◆ If drug therapy is used, monitor serum drug levels and observe the patient for evidence of toxicity.
◆ If the patient isn't on a cardiac monitor, be alert for an irregular pulse and differences in the radial and apical pulse rates.
◆ Monitor the patient's peripheral and apical pulses; watch for evidence of decreased cardiac output and heart failure.
◆ Tell the patient to report changes in pulse rate, dizziness, feeling faint, chest pain, and signs of heart failure, such as dyspnea and peripheral edema.

◆ Administer supplemental oxygen and mechanical ventilation.
◆ Place the patient in Fowler's position.
◆ Administer diuretics, inotropic drugs, vasodilators, angiotensin-converting enzyme inhibitors, angiotensin receptor blockers, cardiac glycosides, beta-adrenergic blockers, or electrolyte supplements.
◆ Initiate cardiac monitoring.
◆ Recurrent heart failure from valvular dysfunction may require surgery.
◆ A ventricular assist device may be needed.
◆ Maintain adequate cardiac output, and monitor hemodynamic stability.
◆ Assess for deep vein thrombosis, and apply antiembolism stockings.

◆ Give oxygen by nasal cannula or mask.
◆ Check ABG levels if the patient develops fresh emboli or worsening dyspnea.
◆ Be prepared to provide endotracheal intubation with assisted ventilation if breathing is severely compromised.
◆ Administer heparin through I.V. push or continuous drip. Monitor coagulation studies daily. Watch closely for nosebleed, petechiae, and other signs of abnormal bleeding; check stools for occult blood. Patients should be protected from trauma and injury; avoid I.M. injections and maintain pressure over venipuncture sites for 5 minutes, or until bleeding stops, to reduce hematoma.
◆ After the patient is stable, encourage him to move about often and assist him with isometric and range-of-motion exercises. Check pedal pulses, temperature, and color of feet to detect venostasis. *Never* massage the patient's legs.
◆ Offer diversional activities to promote rest and relieve restlessness.
◆ Help the patient walk as soon as possible after surgery to prevent venostasis.
◆ Maintain adequate nutrition and fluid balance to promote healing.
◆ Report frequent pleuritic chest pain so that analgesics can be prescribed.
◆ Incentive spirometry can assist in deep breathing.
◆ Warn the patient not to cross his legs; this promotes thrombus formation.

(continued)

DISORDERS AFFECTING
MANAGEMENT OF CARDIOMYOPATHY *(continued)*

DISORDER	SIGNS AND SYMPTOMS	DIAGNOSTIC TEST RESULTS
Systemic or pulmonary embolization *(continued)*	*With a large embolus* ◆ Cyanosis ◆ Syncope ◆ Jugular vein distention ◆ Right ventricular S_3 gallop ◆ Increased intensity of a pulmonic component of second heart sound ◆ Crackles	◆ ECG may show right-axis deviation; right bundle-branch block; tall, peaked P waves; depression of ST segments and T-wave inversions (indicating right-sided heart strain); and supraventricular tachyarrhythmias in extensive pulmonary embolism. A pattern sometimes observed is S wave in lead I, Q wave in lead III, and inverted T wave in lead III. ◆ Arterial blood gas (ABG) analysis showing decreased partial pressure of arterial oxygen and partial pressure of arterial carbon dioxide are characteristic but don't always occur.

■ tachycardia as a compensatory response to low cardiac output
■ pansystolic murmur associated with mitral and tricuspid insufficiency secondary to cardiomegaly and weak papillary muscles
■ third (S_3) and fourth (S_4) heart sound gallop rhythms associated with heart failure
■ irregular pulse, if atrial fibrillation exists
■ worsening renal function as decreased cardiac output produces decreased renal perfusion.

Findings associated with *nonobstructive hypertropic cardiomyopathy* may include:
■ dyspnea caused by elevated left ventricular filling pressure
■ fatigue associated with a reduced cardiac output
■ angina caused by the inability of the intramural coronary arteries to supply enough blood to meet the increased oxygen demands of the hypertrophied heart
■ peripheral pulse with a characteristic double impulse (pulsus biferiens) caused by powerful left ventricular contractions and rapid ejection of blood during systole
■ abrupt arterial pulse resulting from vigorous left ventricular contractions
■ irregular pulse if an enlarged atrium causes atrial fibrillation.

Findings associated with *HOCM* may include:
■ systolic ejection murmur along the left sternal border and at the apex caused by mitral insufficiency

■ angina caused by the inability of the intramural coronary arteries to supply enough blood to meet the increased oxygen demands of the hypertrophied heart
■ syncope resulting from arrhythmias or reduced ventricular filling leading to a reduced cardiac output
■ activity intolerance caused by worsening of outflow-tract obstruction from exercise-induced catecholamine release
■ abrupt arterial pulse resulting from vigorous left ventricular contractions and early termination of left ventricular ejection
■ irregular pulse if an enlarged atrium causes atrial fibrillation
■ displacement of point of maximum impulse inferiorly and laterally because of increased cardiac size.

Findings associated with *restrictive cardiomyopathy* may include:
■ fatigue, dyspnea, orthopnea, chest pain, edema, liver engorgement, peripheral cyanosis, pallor, and S_3 or S_4 gallop rhythms, and jugular vein distention caused by heart failure
■ systolic murmurs caused by mitral and tricuspid insufficiency.

Diagnostic test results
■ *Echocardiography* may reveal asymmetry of the left ventricle and hypertrophy, obstruction of outflow of the left ventricle, decreased ejection fraction, endocardial thickening, and decreased cardiac output.

■ *Chest X-ray* may reveal cardiomegaly associated with any of the cardiomyopathies.
■ *Cardiac catheterization* with possible heart biopsy reveals endocardial fibrosis and thickening. It may also show decreased ejection fraction. (See *Comparing diagnostic tests in cardiomyopathy*, page 77.)

COLLABORATIVE MANAGEMENT
A cardiothoracic surgeon is usually consulted if the patient is considered a candidate for cardiac transplantation. The services of a nutritionist may be necessary to help with dietary measures. Physical and occupational therapists may be consulted to help establish a course of rehabilitation, planning for activity limitations and energy conservation.

TREATMENT AND CARE
Management of *dilated cardiomyopathy* may involve:
■ treatment of the underlying cause, if identifiable
■ angiotensin-converting enzyme (ACE) inhibitors, as first-line therapy, to reduce afterload through vasodilation
■ diuretics, taken with ACE inhibitors, to reduce fluid retention
■ hydralazine (Apresoline) and isosorbide (Isordil) dinitrate, in combination, to produce vasodilation
■ beta-adrenergic blockers for the patient with New York Heart Association (NYHA) class II or III heart failure.

■ antiarrhythmics, such as amiodarone (Cardarone) (used cautiously), to control arrhythmias
■ an implantable cardioverter-defibrillator to prevent and treat ventricular arrhythmias (because of the high incidence of sudden death in patients with NYHA class III or IV heart failure)
■ cardioversion to convert atrial fibrillation to sinus rhythm
■ pacemaker insertion to correct arrhythmias
■ biventricular pacemaker for cardiac resynchronization therapy, if symptoms continue despite optimal drug therapy, for the patient with NYHA class III or IV heart failure, if the QRS complex duration is 0.13 second or more, or if the ejection fraction is 35% or less
■ revascularization, such as coronary artery bypass graft surgery, if dilated cardiomyopathy is from ischemia
■ valve repair or replacement, if dilated cardiomyopathy is from valve dysfunction
■ heart transplantation in cases resistant to medical therapy
■ lifestyle modifications, such as smoking cessation; low-fat, low-sodium diet; physical activity; and abstinence from alcohol
■ anticoagulants (controversial) to reduce the risk of emboli.
Management of *hypertrophic cardiomyopathy* may involve:
■ control of hypertension

- aortic valve replacement, if the valve is stenotic
- verapamil (Calan) or diltiazem (Cardizem) to reduce ventricular stiffness and elevated diastolic pressures
- cardioversion to treat atrial fibrillation
- anticoagulant therapy to reduce the risk of systemic embolism with atrial fibrillation.

Management of *HOCM* may involve:
- beta-adrenergic blockers to slow the heart rate, reduce myocardial oxygen demands, and increase ventricular filling by relaxing the obstructing muscle, thereby increasing cardiac output
- antiarrhythmic drugs, such as amiodarone, to reduce arrhythmias
- cardioversion to treat atrial fibrillation
- anticoagulant therapy to reduce the risk of systemic embolism with atrial fibrillation
- verapamil or diltiazem to reduce septal stiffness and elevated diastolic pressures
- an implantable cardioverter-defibrillator to treat ventricular arrhythmias
- ventricular myotomy or myectomy (resection of the hypertrophied septum) to ease outflow tract obstruction and relieve symptoms
- heart transplantation for symptoms not easily controlled
- mitral valve replacement to treat mitral insufficiency (controversial)
- ablation of the atrioventricular node and implantation of a dual-chamber pacemaker (controversial) in the patient with HOCM and ventricular tachycardia to reduce the outflow gradient by altering the pattern of ventricular contractions.

Management of *restrictive cardiomyopathy* may involve:
- treatment of the underlying cause, such as giving deferoxamine (Desferal) to bind iron in restrictive cardiomyopathy caused by hemochromatosis
- cardiac glycosides, diuretics, and a restricted sodium diet to ease the symptoms of heart failure
- oral vasodilators to decrease afterload and facilitate ventricular ejection.

RED FLAG *Digoxin isn't used in patients with cardiomyopathies because it predisposes them to arrhythmias. Additionally, in patients with restrictive cardiomyopathy caused by amyloidosis, digoxin binds to the heart's amyloid fibers.*

Cerebral contusion

More serious than a concussion, a cerebral contusion is an ecchymosis of brain tissue that results from a severe blow to the head. A cerebral contusion disrupts normal nerve functions in the bruised area and may cause loss of consciousness, hemorrhage, edema, and even death.

ETIOLOGY

A cerebral contusion results from acceleration-deceleration or coup-contrecoup injuries. It's also seen in cases of abuse.

A cerebral contusion can occur directly beneath the site of impact (coup) when the brain rebounds against the skull from the force of a blow (for example, from a blunt instrument), when the force of the blow drives the brain against the opposite side of the skull (contrecoup), or when the head is hurled forward and stopped abruptly (as in a motor vehicle crash when the driver's head strikes the windshield); the brain continues moving and slaps against the skull (acceleration) and then rebounds (deceleration), striking the opposite side of the skull.

PATHOPHYSIOLOGY

Cerebral contusion causes brain tissue to bruise. Although major body systems can be affected because the brain functions as the control center, the most serious problems occur in the neurologic system.

Neurologic system

- When injuries cause the brain to strike against bony prominences inside the skull (especially to the sphenoidal ridges), intracranial hemorrhage or hematoma can occur.
- The patient may suffer brain herniation (shifting of tissue from areas of high pressure to areas of lower pressure) as the tissue attempts to compensate for the increased pressure. This shifting, however, causes the blood supply to the shifted area to close off. (See *Disorders affecting management of cerebral contusion,* pages 86 and 87.)
- Secondary effects, such as brain swelling, may accompany serious contusions, resulting in increased intracranial pressure (ICP) and herniation.

ASSESSMENT

The patient's history (obtained from family, friends, other witnesses, and emergency personnel, if necessary) reveals a severe traumatic impact to the head. Clinical findings depend on the location of the contusion and the extent of the damage.

Clinical findings

■ Depending on the area of the brain affected, hemiparesis, decorticate or decerebrate posturing, or unequal pupillary response
■ A period of unconsciousness after the trauma, possibly lasting 6 hours or more
■ Pale appearance and motionless (unconscious patient)
■ Drowsy, easily disturbed by any form of stimulation (such as noise or light), agitated, and possibly violent (conscious patient)
■ Below-normal blood pressure and temperature
■ Pulse rate within normal levels but feeble
■ Shallow respirations
■ Possible severe scalp wounds
■ Labored respirations and, possibly, involuntary evacuation of the bowels and bladder
■ Less obvious head injuries such as hematoma
■ Cold skin (unconscious patient)
■ Hemiparesis
■ Decorticate or decerebrate posturing
■ Unequal pupillary response
■ Temporary rousing during examination (if the patient is unconscious)
■ Relatively alert state upon neurologic examination after the acute stage of the injury, perhaps with temporary aphasia, slight hemiparesis, or unilateral numbness

Diagnostic test results

■ *Cerebral angiography* outlines vasculature.
■ *Computed tomography (CT) scan* shows ischemic or necrotic tissue, cerebral edema, areas of petechial hemorrhage, and subdural, epidural, and intracerebral hematomas. CT scan may also reveal a shift in brain tissue.

COLLABORATIVE MANAGEMENT

A neurosurgeon may coordinate care if the patient's head trauma is severe enough to require surgery or invasive ICP monitoring. Physical therapy, occupational therapy, and social services may be necessary if the patient has physical or cognitive deficits from the injury and requires assistance with activities of daily living. For children with head injury, a child-life therapist may help facilitate normal growth and development through the use of play and self-expression therapy. In cases of extremely severe injury, the family may require spiritual support as well as help in considering whether the patient may be a candidate for organ donation.

TREATMENT AND CARE

■ Immediate treatment may include establishing and maintaining a patent airway and, if necessary, a tracheotomy or endotracheal intubation.
■ Treatment may consist of careful administration of I.V. fluids (lactated Ringer's or normal saline solution), I.V. mannitol to reduce ICP, and restricted fluid intake to decrease intracerebral edema. Dexamethasone may be given I.M. or I.V. for several days to control cerebral edema.
■ The patient's ICP may be reduced by maintaining his partial pressure of arterial carbon dioxide ($Paco_2$) between 30 and 35 mm Hg. This can be accomplished by adjusting the ventilator settings for an intubated patient. A decreased $Paco_2$ constricts cerebral blood vessels and reduces cerebral blood flow, thus reducing ICP.
■ If necessary, additional treatments may include blood transfusion and craniotomy to control bleeding and to aspirate blood.
■ Neurologic examinations should be performed, focusing on level of consciousness, motor responses, and ICP.
■ Vital signs and respirations should be monitored regularly (usually every 15 minutes). Abnormal respirations could indicate a breakdown in the patient's respiratory center in the brain stem and, possibly, an impending brain herniation, which is a neurologic emergency.
■ Administer short-acting analgesics or diuretics.
■ To decrease the patient's anxiety, speak calmly to him and explain your actions, even if he's unconscious.
■ Insert an indwelling urinary catheter. Monitor intake and output.
■ If the patient is unconscious, insert a nasogastric tube to prevent aspiration, but only after a basilar skull fracture has been ruled out. Otherwise, the tube may be inserted into the cranial vault.

DISORDERS AFFECTING
MANAGEMENT OF CEREBRAL CONTUSION

This chart highlights disorders that affect the management of cerebral contusion.

DISORDER	SIGNS AND SYMPTOMS	DIAGNOSTIC TEST RESULTS
Brain herniation (complication)	*Intracerebral hemorrhage or hematoma* ◆ Nuchal rigidity ◆ Photophobia ◆ Nausea and vomiting ◆ Dizziness ◆ Seizures ◆ Decreased respiratory rate ◆ Progressive obtundation *Epidural hemorrhage or hematoma* ◆ Contralateral hemiparesis ◆ Progressively severe headache ◆ Ipsilateral pupillary dilation ◆ Signs of increased intracranial pressure (ICP) ◆ Decrease in pulse and respiratory rates ◆ Increase in systolic blood pressure *Epidural hematoma* ◆ Drowsiness and confusion ◆ Dilation of one or both pupils ◆ Hyperventilation ◆ Nuchal rigidity ◆ Bradycardia ◆ Decorticate or decerebrate posturing	◆ Computed tomography (CT) scan may reveal herniation.
Intracranial hemorrhage or hematoma (complication)	*Subacute or chronic subdural hemorrhage or hematoma* ◆ May not occur until days after the injury *Acute subdural hematoma* ◆ Loss of consciousness ◆ Weakness ◆ Paralysis	◆ Computed tomography (CT) scan may reveal a mass confirming a hematoma or hemorrhage. ◆ Skull X-ray may reveal a mass confirming a hematoma or hemorrhage. ◆ Arteriography may reveal altered blood flow in the area.

■ Carefully observe the patient for leakage of cerebrospinal fluid (CSF). Check the bed sheets for a blood-tinged spot surrounded by a lighter ring (halo sign). If CSF leakage develops and spinal injury is ruled out, raise the head of the bed 30 degrees. If you detect CSF leakage from the nose, place a gauze pad under the nostrils. If CSF leaks from the ear, position the patient so that his ear drains naturally; don't pack the ear or nose.

RED FLAG To prevent central nervous system (CNS) infection, avoid cleaning or suctioning the ears or nose of a patient with a head injury. Doing so could introduce microorganisms into the CNS.

■ If the patient is unconscious and spinal injury is ruled out, elevate the head of the bed and maintain the patient's head in the midline position to decrease ICP. If his head is turned to the side, he may have poor jugular venous return, which can increase ICP.

■ Restrict total fluid intake to reduce volume and intracerebral swelling.

TREATMENT AND CARE

◆ Check vital signs, level of consciousness, and pupil size every 15 minutes.

◆ Establish and maintain a patent airway. Intubation may be needed.

◆ Observe for cerebrospinal fluid (CSF) drainage from the patient's ears, nose, or mouth. If the patient's nose is draining CSF, wipe it—don't let him blow. If an ear is draining, cover it lightly with sterile gauze; don't pack it.

◆ Take seizure precautions, but don't restrain the patient.

◆ Agitated behavior may be caused by hypoxia or increased ICP, so check for these symptoms. Speak in a calm voice, and touch the patient gently. Don't make any sudden, unexpected moves.

◆ Restrict total fluid intake to 1,200 to 1,500 ml/day to reduce fluid volume and intracellular swelling.

◆ A craniotomy may be necessary to locate and control bleeding and to aspirate blood.

◆ Epidural and subdural hematomas may be drained through burr holes in the skull.

◆ Administer I.V. mannitol, steroids, or diuretics to control decreased ICP.

◆ Follow treatment and care for brain herniation.

■ After the patient is stabilized, clean and dress any superficial scalp wounds. (If the skin has been broken, the patient may need tetanus prophylaxis.) Assist with suturing, if needed.

■ If the patient develops temporary aphasia, provide an alternative means of communication.

Chronic glomerulonephritis is a slow, progressive disease characterized by inflammation of the glomeruli structure of the kidney. This inflammation results in sclerosis and scarring and may progress to renal failure.

Chronic glomerulonephritis develops insidiously, usually going undetected until the progressive phase begins. By the time symptoms of proteinuria, granular tube casts, and hematuria develop, chronic glomerulonephritis is generally irreversible.

ETIOLOGY

Common causes of chronic glomerulonephritis include such renal disorders as membranoproliferative glomerulonephritis, membranous glomerulopathy, focal glomerulosclerosis, rapidly progressive glomerulonephritis and poststreptococcal glomerulonephritis. Systemic disorders, such as lupus erythematosus, Goodpasture's syndrome, and diabetes, may also cause chronic glomerulonephritis.

PATHOPHYSIOLOGY

In nearly all types of glomerulonephritis, the epithelial layer of the glomerular membrane is disturbed, causing a loss of the negative charge.

Renal system

■ Chronic glomerulonephritis progresses slowly — over a period of 20 to 30 years— leading to changes in the renal parenchyma.

■ Kidney tissue atrophies and the functional mass of nephrons decreases significantly, resulting in decreased glomerular filtration.

■ The cortex of the parenchyma thins, but the calices and pelves remain normal.

■ Renal biopsy of the kidney tissue in the late stages of glomerulonephritis shows hyalinization of the glomeruli, loss of tubules, and fibrosis of kidney tissue.

■ The late stages of the disease produce symptoms related to uremia, which requires dialysis or renal transplantation.

■ Glomerular injury causes proteinuria because of the increased permeability of the glomerular capillaries.

DISORDERS AFFECTING MANAGEMENT OF CHRONIC GLOMERULONEPHRITIS

This chart highlights disorders that affect the management of chronic glomerulonephritis.

DISORDER	SIGNS AND SYMPTOMS	DIAGNOSTIC TEST RESULTS
Heart failure (complication)	◆ Cough that produces pink, frothy sputum ◆ Cyanosis of the lips and nail beds ◆ Pale, cool, clammy skin ◆ Diaphoresis ◆ Jugular vein distention ◆ Ascites ◆ Pulsus alternans ◆ Tachycardia ◆ Hepatomegaly ◆ Decreased pulse pressure ◆ Third and fourth heart sounds ◆ Moist, basilar crackles ◆ Rhonchi ◆ Expiratory wheezing ◆ Decreased pulse oximetry ◆ Peripheral edema ◆ Decreased urinary output	◆ B-type natriuretic peptide immunoassay is elevated. ◆ Chest X-ray shows increased pulmonary vascular markings, interstitial edema, or pleural effusions and cardiomegaly. ◆ Electrocardiogram (ECG) reveals heart enlargement or ischemia, tachycardia, extrasystole, or atrial fibrillation. ◆ Pulmonary artery pressure, pulmonary artery wedge pressure, and left ventricular end-diastolic pressure are elevated in the presence of left-sided heart failure; right atrial or central venous pressure is elevated in right-sided heart failure.
Hyperkalemia (complication)	◆ Nausea ◆ Muscle weakness ◆ Paresthesia ◆ Diarrhea ◆ Abdominal cramps ◆ Irritability ◆ Hypotension ◆ Irregular heart rate ◆ Possible cardiac arrhythmias	◆ Serum potassium level is greater than 5 mEq/L. ◆ Arterial pH is decreased. ◆ ECG shows tall, peaked T waves, and possibly flattened P waves, prolonged PR intervals, widened QRS complexes, and depressed ST segments.

■ Chronic glomerulonephritis eventually progresses to chronic renal failure.

Cardiovascular system
■ Hypertension results from the sclerosis of renal arterioles; severe hypertension may cause cardiac hypertrophy, leading to heart failure.
■ Fluid overload may result from oliguria leading to peripheral edema and heart failure.
■ Severe hyperkalemia can result in cardiac arrest and should be treated as a medical emergency.

Endocrine and metabolic systems
■ Renal failure leads to electrolyte, fluid, and acid-base imbalances.
■ Proteinuria leads to serum protein loss.

Gastrointestinal system
■ Accumulation of toxins results in nausea, vomiting, and anorexia.
■ Coagulopathies increase the risk of GI bleeding.

Immune and hematologic systems
■ Renal failure compromises the immune system, leading to an increased risk of infection.
■ Decreased erythropoiesis related to renal failure leads to anemia resulting in fatigue, malaise, and dyspnea.

Integumentary system
■ The accumulation of waste products leads to dry skin, brittle hair, and pruritus.

TREATMENT AND CARE

- Administer supplemental oxygen and mechanical ventilation, if needed.
- Place the patient in Fowler's position.
- Administer diuretics, inotropic drugs, vasodilators, angiotensin-converting enzyme inhibitors, angiotensin receptor blockers, cardiac glycosides, beta-adrenergic blockers, and electrolyte supplements.
- Initiate cardiac monitoring.
- Recurrent heart failure from valvular dysfunction may require surgery.
- A ventricular assist device may be needed.
- Maintain adequate cardiac output, and monitor hemodynamic stability.
- Assess for deep vein thrombosis, and apply antiembolism stockings.

- Determine and remove the underlying cause, if possible.
- Administer a rapid infusion of 10% calcium gluconate to decrease myocardial irritability.
- Administer insulin and 10% to 50% glucose I.V. for severe hyperkalemia.
- Administer sodium polystyrene sulfonate orally or rectally using an enema for mild hyperkalemia.
- Initiate dialysis as a final treatment option, or if the hyperkalemia is related to renal failure.
- Discontinue medications that may cause hyperkalemia.
- Monitor cardiac rhythm and response to treatment.
- Implement a potassium-restricted diet.

■ Hyperphosphatemia worsens pruritus and can cause the patient to scratch until the skin integrity is compromised.

■ Coagulation abnormalities may cause ecchymoses or petechiae.

■ Deposition of uremic toxins in the skin results in darkened or yellow skin tones.

Musculoskeletal system

■ Alterations in calcium and phosphorous balance lead to hypocalcemia, placing the patient at risk for pathological fractures.

■ Hyperkalemia, a medical emergency, may result in muscle weakness. (See *Disorders affecting management of chronic glomerulonephritis.*)

Neurologic system

■ Nerve cells are affected by the accumulation of waste products leading to irritability, changes in mental status, peripheral neuropathies, ataxia, asterixis seizures and, if left untreated, coma.

Respiratory system

■ Hypervolemia may result in fluid accumulation in the lungs leading to crackles, dyspnea, orthopnea, and pulmonary edema.

■ Hyperventilation occurs as a result of metabolic acidosis.

ASSESSMENT

Diagnosis of chronic glomerulonephritis is usually delayed until the condition has progressed to an advanced stage. Urine output may decrease, but gross visual changes in the urine are uncommon unless the patient has a urinary tract infection.

Clinical findings
- Irritability, drowsiness, or confusion
- Altered level of consciousness
- Dry, pruritic skin
- Infection related to an altered immune status
- Hematuria, petechiae, and ecchymosis related to bleeding abnormalities
- Proteinuria
- In children, encephalopathy with seizures and local neurologic deficits
- In elderly patients, vague, nonspecific symptoms, such as nausea, fatigue, and arthralgia
- Altered urinary elimination (oliguria)
- Edema related to fluid retention
- Tachycardia
- Bibasilar crackles
- Uremic breath odor
- Hypertension related to hypervolemia
- Anorexia, nausea, and vomiting related to excessive uremic toxin accumulation
- Dry skin and brittle hair

Diagnostic test results
- *Urinalysis* commonly reveals proteinuria; red blood cells and casts may be in the urine, indicating chronic renal disease processes.
- *Creatinine clearance* is reduced.
- *Blood studies* reveal elevated blood urea nitrogen and serum creatinine levels, low hemoglobin and hematocrit levels, platelet abnormalities, metabolic acidosis, mild hypocalcemia, hyperphosphatemia, and hyperkalemia.
- *Electrocardiography (ECG)* may show arrhythmias due to electrolyte imbalances.

RED FLAG *Hyperkalemia is a medical emergency. ECG changes consistent with hyperkalemia include a widening QRS segment, disappearing P waves, and tall, peaked T waves.*
- *X-ray, I.V. urography, ultrasonography,* or *computed tomography* reveals kidneys that are smaller than normal.
- *Renal biopsy* performed in the early stages when proteinuria and hematuria are present shows an increase in the number and types of cells infiltrating the glomerular tissue, deposition of immune complexes, and vessel sclerosis.

COLLABORATIVE MANAGEMENT
A renal specialist or a nephrologist can help evaluate, treat, and manage the patient's kidney function. Respiratory and cardiology specialists may be consulted depending on the patient's history and possible complications. Nutritional therapy may be involved to help institute necessary restrictions or supplementation. Physical and occupational therapy may be needed to help with energy conservation and rehabilitation depending on the patient's condition and length of stay. If a prolonged hospital stay is expected and the patient requires long-term care or home care, social services may be consulted early on in the patient's care. The patient may also benefit from spiritual or psychological counseling if he's acutely ill or will require continued care even after discharge.

TREATMENT AND CARE
- Treatment focuses on slowing the progression of the disease and managing complications.
- Nutritional management may include the restriction of potassium, sodium, phosphorus, and fluids. To achieve an anabolic state, adequate calories and essential amino acids must be maintained and protein may need to be restricted.
- Monitoring includes assessing intake and output, vital signs, hemoglobin and hematocrit levels, electrolyte balance, and ECG changes.
- Blood transfusions may be required for anemia.
- Antibiotics may be ordered for infection.
- Hyperkalemia requires immediate management with I.V. glucose, insulin, and sodium bicarbonate, or oral or rectal sodium polystyrene sulfonate to reduce extracellular potassium levels.
- Hemodialysis, peritoneal dialysis, or continuous renal replacement therapy may be required for severe catabolism.
- Diuretic therapy has little benefit after the patient has progressed to chronic renal failure because of limited nephron function.

■ Provide emotional support and supply information on the disease process to the patient and his family.

■ Assist the patient in locating a facility that will provide chronic hemodialysis or peritoneal dialysis training if chronic renal failure develops.

Chronic obstructive pulmonary disease

Chronic obstructive pulmonary disease (COPD) is the most common chronic lung disease, affecting about 17 million Americans, and its prevalence is rising. COPD affects more men than women and more Whites than Blacks. Although COPD doesn't always produce symptoms and causes only minimal disability in many patients, it tends to worsen with time.

ETIOLOGY
Predisposing factors include cigarette smoking, recurrent or chronic respiratory tract infections, air pollution, occupations involving exposure to dusts or noxious gases, and allergies. Familial and hereditary factors (for example, deficiency of alpha$_1$-antitrypsin) may also predispose a person to COPD.

PATHOPHYSIOLOGY
COPD results from emphysema, chronic bronchitis, asthma, or any combination of these disorders. Usually, more than one of these underlying conditions coexist; most commonly, bronchitis and emphysema occur together.

Respiratory system
■ Smoking impairs ciliary action and macrophage functions, causing airway inflammation, increased mucus production, destruction of alveolar septae, and peribronchiolar fibrosis. Early inflammatory changes may reverse if the patient stops smoking before lung destruction becomes extensive.

■ Mucus plugs and narrowed airways cause air trappings, as in asthma, chronic bronchitis, and emphysema.

■ Alveoli hyperinflate on expiration.

■ On inspiration, airways enlarge, allowing air to pass beyond the obstruction; on expiration, airways narrow and gas flow is prevented.

Cardiovascular system
■ Chronic hypoxemia and acidosis may result in constriction of the pulmonary vasculature, which eventually leads to increased pulmonary pressure and ventricular hypertrophy or cor pulmonale.

ASSESSMENT
Typically, the patient with COPD is a middle-age, long-term cigarette smoker who's asymptomatic or has mild symptoms. As the disease progresses, the patient is likely to state that he can't exercise or do strenuous work as easily as he used to. Symptoms become more pronounced as the patient ages and the disease progresses.

Clinical findings
■ Productive cough due to stimulation of the reflex by mucus
■ Dyspnea on minimal exertion
■ Frequent respiratory tract infections
■ Intermittent or continuous hypoxemia
■ Thoracic deformities in advanced form with overwhelming disability
■ Cor pulmonale
■ Severe respiratory failure (see *Disorders affecting management of COPD*, pages 92 to 95)

Diagnostic test results
■ *Arterial blood gas analysis* reveals decreased partial pressure of arterial oxygen and normal or increased partial pressure of arterial carbon dioxide.
■ *X-ray* may show advanced emphysema, flattened diaphragm, reduced vascular markings at lung periphery, vertical heart, enlarged anteroposterior chest diameter and large retrosternal airspace. *In asthma:* hyperinflation and air trapping during an attack. (See *Air trapping in COPD*, page 96.) *In*

(Text continues on page 94.)

DISORDERS AFFECTING MANAGEMENT OF COPD

This chart highlights disorders that affect the management of chronic obstructive pulmonary disease (COPD).

DISORDER	SIGNS AND SYMPTOMS	DIAGNOSTIC TEST RESULTS
Acute respiratory failure (complication)	◆ Increased respiratory rate ◆ Cyanosis ◆ Crackles ◆ Rhonchi ◆ Wheezing ◆ Diminished breath sounds ◆ Restlessness ◆ Confusion ◆ Loss of concentration ◆ Irritability ◆ Coma ◆ Tachycardia ◆ Increased cardiac output ◆ Increased blood pressure ◆ Cardiac arrhythmias	◆ Arterial blood gas (ABG) analysis shows deteriorating values and a pH below 7.35. ◆ Chest X-rays identify a pulmonary disease or condition. ◆ Electrocardiogram (ECG) may show ventricular arrhythmias or right ventricular hypertrophy. ◆ Pulse oximetry reveals decreasing arterial oxygen saturation. ◆ White blood cell (WBC) count detects underlying infection.
Cor pulmonale (complication)	◆ Progressive dyspnea worsening on exertion ◆ Tachypnea ◆ Orthopnea ◆ Edema ◆ Weakness ◆ Dependent edema ◆ Distended neck veins ◆ Enlarged, tender liver ◆ Tachycardia ◆ Hypotension ◆ Weak pulse	◆ Pulmonary artery pressure (PAP) shows increased right ventricular pressures. ◆ Echocardiography or angiography indicates right ventricular enlargement. ◆ Chest X-ray suggests right ventricular enlargement. ◆ ABG analysis shows a partial pressure of arterial oxygen of less than 70 mm Hg. ◆ ECG may show various arrhythmias. ◆ Pulmonary function tests are consistent with the underlying disorder.
Heart failure (complication)	*Left-sided heart failure* ◆ Dyspnea ◆ Orthopnea ◆ Paroxysmal nocturnal dyspnea ◆ Fatigue ◆ Nonproductive cough ◆ Crackles ◆ Hemoptysis ◆ Tachycardia ◆ Third (S_3) and fourth (S_4) heart sounds ◆ Cool, pale skin ◆ Restlessness and confusion *Right-sided heart failure* ◆ Jugular vein distention ◆ Positive hepatojugular reflux ◆ Right-upper-quadrant pain ◆ Anorexia ◆ Nausea ◆ Nocturia	◆ Chest X-rays may show pulmonary vascular markings, interstitial edema, or pleural effusion and cardiomegaly. ◆ ECG may indicate hypertrophy, ischemic changes, or infarction, and may reveal tachycardia and extrasystoles. ◆ Liver function tests are abnormal; blood urea nitrogen (BUN) and creatinine levels are elevated. ◆ Prothrombin time is prolonged. ◆ Brain natriuretic peptide assay may be elevated. ◆ Echocardiography may reveal left ventricular hypertrophy, dilation, and abnormal contractility. ◆ PAP, pulmonary artery wedge pressure, and left ventricular end-diastolic pressure are elevated in the presence of left-sided heart failure; right atrial or central venous pressure is elevated in right-sided heart failure. ◆ Radionuclide ventriculography may reveal ejection fraction of less than 40% in diastolic dysfunction.

TREATMENT AND CARE

- ◆ Monitor the effects of oxygen therapy.
- ◆ Maintain a patent airway; prepare for endotracheal intubation if indicated.
- ◆ For the intubated patient, suction as needed after hyperoxygenation. Observe for change in quantity, consistency, and color of sputum. Provide humidification to liquefy secretions.
- ◆ Observe closely for respiratory arrest.
- ◆ Auscultate for chest sounds.
- ◆ Monitor ABG levels and report changes immediately.
- ◆ Monitor serum electrolyte levels and correct imbalances.
- ◆ Monitor fluid balance by recording input and output or daily weight.
- ◆ Check the cardiac monitor for arrhythmias.
- ◆ Administer antibiotics, bronchodilators, corticosteroids, positive inotropic agents, vasopressors, or diuretics.

- ◆ Provide meticulous respiratory care, including oxygen therapy, suctioning as needed, and deep-breathing and coughing exercises.
- ◆ Monitor ABG values and monitor for signs of respiratory failure (change in pulse rate; deep, labored respirations; and increased fatigue on exertion).
- ◆ Monitor fluid status carefully; limit fluid intake to 1,000 to 2,000 ml/day and provide a low-sodium diet.
- ◆ Monitor serum potassium levels if the patient is receiving diuretics; low serum potassium levels can potentiate arrhythmias.
- ◆ Encourage bedrest.
- ◆ Administer digoxin, diazoxide, nitroprusside, hydralazine, angiotensin-converting enzyme inhibitors, calcium channel blockers, prostaglandins, heparin, or corticosteroids.

- ◆ Place patient in Fowler's position and give supplemental oxygen.
- ◆ Weigh the patient daily.
- ◆ Check for peripheral edema.
- ◆ Administer diuretics, beta-adrenergic blockers, digoxin, inotropics (doputamine or milrinone), nesiritide, nitrates, or morphine.
- ◆ Monitor intake and output, vital signs, and mental status.
- ◆ Auscultate for S_3 and crackles or rhonchi.
- ◆ Prepare the patient for coronary artery bypass surgery, angioplasty, or heart transplantation.
- ◆ Monitor BUN; creatinine; and serum potassium, sodium, chloride, and magnesium levels.
- ◆ Institute continuous cardiac monitoring to identify and treat arrhythmias promptly.
- ◆ Encourage lifestyle modifications or changes.

(continued)

DISORDERS AFFECTING MANAGEMENT OF COPD *(continued)*

DISORDER	SIGNS AND SYMPTOMS	DIAGNOSTIC TEST RESULTS
Heart failure *(continued)*	◆ Weight gain ◆ Edema ◆ Ascites or anasarca	
Hypertension (complication)	◆ Usually asymptomatic ◆ Elevated blood pressure readings on at least two consecutive occasions ◆ Occipital headache ◆ Epistaxis ◆ Bruits ◆ Dizziness ◆ Confusion ◆ Fatigue ◆ Blurry vision ◆ Nocturia ◆ Edema	◆ Serial blood pressure measurements reveal elevations of 140/90 mm Hg or greater on two or more separate occasions. ◆ Urinalysis may show protein, casts, red blood cells, or WBCs. ◆ BUN and serum creatinine levels are elevated, suggesting renal disease. ◆ Complete blood count may reveal polycythemia or anemia. ◆ Excretory urography may reveal renal atrophy. ◆ ECG may show left ventricular hypertrophy or ischemia. ◆ Chest X-rays may show cardiomegaly. ◆ Echocardiography may reveal left ventricular hypertrophy.
Respiratory acidosis (complication)	◆ Restlessness ◆ Confusion ◆ Apprehension ◆ Somnolence ◆ Fine or flapping tremor ◆ Coma ◆ Headaches ◆ Dyspnea ◆ Tachypnea ◆ Papilledema ◆ Depressed reflexes ◆ Hypoxemia ◆ Tachycardia ◆ Hypertension or hypotension ◆ Atrial and ventricular arrhythmias	◆ ABG analysis reveals a partial pressure of arterial carbon dioxide greater than 45 mm Hg, a pH less than 7.35, normal HCO_3^- level in the acute stage, and elevated HCO_3^- in the chronic stage. ◆ Chest X-ray may reveal the pulmonary cause (for example, heart failure, pneumonia, COPD, or pneumothorax). ◆ Potassium level is greater than 5 mEq/L. ◆ Serum chloride is low.

chronic bronchitis: hyperinflation and increased bronchovascular markings.

■ *Pulmonary function studies* show increased residual volume, total lung capacity, and compliance; and decreased vital capacity, diffusing capacity, and expiratory volumes. During an asthma attack, the forced expiratory volume will be decreased. In chronic bronchitis, the forced expiratory volume will be decreased and the diffusing capacity will be normal.

■ *Electrocardiography* may show arrhythmias consistent with hypoxemia.

COLLABORATIVE MANAGEMENT

Pulmonary and rehabilitation specialists may be helpful in managing dyspnea, improving functional performance, increasing exercise tolerance, decreasing oxygen consumption, and improving oxygen utilization. Nutritional support may be needed if the patient shows signs of debilitation and malnourishment.

TREATMENT AND CARE

◆ Monitor the patient's blood pressure, his response to antihypertensive medications, and laboratory studies.
◆ Encourage lifestyle modifications or changes (such as a reduced-sodium diet).
◆ Monitor for complications of hypertension such as stroke, myocardial infarction, and renal disease.
◆ Administer thiazide diuretics, angiotensin-converting enzyme inhibitors, angiotensin receptor blockers, beta-adrenergic blockers, or calcium channel blockers.

◆ Be alert for critical changes in the patient's respiratory, central nervous system, and cardiovascular functions. Report changes in function, ABG levels, and electrolyte status immediately.
◆ Maintain adequate hydration.
◆ Maintain a patent airway and provide adequate humidification if acidosis requires mechanical ventilation. Perform tracheal suction regularly and chest physiotherapy if ordered. Continuously monitor ventilator settings and respiratory status.
◆ Monitor patients with COPD and chronic carbon dioxide retention for signs of acidosis.
◆ Administer oxygen at low flow rates as indicated.
◆ Monitor patients who receive opioids and sedatives carefully.

Physical therapists may help with energy conservation measures (to enhance respiratory function), and respiratory therapists may assist with respiratory treatments. Home health care may be necessary for the patient.

TREATMENT AND CARE

■ Most patients are treated with beta-agonist bronchodilators (such as albuterol or salmeterol), anticholinergic bronchodilators (such as ipratropium), and corticosteroids (such as beclomethasone or triamcinolone). Because these are usually administered by metered-dose inhaler, the patient must be taught the correct administration technique.
■ Antibiotics are used to treat respiratory infections. Emphasize to the patient the need to complete the prescribed course of antibiotic therapy.

AIR TRAPPING IN COPD

In chronic obstructive pulmonary disease (COPD), mucus plugs and narrowed airways trap air (also called *ball-valving*). During inspiration, the airways enlarge and gas enters; on expiration, the airways narrow and air can't escape. This process commonly occurs in asthma and chronic bronchitis.

Inspiration: Air is allowed to flow freely in.

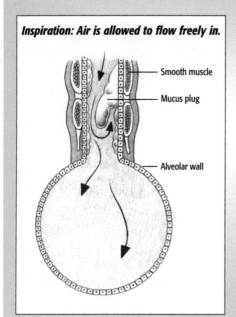

Smooth muscle

Mucus plug

Alveolar wall

Expiration: Air is trapped.

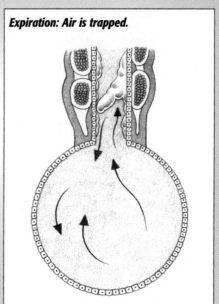

Cirrhosis

Cirrhosis is a chronic disease characterized by diffuse destruction and fibrotic regeneration of hepatic cells. As necrotic tissue yields to fibrosis, the disease damages liver tissue and normal vasculature, impairs blood and lymph flow, and ultimately causes hepatic insufficiency. It's twice as common in men as in women, and is especially prevalent among malnourished individuals older than age 50 with chronic alcoholism. Mortality is high; many patients die within 5 years of onset.

ETIOLOGY

Laennec's cirrhosis (portal, nutritional, or al-coholic cirrhosis) is the most common type of cirrhosis. It's primarily caused by hepatitis C and alcoholism. Liver damage results from malnutrition and chronic alcohol use, and fibrous tissue forms in portal areas and around central veins.

Postnecrotic cirrhosis accounts for 10% to 30% of cirrhosis cases. It stems from various types of hepatitis or toxic exposures. Autoimmune disease, such as sarcoidosis or chronic inflammatory bowel disease, is another hepatocellular cause of cirrhosis.

Cholestatic diseases that may cause cirrhosis include diseases of the biliary tree (biliary cirrhosis resulting from bile duct diseases suppressing bile flow) and sclerosing cholangitis. Metabolic diseases that may cause cirrhosis include Wilson's disease, alpha$_1$-antitrypsin deficiency, and hemochromatosis (pigment cirrhosis).

WHAT HAPPENS IN PORTAL HYPERTENSION

Portal hypertension (elevated pressure in the portal vein) occurs when blood flow meets increased resistance. This common result of cirrhosis may also stem from mechanical obstruction and occlusion of the hepatic veins (Budd-Chiari syndrome).

As the pressure in the portal vein rises, blood backs up into the spleen and flows through collateral channels to the venous system, bypassing the liver. Thus, portal hypertension causes:

◆ splenomegaly with thrombocytopenia

◆ dilated collateral veins (esophageal varices, hemorrhoids, or prominent abdominal veins)
◆ ascites.

In many patients, the first sign of portal hypertension is bleeding esophageal varices (dilated tortuous veins in the submucosa of the lower esophagus).

Esophageal varices commonly cause massive hematemesis, requiring emergency care to control hemorrhage and prevent hypovolemic shock.

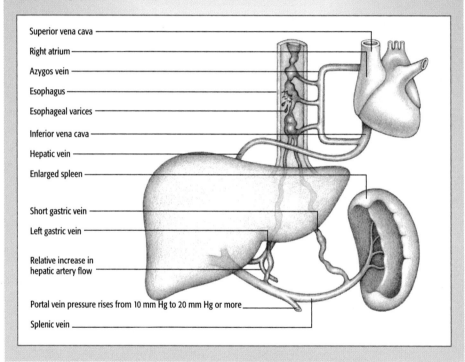

Superior vena cava
Right atrium
Azygos vein
Esophagus
Esophageal varices
Inferior vena cava
Hepatic vein
Enlarged spleen
Short gastric vein
Left gastric vein
Relative increase in hepatic artery flow
Portal vein pressure rises from 10 mm Hg to 20 mm Hg or more
Splenic vein

Other types of cirrhosis include Budd-Chiari syndrome (see *What happens in portal hypertension*) (which involves epigastric pain, liver enlargement, and ascites caused by hepatic vein obstruction), cryptogenic cirrhosis (cirrhosis of unknown etiology), and, rarely, cardiac cirrhosis (resulting from right-sided heart failure).

PATHOPHYSIOLOGY

Cirrhosis begins with hepatic scarring or fibrosis. The scar begins as an increase in extracellular matrix components — fibril-forming collagens, proteoglycans, fibronectin, and hyaluronic acid. The site of collagen deposition varies with the cause. Hepatocyte function is eventually impaired as the matrix changes. Fat-storing cells are believed to be the source of new matrix components. Contraction of these cells may also contribute to

DISORDERS AFFECTING MANAGEMENT OF CIRRHOSIS

This chart highlights disorders that affect the management of cirrhosis.

DISORDER	SIGNS AND SYMPTOMS	DIAGNOSTIC TEST RESULTS
Esophageal varices (complication)	◆ Massive hematemesis ◆ Tachycardia ◆ Tachypnea ◆ Hypotension ◆ Decreased pulses ◆ Dry mucous membranes ◆ Poor skin turgor ◆ Altered level of consciousness	◆ Endoscopy identifies ruptured varix as the bleeding site and excludes other potential sources in the upper GI tract. ◆ Complete blood count reveals decreased hemoglobin level; hematocrit; and red blood cell, white blood cell, and platelet counts. ◆ Coagulation studies reveal prolonged prothrombin time secondary to hepatocellular disease. ◆ Serum chemistry tests may reveal elevated blood urea nitrogen, sodium, total bilirubin and ammonia levels, and decreased serum albumin resulting from liver damage and elevated liver enzyme levels.
Portal hypertension (complication)	◆ Bleeding from esophageal varices	◆ Portal venous pressures exceed 10 mm Hg. ◆ Angiography helps to identify patency of the portal vein and development of collateral vessels.

disruption of the lobular architecture and obstruction of blood or bile flow. Cellular changes producing bands of scar tissue also disrupt the lobular structure.

Endocrine system
■ Testicular atrophy, menstrual irregularities, gynecomastia, and loss of chest and axillary hair result from decreased hormone metabolism.

Hematologic system
■ Bleeding tendencies (nosebleeds, easy bruising, bleeding gums), splenomegaly, and anemia resulting from thrombocytopenia

(secondary to splenomegaly and decreased vitamin K absorption) may develop.
■ Portal hypertension may occur, which can result in enlarged superficial abdominal veins, hemorrhoids, and hemorrhage from esophageal varices. (See *Disorders affecting management of cirrhosis.*)

Hepatic system
■ Jaundice results from decreased bilirubin metabolism.
■ Hepatomegaly occurs secondary to liver scarring and portal hypertension.
■ Ascites and edema of the legs result from portal hypertension and decreased plasma proteins.

TREATMENT AND CARE

- Assess the patient for the extent of blood loss.
- Ensure a patent airway and assess breathing and circulation.
- Monitor cardiac and respiratory status.
- Administer supplemental oxygen and monitor its effects.
- Monitor oxygen saturation and arterial blood gas (ABG) levels.
- Prepare for endotracheal intubation as indicated.
- Monitor vital signs continuously.
- Perform hemodynamic and cardiac monitoring.
- Administer fluid replacement and blood component therapy.
- Obtain serial hemoglobin level and hematocrit.
- Monitor input and output closely; assess all losses from the GI tract.
- Assist with balloon tamponade, as necessary, and maintain pressure; monitor for vomiting and respiratory distress closely.
- Prepare for surgery as necessary.
- Provide emotional support.
- Administer sclerosing agents or vasopressin.

- Assess the patient for the extent of blood loss.
- Ensure a patent airway and assess breathing and circulation.
- Monitor cardiac and respiratory status.
- Prepare the patient for surgery to insert a portosystemic shunt to decrease portal hypertension.
- Administer supplemental oxygen and monitor its effects.
- Monitor oxygen saturation and ABG levels.
- Prepare for endotracheal intubation as indicated
- Monitor vital signs continuously.
- Perform hemodynamic and cardiac monitoring.
- Administer fluid replacement and blood component therapy.
- Obtain serial hemoglobin level and hematocrit.
- Monitor input and output; assess all losses from the GI tract.

■ Hepatic encephalopathy may occur from ammonia toxicity.

■ Hepatorenal syndrome results from advanced liver disease and subsequent renal failure.

Integumentary system

■ Abnormal pigmentation, spider nevi, palmar erythema, and jaundice are related to impaired hepatic function.

■ Severe pruritus develops secondary to jaundice from bilirubinemia.

■ Extreme dryness and poor tissue turgor are related to malnutrition.

Neurologic system

■ Progressive signs or symptoms of hepatic encephalopathy, including lethargy, mental changes, slurred speech, asterixis, peripheral neuritis, paranoia, hallucinations, extreme obtundation, and coma may be secondary to urea conversion and consequent delivery of toxic ammonia to the brain.

Respiratory system

■ Pleural effusion and limited thoracic expansion occur because of abdominal ascites.

■ Interference with efficient gas exchange causes hypoxia.

ASSESSMENT

In addition to signs and symptoms of cirrhosis, examination may reveal related complications, such as portal hypertension and esophageal varices.

Clinical findings

- Anorexia from distaste for certain foods
- Nausea and vomiting from inflammatory response and systemic effects of liver inflammation
- Diarrhea from malabsorption
- Dull abdominal ache from liver inflammation
- Muscle cramps
- Fatigue
- Weight loss
- Abdominal pain
- Auscultation of pleural rub in pleural effusion
- Ascites
- Altered mentation
- Bleeding
- Gynecomastia
- Testicular atrophy
- Loss of chest and axillary hair
- Extremely dry skin
- Poor skin turgor
- Spider nevi
- Palmar erythema
- Jaundice
- Hepatomegaly
- Musty breath
- Enlarged superficial abdominal veins
- Hemorrhoids

Diagnostic test results

- *Liver biopsy* reveals tissue destruction and fibrosis.
- *Abdominal X-ray* shows enlarged liver, cysts, or gas within the biliary tract or liver; liver calcification; and massive fluid accumulation (ascites).
- *Computed tomography* and *liver scans* show liver size, abnormal masses, and hepatic blood flow and obstruction.
- *Esophagogastroduodenoscopy* reveals bleeding esophageal varices, stomach irritation or ulceration, and duodenal bleeding and irritation.
- *Blood studies* reveal elevated liver enzyme, total serum bilirubin, and indirect bilirubin levels; decreased total serum albumin and protein levels; prolonged prothrombin time; decreased hemoglobin level, hema-

tocrit, and serum electrolytes; and deficiency of vitamins A, C, and K.

- *Urine studies* show increased bilirubin and urobilirubinogen level.
- *Fecal studies* show decreased fecal urobilirubinogen level.

COLLABORATIVE MANAGEMENT

Respiratory therapy is needed for airway and ventilation maintenance, especially if the patient is experiencing problems such as impaired gag reflex, aspiration, or difficulty with respirations because of ascites. Nutritional therapy is crucial in providing a high-calorie, protein-restricted, and possibly sodium-restricted diet (enteral or parenteral nutritional therapy may be necessary). Physical therapy may be required to maintain joint function while the patient is on strict bed rest.

TREATMENT AND CARE

- The patient and his family may benefit from referrals for supportive counseling and social services.
- Aldosterone agonists, such as spironolactone, may be administered to reduce ascites.

Cushing's syndrome

Cushing's syndrome is a cluster of clinical abnormalities caused by excessive adrenocortical hormones, particularly cortisol, or related corticosteroids and, to a lesser extent, androgens and aldosterone. Cushing's disease (pituitary corticotropin excess) accounts for about 80% of endogenous cases of Cushing's syndrome. Cushing's disease occurs most commonly between ages 20 and 40 and is three to eight times more common in females. The annual incidence of endogenous cortisol excess in the United States is two to four cases per one million people per year.

ETIOLOGY

Causes of Cushing's syndrome include:

- anterior pituitary hormone excess
- autonomous, ectopic corticotropin secretion by a tumor outside the pituitary — usually a malignant, oat-cell carcinoma of the lung

■ excessive or prolonged use of glucocorticoids.

PATHOPHYSIOLOGY

Cushing's syndrome can be exogenous, resulting from excessive or prolonged glucocorticoid use, or endogenous, resulting from increased cortisol or corticotropin secretion. Cortisol excess results in anti-inflammatory effects and excess catabolism of protein and peripheral fat to support hepatic glucose production. The mechanism that triggers the secretion may be corticotropin dependent (elevated plasma corticotropin levels stimulate the adrenal cortex to produce excess cortisol), or corticotropin independent (excess cortisol is produced by the adrenal cortex or exogenously administered). Excess cortisol suppresses the hypothalamic-pituitary-adrenal axis.

Cardiovascular system

■ Sodium and secondary fluid retention leads to hypertension, possibly leading to heart failure and left ventricular hypertrophy.
■ Capillary weakness may occur from protein loss, leading to bleeding and ecchymosis.

Endocrine system

■ Diabetes mellitus develops because of cortisol-induced insulin resistance and increased gluconeogenesis in the liver. (See *Disorders affecting management of Cushing's syndrome,* pages 102 to 105.)

Gastrointestinal system

■ Peptic ulcer may occur because of an increase in gastric secretions and pepsin production and a decrease in gastric mucus.

Immunologic system

■ The patient's susceptibility to infection is increased as a result of decreased lymphocyte production and suppressed antibody formation. Resistance to stress is decreased.

Integumentary system

■ Decreased collagen and weakened tissues result in integumentary changes, such as increased body hair, purple striae, acne, facial plethora, and poor wound healing.

Musculoskeletal system

■ Muscle weakness caused by hypokalemia or loss of muscle mass from increased catabolism may occur.
■ Pathologic fractures may occur because of decreased bone mineral ionization, osteopenia, osteoporosis, and skeletal growth retardation in children.

Neurologic system

■ The patient may have insomnia as a result of cortisol's role in neurotransmission.

Renal and urologic systems

■ Fluid retention occurs secondary to sodium restriction.
■ Potassium excretion increases.
■ Ureteral calculi result from increased bone demineralization associated with hypercalciuria.

ASSESSMENT

Signs and symptoms depend on the degree and duration of hypercortisolism, the presence or absence of androgen excess, and the additional tumor-related effects of adrenal carcinoma or ectopic corticotropin syndrome.

Clinical findings

■ Complaints of muscle weakness, irritability, emotional lability ranging from euphoric behavior to depression or psychosis
■ History of susceptibility to infection
■ Possible diabetes mellitus
■ Purple striae; facial plethora (edema and blood vessel distention); acne; fat pads above the clavicles, over the upper back (buffalo hump), on the face (moon facies), and throughout the trunk (truncal obesity) with slender arms and legs
■ Little or no scar formation, poor wound-healing, ecchymosis, hyperpigmentation, fungal skin infections
■ Hypertension
■ Edema
■ Increased androgen production with clitoral hypertrophy, mild virilism, hirsutism, and amenorrhea or oligomenorrhea in women; sexual dysfunction; impotence

Diagnostic test results

■ *Blood glucose levels* may reveal hyperglycemia.

(Text continues on page 104.)

DISORDERS AFFECTING MANAGEMENT OF CUSHING'S SYNDROME

This chart highlights disorders that affect the management of Cushing's syndrome.

DISORDER	SIGNS AND SYMPTOMS	DIAGNOSTIC TEST RESULTS
Diabetes mellitus (coexisting)	◆ Weight loss despite voracious hunger ◆ Weakness ◆ Vision changes ◆ Frequent skin and urinary tract infections ◆ Dry, itchy skin ◆ Poor skin turgor ◆ Dry mucous membranes ◆ Dehydration ◆ Decreased peripheral pulses ◆ Cool skin temperature ◆ Decreased reflexes ◆ Orthostatic hypotension ◆ Muscle wasting ◆ Loss of subcutaneous fat ◆ Fruity breath odor because of keto-acidosis	◆ Fasting plasma glucose is 126 mg/dl or greater on at least two occasions; a random blood glucose level is 200 mg/dl or greater. ◆ Blood glucose level is 200 mg/dl or greater 2 hours after ingesting 75 grams of oral dextrose. ◆ Ophthalmologic examination may show diabetic retinopathy.
Hypertension (coexisting)	◆ Usually asymptomatic ◆ Elevated blood pressure readings on at least two consecutive occasions ◆ Occipital headache ◆ Epistaxis ◆ Bruits ◆ Dizziness ◆ Confusion ◆ Fatigue ◆ Blurry vision ◆ Nocturia ◆ Edema	◆ Serial blood pressure measurements reveal elevations of 140/90 mm Hg or greater on two or more separate occasions. ◆ Urinalysis may show protein, casts, red blood cells or white blood cells (WBCs). ◆ Blood urea nitrogen and serum creatinine levels are elevated. ◆ Complete blood count may reveal polycythemia or anemia. ◆ Excretory urography may reveal renal atrophy. ◆ Electrocardiography may show left ventricular hypertrophy or ischemia. ◆ Chest X-rays may show cardiomegaly. ◆ Echocardiography may reveal left ventricular hypertrophy.
Peptic ulcer (coexisting)	◆ Recent loss of weight or appetite ◆ Anorexia ◆ Feeling of fullness or distention ◆ Pain may be worsened by eating or may be relieved by it ◆ Sharp, burning or gnawing, epigastric pain ◆ Hyperactive bowel sounds ◆ Possible epigastric tenderness in the midline and midway between the umbilicus and the xiphoid process ◆ Anemic pallor	◆ Barium swallow or upper GI and small-bowel series may reveal the presence of the ulcer. ◆ Upper GI endoscopy or esophagogastroduodenoscopy confirms the presence of an ulcer and permits cytologic studies and biopsy to rule out *Helicobacter pylori* or cancer. ◆ Upper GI tract X-rays reveal mucosal abnormalities. ◆ Laboratory analysis may disclose occult blood in stools. ◆ Immunoglobin A anti-H. pylori test on a venous blood sample can be used to detect antibodies to *H. pylori*.

TREATMENT AND CARE

◆ Check blood glucose levels periodically because steroid replacement may necessitate adjustment of the insulin dosage.
◆ Keep a late-morning snack available in case the patient becomes hypoglycemic.
◆ Keep accurate records of vital signs, weight, fluid intake, urine output, and calorie intake.
◆ Monitor serum glucose and urine acetone levels.
◆ Monitor for acute complications of diabetic therapy, especially hypoglycemia (vagueness, slow cerebration, dizziness, weakness, pallor, tachycardia, diaphoresis, seizures, and coma); immediately give carbohydrates in the form of fruit juice, hard candy, honey or, if the patient is unconscious, glucagon or I.V. dextrose.
◆ Be alert for signs of hyperosmolar coma (polyuria, thirst, neurologic abnormalities, and stupor). This hyperglycemic crisis requires I.V. fluids and insulin replacement.
◆ Monitor the patient for the effects of diabetes on the cardiovascular system (such as cerebrovascular, coronary artery, and peripheral vascular impairment) and on the peripheral and autonomic nervous systems.
◆ Provide meticulous skin care, especially to the feet and legs. Treat all injuries, cuts, and blisters.
◆ Administer insulin replacement or oral antidiabetics.
◆ Observe for signs of urinary tract and vaginal infections.
◆ Encourage adequate fluid intake.

◆ Monitor blood pressure, response to antihypertensive medication, and laboratory studies.
◆ Maintain a reduced-sodium diet.
◆ Monitor for complications of hypertension, such as signs of stroke or myocardial infarction.
◆ Administer thiazide diuretics, angiotensin-converting enzyme inhibitors, angiotensin receptor blockers, or calcium channel blockers.

◆ Support the patient emotionally and offer reassurance.
◆ Administer antacids, antimicrobials, misoprostol, anticholinergics, histamine-2-blockers, or proton gastric pump inhibitors, and monitor the patient for the desired effects. Also watch for adverse reactions. Most medications should alleviate the patient's discomfort, so ask whether his pain is relieved.
◆ Provide six small meals or small hourly meals as ordered. Advise the patient to eat slowly, chew thoroughly, and have small snacks between meals.
◆ Schedule the patient's care so that he can get plenty of rest.

(continued)

DISORDERS AFFECTING
MANAGEMENT OF CUSHING'S SYNDROME *(continued)*

DISORDER	SIGNS AND SYMPTOMS	DIAGNOSTIC TEST RESULTS
Peptic ulcer *(continued)*		◆ Serologic testing may disclose clinical signs of infection such as an elevated WBC count. ◆ Gastric secretory studies show hyperchlorhydria. ◆ Carbon 13 urea breath test results reflect activity of *H. pylori.*
Urinary calculi (complication)	◆ Pain that travels from the costovertebral angle to the flank and then to the suprapubic region and external genitalia (classic renal colic pain) ◆ Constant, dull pain and possible back pain (if calculi are in the renal pelvis and calyces) ◆ Severe abdominal pain ◆ Nausea and vomiting ◆ Fever and chills ◆ Hematuria ◆ Abdominal distention ◆ Anuria (rare)	◆ Kidney-ureter-bladder radiography reveals most renal calculi. ◆ Excretory urography helps confirm the diagnosis and determine the size and location of calculi. ◆ Kidney ultrasonography detects obstructive changes. ◆ Urine culture of a midstream specimen may indicate pyuria, a sign of urinary tract infection. ◆ A 24-hour urine collection reveals evaluated calcium oxalate, phosphorus, and uric acid excretion levels. ◆ Calculus analysis shows mineral content.

■ *Serum electrolyte levels* may show hypernatremia and hypokalemia.

■ *Arterial blood gas analysis* may reveal metabolic alkalosis.

■ *Urinary free cortisol levels* are more than 150 µg/24 hours.

■ *Dexamethasone suppression test* determines the cause.

■ *Computed tomography (CT)* scan and *magnetic resonance imaging* of the head may identify pituitary tumors.

■ *Blood studies* detect levels of corticotropin-releasing hormone, corticotropin, and different glucocorticoids to diagnose and localize cause to pituitary or adrenal gland.

■ *Ultrasound, CT,* or *angiography* may show location of adrenal tumors.

COLLABORATIVE MANAGEMENT

As other body systems become involved, the patient may need the assistance of a cardiologist, nephrologist, and endocrinologist. Nutritional consults and reproductive specialists may also be needed to assist the patient.

TREATMENT AND CARE

Treatment to restore hormone imbalance and reverse Cushing's syndrome may include:

■ radiation

■ drug therapy (aminoglutethimide and ketoconazole or aminoglutethimide alone or in combination with metyrapone in metastatic adrenal carcinoma)

◆ To aid diagnosis, maintain a 24- to 48-hour record of urine pH using nitrazine pH paper. Strain all urine through gauze or a tea strainer, and save all solid material recovered for analysis.
◆ To facilitate spontaneous passage of calculi, encourage the patient to walk, if possible. Also force fluids to maintain a urine output of 3 to 4 L/day (urine should be very dilute and colorless).
◆ If the patient can't drink the required amount of fluid, give supplemental I.V. fluids.
◆ Record intake and output and daily weight to assess fluid status and renal function.
◆ Medicate the patient generously for pain when he's passing a calculus.
◆ To help acidify urine, offer fruit juices, especially cranberry juice.

If the patient had calculi surgically removed
◆ Anticipate that the patient will have an indwelling catheter or a nephrostomy tube.
◆ Unless one of his kidneys was removed, expect bloody drainage from the catheter.
◆ Never irrigate the catheter without a physician's order.
◆ Check dressings regularly for bloody drainage, and know how much drainage to expect.
◆ Immediately report excessive drainage or a rising pulse rate, which are symptoms of hemorrhage.
◆ Use sterile technique when changing dressings or providing catheter care.
◆ Watch for signs of infection, such as a rising temperature or chills.
◆ Administer antibiotics, meperidine, morphine, antimicrobials or allopurinol.

■ surgery (partial or complete hypophysectomy, or bilateral adrenalectomy).

Cystic fibrosis

Cystic fibrosis involves dysfunction of the exocrine glands, which affects multiple organ systems. The disease affects males as well as females, and is the most common fatal genetic disease in White children. Accompanied by many complications, it carries an average life expectancy of only 32 years. The disease is characterized by chronic airway infection, leading to bronchiectasis, bronchiolectasis, exocrine pancreatic insufficiency, intestinal dysfunction, abnormal sweat gland function, and reproductive dysfunction. (See *Disorders affecting management of cystic fibrosis*, pages 106 to 109.)

The incidence of cystic fibrosis varies with ethnic origin. It occurs in one of 2,000 births in whites of North America and northern European descent, one in 17,000 births in Blacks, and one in 90,000 births in the Asian population in Hawaii.

ETIOLOGY
The responsible gene is on chromosome 7q; it encodes a membrane-associated protein called the *cystic fibrosis transmembrane regulator (CFTR)*. The exact function of CFTR

(Text continues on page 110.)

DISORDERS AFFECTING
MANAGEMENT OF CYSTIC FIBROSIS

This chart highlights disorders that affect the management of cystic fibrosis.

DISORDER	SIGNS AND SYMPTOMS	DIAGNOSTIC TEST RESULTS
Acute respiratory failure (complication)	◆ Changes in respiratory rate (may be increased, decreased, or normal depending on the cause) ◆ Cyanosis ◆ Crackles ◆ Rhonchi ◆ Wheezing ◆ Diminished breath sounds ◆ Restlessness ◆ Confusion ◆ Loss of concentration ◆ Irritability ◆ Coma ◆ Tachycardia ◆ Increased cardiac output ◆ Elevated blood pressure ◆ Arrhythmias	◆ Arterial blood gas (ABG) analysis indicates respiratory failure by deteriorating values and a pH below 7.35. ◆ Chest X-rays identify pulmonary disease. ◆ Electrocardiogram (ECG) may show ventricular arrhythmias or right ventricular hypertrophy. ◆ Pulse oximetry reveals decreasing arterial oxygen saturation. ◆ White blood cell count detects underlying infection.
Diabetes mellitus (complication)	◆ Weight loss despite voracious hunger ◆ Weakness ◆ Vision changes ◆ Frequent skin and urinary tract infections ◆ Dry, itchy skin ◆ Poor skin turgor ◆ Dry mucous membranes ◆ Dehydration ◆ Decreased peripheral pulses ◆ Cool skin ◆ Decreased reflexes ◆ Orthostatic hypotension ◆ Muscle wasting ◆ Loss of subcutaneous fat ◆ Fruity breath odor because of ketoacidosis	◆ Two-hour postprandial blood glucose is 200 mg/dl or greater. ◆ Fasting blood glucose is 126 mg/dl or higher after at least an 8-hour fast.
Heart failure (complication)	*Left-sided heart failure* ◆ Dyspnea ◆ Orthopnea ◆ Paroxysmal nocturnal dyspnea ◆ Fatigue ◆ Nonproductive cough ◆ Crackles ◆ Hemoptysis ◆ Tachycardia ◆ Third (S_3) and fourth (S_4) heart sounds ◆ Cool, pale skin ◆ Restlessness ◆ Confusion	◆ Chest X-rays may show pulmonary vascular markings, interstitial edema, or pleural effusion and cardiomegaly. ◆ ECG may indicate hypertrophy, ischemic changes, or infarction, and may reveal tachycardia and extrasystoles. ◆ Liver function tests are abnormal. ◆ Blood urea nitrogen (BUN) creatinine levels are elevated. ◆ Prothrombin time is prolonged. ◆ Brain natriuretic peptide assay may be elevated. ◆ Echocardiography may reveal left ventricular hypertrophy, dilation, and abnormal contractility.

TREATMENT AND CARE

- ◆ Monitor the patient for effects of oxygen therapy.
- ◆ Maintain a patent airway; prepare for endotracheal intubation if indicated.
- ◆ In the intubated patient, suction as needed after hyperoxygenation. Observe for change in quantity, consistency, and color of sputum. Provide humidification to liquefy secretions.
- ◆ Observe closely for respiratory arrest.
- ◆ Auscultate for chest sounds.
- ◆ Provide high-frequency ventilation.
- ◆ Monitor ABG levels and report changes immediately.
- ◆ Monitor serum electrolyte levels and correct imbalances.
- ◆ Monitor fluid balance by recording intake and output or daily weight.
- ◆ Check cardiac monitor for arrhythmias.
- ◆ Administer antibiotics, corticosteroids, bronchodilators, vasopressors, and diuretics.

- ◆ Monitor the patient's blood glucose level because beta-adrenergic blockers can cause hyperglycemia.
- ◆ Watch for signs of diabetic neuropathy (numbness or pain in the hands and feet, footdrop, impotence, neurogenic bladder).
- ◆ Watch for signs of infection (increased temperature), signs of cardiac distress (chest pain, palpitations, dyspnea, confusion), changes in vision, peripheral numbness or tingling, constipation, anorexia, and blisters or skin openings (particularly on the feet).
- ◆ Monitor serum potassium levels when administering diuretics because thiazide and loop diuretics promote potassium excretion.
- ◆ Monitor intake and output and watch for signs of dehydration.
- ◆ Review with the patient foods that are high and low in sodium and potassium.
- ◆ Administer oral antidiabetics and injectable insulin.

- ◆ Place patient in Fowler's position and give supplemental oxygen.
- ◆ Administer angiotensin-converting inhibitors, digoxin, diuretics, beta-adrenergic blockers, inotropic agents, nesiritide, nitrates, and morphine.
- ◆ Weigh the patient daily.
- ◆ Check for peripheral edema.
- ◆ Monitor intake and output, vital signs, and mental status.
- ◆ Auscultate for S_3 and crackles or rhonchi.
- ◆ Monitor BUN; creatinine; and serum potassium, sodium, chloride, and magnesium levels.
- ◆ Institute continuous cardiac monitoring to identify and treat arrhythmias promptly.

(continued)

DISORDERS AFFECTING
MANAGEMENT OF CYSTIC FIBROSIS *(continued)*

DISORDER	SIGNS AND SYMPTOMS	DIAGNOSTIC TEST RESULTS
Heart failure *(continued)*	*Right-sided heart failure* ◆ Jugular vein distention ◆ Positive hepatojugular reflux ◆ Right-upper-quadrant pain ◆ Anorexia, nausea ◆ Nocturia ◆ Weight gain ◆ Edema ◆ Ascites or anasarca	◆ Pulmonary artery pressure, pulmonary artery wedge pressure, and left ventricular end-diastolic pressure are elevated in the presence of left-sided heart failure; right atrial or central venous pressure is elevated in right-sided heart failure. ◆ Radionuclide ventriculography may reveal ejection fraction less than 40% in diastolic dysfunction.
Liver failure (complication)	◆ Ascites ◆ Shortness of breath ◆ Right-upper-quadrant tenderness ◆ Jaundice ◆ Nausea and anorexia ◆ Fatigue and weight loss ◆ Pruritus ◆ Oliguria ◆ Splenomegaly ◆ Peripheral edema ◆ Varices ◆ Weight loss	◆ Liver function studies reveal elevated aspartate aminotransferase, alanine aminotransferase, alkaline phosphatase, and bilirubin levels. ◆ Blood studies reveal anemia, impaired red blood cell production, elevated bleeding and clotting times, low blood glucose levels, and increased serum ammonia levels. ◆ Urine osmolarity is increased. ◆ Liver scan may show filling defects.
Malnutrition (complication)	◆ Generalized malnutrition ◆ Diarrhea ◆ Steatorrhea ◆ Flatulence and abdominal discomfort ◆ Nocturia ◆ Weakness and fatigue ◆ Edema ◆ Amenorrhea ◆ Anemia ◆ Glossitis ◆ Peripheral neuropathy ◆ Bruising ◆ Bone pain ◆ Skeletal deformities ◆ Fractures ◆ Tetany ◆ Paresthesias	◆ Stool specimen for fat reveals excretion of greater than 6 g of fat per day. ◆ D-xylose absorption test shows less than 20% of 25 g of D-xylose in the urine after 5 hours. ◆ Schilling test reveals deficiency of vitamin B_{12} absorption. ◆ Culture of duodenal and jejunal contents confirms bacterial overgrowth in the proximal bowel. ◆ GI barium studies show characteristic features of the small intestine. ◆ Small intestine biopsy reveals atrophy of the mucosal villi.

TREATMENT AND CARE

- Provide meals low in protein and high in carbohydrate
- Auscultate lung sounds for crackles, rhonchi, or stridor. Observe for any signs of airway obstruction including labored breathing, severe hoarseness, and dyspnea.
- Administer supplemental humidified oxygen.
- Monitor oxygen saturation with continuous pulse oximetry and serial ABG studies for evidence of hypoxemia.
- Anticipate the need for endotracheal intubation and mechanical ventilation should the patient's respiratory status deteriorate.
- Monitor ABG levels for increasing partial pressure of arterial carbon dioxide and decreasing pH. These suggest respiratory acidosis.
- Administer I.V. fluid therapy. Obtain laboratory specimens to assess for drug, electrolytes, and glucose levels. Anticipate administering normal saline solution and vasopressors if the patient is hypotensive, or dextrose 5% in water if the patient is hypoglycemic.
- Maintain salt restriction, and administer potassium-sparing diuretics if the patient has ascites.
- For the patient who has a history of chronic alcohol abuse, use of dextrose solutions may precipitate Wernicke-Korsakoff syndrome, a thiamine deficiency with severe neurologic impairment.
- Place the patient in semi-Fowler's position to maximize chest expansion. Keep the patient as quiet and comfortable as possible to minimize oxygen demands.
- Monitor for encephalopathy; lactulose may provide palliative treatment.

- Observe nutritional status and progress with daily calorie counts and weight checks.
- Evaluate the patient's tolerance to foods.
- Assess fluid status; record intake and output and the number of stools.
- Administer dietary supplements and vitamins.
- Assess for signs and symptoms of dehydration, such as dry skin and mucous membranes and poor skin turgor.
- Check serum electrolyte levels, and monitor coagulation studies.
- Assist with nutritional therapy, such as peripheral parenteral nutrition or total parenteral nutrition, and monitor for effects.

remains unknown, but it appears to help regulate chloride and sodium transport across epithelial membranes. Causes of cystic fibrosis include abnormal coding found on as many as 350 CFTR alleles as well as autosomal recessive inheritance.

PATHOPHYSIOLOGY

Most cases arise from the mutation that affects the genetic coding for a single amino acid, causing CFTR to malfunction. CFTR resembles other transmembrane transport proteins, but it lacks the phenylalanine that's present in the protein produced by normal genes. This regulator interferes with cyclic adenosine monophosphate–regulated chloride channels and transport of other ions by preventing adenosine triphosphate from binding to the protein or by interfering with activation by protein kinase.

The mutation affects volume-absorbing epithelia (in the airways and intestines), salt-absorbing epithelia (in sweat ducts), and volume-secretory epithelia (in the pancreas). Lack of phenylalanine leads to dehydration and, ultimately, to glandular duct obstruction.

Respiratory system
■ Thick secretions and dehydration occur as a result of ionic imbalance.
■ Chronic airway infections by *Staphylococcus aureus, Pseudomonas aeruginosa,* and *Pseudomonas cepacia* may develop, possibly due to abnormal airway surface fluids and failure of lung defenses.
■ Accumulation of thick secretions in the bronchioles and alveoli results in dyspnea.
■ Stimulation of the secretion-removal reflex produces a paroxysmal cough.
■ Barrel chest, cyanosis, and clubbing of fingers and toes result from chronic hypoxia.
■ Obstructed glandular ducts occur leading to peribronchial thickening; this obstruction is due to increased viscosity of bronchial, pancreatic, and other mucous gland secretions.

Cardiovascular system
■ Fatal shock and arrhythmias may result from hyponatremia and hypochloremia from sodium lost in sweat.
■ Pulmonary hypertension can result in cardiac dysfunction in adult cystic fibrosis patients with severe lung disease.

■ Pulmonary hypertension and cor pulmonale in cystic fibrosis are thought to be related to progressive destruction of the lung parenchyma and pulmonary vasculature and to pulmonary vasoconstriction secondary to hypoxemia.

Endocrine system
■ Retention of bicarbonate and water due to the absence of CFTR chloride channel in the pancreatic ductile epithelia limits membrane function and leads to retention of pancreatic enzymes, chronic cholecystitis and cholelithiasis, and the ultimate destruction of the pancreas.
■ Diabetes, pancreatitis, and hepatic failure can develop because of the disease's effects on the intestines, pancreas, and liver.

Gastrointestinal system
■ Obstruction of the small and large intestines results from inhibited secretion of chloride and water and excessive absorption of liquid.
■ Biliary cirrhosis occurs because of retention of biliary secretions.
■ Malnutrition and malabsorption of fat-soluble vitamins (A, D, E, and K) are caused by deficiencies of trypsin, amylase, and lipase from obstructed pancreatic ducts, preventing the conversion and absorption of fat and protein in the intestinal tract.

Genitourinary system
■ In males, a bilateral congenital absence of the vas deferens is accompanied by a lack of sperm in the semen.
■ In females, secondary amenorrhea and increased mucus in the reproductive tracts block the passage of ova.

ASSESSMENT

In addition to the typical signs and symptoms, patients with cystic fibrosis may have a history of airway infections or pneumonia.

Clinical findings
■ Thick respiratory secretions
■ Coughing
■ Abdominal pain or discomfort
■ Reproductive problems
■ Crackles and wheezes due to constricted airways
■ Clubbing of fingers and toes
■ Barrel chest

- Salty-tasting skin
- Greasy, foul-smelling stools (steatorrhea)
- Cyanosis
- Arrhythmias
- Failure to thrive (poor weight gain, poor growth, distended abdomen, thin extremities, and sallow skin with poor turgor due to malabsorption)
- Clotting problems, retarded bone growth, and delayed sexual development due to deficiency of fat-soluble vitamins
- Rectal prolapse in infants and children due to malnutrition and wasting of perirectal supporting tissues
- Esophageal varices due to cirrhosis and portal hypertension

Diagnostic test results
The Cystic Fibrosis Foundation has developed certain criteria for a definitive diagnosis:
- Two *sweat tests* using a pilocarpine solution (a sweat inducer) detect elevated sodium chloride levels; these elevated levels occur along with an obstructive pulmonary disease, confirmed pancreatic insufficiency or failure to thrive, or a family history of cystic fibrosis.
- *Chest X-ray* indicates early signs of obstructive lung disease.
- *Stool specimen analysis* indicates the absence of trypsin, suggesting pancreatic insufficiency.

These tests may also support diagnosis:
- *Deoxyribonucleic acid testing* locates the presence of the Delta F 508 deletion, allowing for prenatal diagnosis.
- *Pulmonary function tests* reveal decreased vital capacity, elevated residual volume due to air entrapments, and decreased forced expiratory volume in 1 second. This test is used if pulmonary exacerbation already exists.
- *Liver enzyme tests* may reveal hepatic insufficiency.
- *Sputum culture* reveals organisms that cystic fibrosis patients typically and chronically colonize, such as *Staphylococcus* and *Pseudomonas*.
- *Serum albumin* measurements help assess nutritional status.
- *Electrolyte analysis* assesses hydration.

COLLABORATIVE MANAGEMENT
Pulmonary specialists and respiratory therapists assist with clearing airway secretions and maintain a patent airway. An endocrinologist may assist with managing diabetes as well as other pancreatic and reproductive disorders. Nutritional specialists may be consulted to help with dietary measures (such as providing high-calorie meals that includes the appropriate level of salt needed) and fluid therapy. Physical and occupational therapists may be needed to help with activity management and energy conservation.

TREATMENT AND CARE
The goal of treatment is to help the child live as normal a life as possible. The type of treatment depends on the organ system involved and may include:
- hypertonic radiocontrast materials delivered by enema to treat acute obstructions caused by meconium ileus
- breathing exercises, postural drainage, and chest percussion to clear pulmonary secretions
- antibiotics to treat lung infection (guided by sputum culture results)
- bronchodilators to increase mucus clearance
- inhaled beta-adrenergic agonists to control airway constriction
- pancreatic enzymes replacements to maintain adequate nutrition
- sodium-channel blockers to decrease sodium reabsorption from secretions and improve viscosity
- uridine triphosphate to stimulate chloride secretion by a non-CFTR
- salt supplements to replace electrolytes lost through sweat
- Dornase alpha (genetically engineered pulmonary enzyme) to help liquefy mucus
- recombinant alpha-anti-trypsin to counteract excessive proteolytic activity produced during airway inflammation
- gene therapy to introduce normal CFTR into affected epithelial cells
- heart and lung transplantation in severe organ failure.

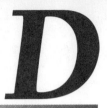

Decompression sickness

Decompression sickness (DCS) involves a complex process called *dysbarism,* which results from changed barometric pressure. Pressure increases as depth under the water increases, such as that experienced in free or assisted dives. This increased pressure affects the gases dissolved in the blood and areas of the body that have hollow spaces and viscous organs. The incidence of DCS ranges from four per 100,000 to 15.4 per 100,000 and can be life-threatening.

DCS may be classified as type I (mild), type II (serious), or as one that results in embolization.

ETIOLOGY
DCS results from ascending from a dive faster than the body can compensate for the pressures (nitrogen bubbles form in the blood, causing symptoms).

Inadequate decompression, surpassing no-decompression limits, increased depth and duration of dives, and repeated dives may predispose the patient to this condition. Failure to take recommended safety stops during a dive may also result in DCS. Other factors include obesity, fatigue, age, poor physical condition, dehydration, illness affecting lung or circulatory efficiency, and previous musculoskeletal injury (scar tissue decreases diffusion). Predisposing environmental factors include cold water (vasoconstriction decreases nitrogen offloading), heavy work (which produces a vacuum effect in which tendon use causes gas pockets), rough sea conditions, and heated diving suits (which can lead to dehydration).

PATHOPHYSIOLOGY
The reduction in pressure that occurs during a too-rapid ascent at the end of a dive can release dissolved gases (in particular, nitrogen) from the tissues and blood. This gas release forms bubbles in the body, which impact organ systems. Indeed, these bubbles can cause loss of cell function, mechanical compression, and stretching of the blood vessels and nerves. These bubbles may also activate the blood coagulation system, releasing vasoactive substances, and act as emboli by blocking circulation.

Cardiovascular system
- Fluid shifts from the intravascular to extravascular spaces resulting in tachycardia and postural hypotension.
- Thrombi may form from activation of blood coagulation and release of vasoactive substances from cells lining the blood vessels
- Bubble formation may result in mechanical stretching, damage and blockage of blood flow from embolization, or activation of the complement and coagulation pathways, resulting in a thrombus.
- Coronary artery embolization of gas bubbles can lead to myocardial infarction or arrhythmia.

Neurologic system
- As the person descends deeper into water, nitrogen increasingly dissolves in the blood and, at higher partial pressures, it alters the electrical properties of cerebral cellular membranes. This causes an anesthetic effect (nitrogen narcosis).
- Every 50′ (15.2 m) of depth is equal to the effects of one drink of alcohol. At 150′ (46 m), divers can experience alterations in reasoning, memory, response time, and problems such as idea fixation, overconfidence, and calculation errors.

■ Cerebral embolization of gas bubbles can result in stroke or seizures.

Respiratory system

■ Descending deeply into water increases the amount of dissolved oxygen. Oxygen toxicity can occur within 30 to 60 minutes of breathing 100% oxygen at 2 atmospheres (33′ [10 m]).

■ With increasing water depth, nitrogen gas bubbles equilibrates from the alveoli into the blood. Over time, more nitrogen dissolves in the lipid part of tissues and accumulates.

■ As the person ascends, lag occurs before saturated tissues release nitrogen back into the blood. Ascending too quickly causes dissolved nitrogen to return to a gaseous state while still in the blood or tissues, causing bubbles to form.

■ Bubbles in the tissues cause local tissue dysfunction; if located in the blood, embolization results.

■ Pulmonary overpressurization can cause large gas emboli to lodge in coronary, cerebral, and other systemic arterioles. These gas bubbles continue to expand as ascending pressure decreases.

ASSESSMENT

Symptoms occur within 10 to 20 minutes after resurfacing. Multiple systems may be involved. Headache, dizziness, and profound anxiousness may occur initially; more dramatic symptoms include unresponsiveness, shock, and seizures.

No specific diagnostic tests exist for DCS; however, hyperbaric oxygen therapy may be useful in differential diagnosis.

Clinical findings
Type I DCS
■ Mild pains resolving within 10 minutes of onset (niggles)
■ Pruritus (skin bends)
■ Skin rash (mottling or marbling of the skin, or a papular or plaquelike rash)
■ Orange-peel skin (rarely)
■ Pitting edema
■ Anorexia
■ Excessive fatigue
■ Dull, deep, throbbing, toothache-type pain in a joint, tendon, or tissue (the bends)

Type II DCS
■ Symptoms mimicking spinal cord trauma (low back pain progressing to paresis, paralysis, paresthesia, loss of sphincter control, girdle pain, or lower trunk pain)
■ Headaches or vision disturbances
■ Dizziness
■ Tunnel vision
■ Changes in mental status
■ Nausea, vomiting, vertigo, nystagmus, tinnitus, and partial deafness
■ Burning substernal discomfort on inspiration, nonproductive coughing that can become paroxysmal, and severe respiratory distress
■ Hypovolemic shock
■ Arterial gas embolization
■ Signs and symptoms dependent on where the gas emboli travel, such as myocardial infarction, stroke, and seizures (see *Disorders affecting management of decompression sickness,* pages 114 and 115.)

Diagnostic test results
■ *Laboratory studies,* including blood glucose, electrolytes, oxygen saturation, ethanol level, and carboxyhemoglobin, can help determine the cause of mental status changes or shock.

■ *Chest X-ray* may identify injuries to lungs and chest and show evidence of pneumothorax, pneumomediastinum, subcutaneous emphysema, pneumocranium, alveolar hemorrhage, and decreased pulmonary blood flow.

■ *Magnetic resonance imaging* may reveal spinal lesions or localize DCS injury.

■ *Electrocardiography* determines cardiac status and identifies possible cardiac arrhythmias.

COLLABORATIVE MANAGEMENT

Prehospital care involves assistance from advanced life support personnel and extrication teams to get the patient to the nearest emergency department that has a hyperbaric facility as soon as possible. If local support isn't available, The Divers Alert Network (DAN) (919-684-8111) is an organization that maintains a database of diving-related injuries. Consultation services are available as well as assistance with appropriate treatment of the patient (similar to that in poison control centers).

DISORDERS AFFECTING MANAGEMENT OF DECOMPRESSION SICKNESS

This chart highlights disorders that affect the management of decompression sickness.

DISORDER	SIGNS AND SYMPTOMS	DIAGNOSTIC TEST RESULTS
Avascular necrosis (complication)	◆ Pain of extremity ◆ Decreased circulation distally ◆ Edema ◆ Warmth to site	◆ X-rays, computed tomography (CT) scan, and magnetic resonance imaging (MRI) may help differentiate diagnosis of avascular necrosis.
Intravascular volume depletion (complication)	◆ Shock (tachycardia, tachypnea, hypotension, decreased urine output)	◆ Elevated potassium, serum lactate, and blood urea nitrogen levels may be present in hypovolemic shock. ◆ Urine specific gravity is greater than 1.020; urine osmolality is increased. ◆ Blood pH and partial pressure of arterial oxygen is decreased; partial pressure of arterial carbon dioxide is increased.
Massive venous air embolism (complication)	◆ If in an extremity: Decreased peripheral circulation, pain, discoloration ◆ If pulmonary or cardiac: Shortness of breath, chest pain, tachycardia, tachypnea, respiratory distress ◆ If in cerebral circulation: Signs of stroke (change in mental status, facial drooping, weakness of one side of the body)	◆ Chest X-ray, CT scan, MRI may show evidence of air embolism. ◆ Arterial blood gas analysis may show decreased partial pressure of oxygen, increased carbon dioxide level, and respiratory acidosis.
Vascular occlusion (complication)	*Peripheral occlusion* ◆ Pain ◆ Pulselessness ◆ Pallor ◆ Paresthesias to extremity *Cardiac occlusion* ◆ Signs of myocardial infarction (chest pain, diaphoresis, shortness of breath) *Neurologic occlusion* ◆ Signs of stroke (change in mental status, facial drooping, weakness on one side of the body)	◆ Cardiac enzymes may reveal elevated CK-MB and troponin levels. ◆ A venogram may detect the specific site of occlusion.

TREATMENT AND CARE

■ Treatment consists of recompression and oxygen administration, followed by gradual decompression. In recompression, which takes place in a hyperbaric chamber, air pressure is increased to 2.8 absolute atmospheric pressure over 1 to 2 minutes. This rapid rise in pressure reduces the size of the circulating nitrogen bubbles and relieves pain and other clinical effects.

■ During recompression, intermittent oxygen administration with periodic maximal exhalations, promotes gas bubble diffusion.

■ Administer fluid replacement in hypovolemic shock.

■ Administer corticosteroids to reduce the risk of spinal edema.

    RED FLAG *Don't administer opioids because they further depress the respiratory system.*

TREATMENT AND CARE

◆ Monitor extremities for adequate circulation, but handle extremity gently to avoid further trauma.
◆ Prepare the patient for surgery to alleviate condition.
◆ Monitor effects of antibiotics; also monitor for sepsis.

◆ Ensure a patent airway and adequate circulation. Begin cardiopulmonary resuscitation (CPR).
◆ Monitor for signs of shock (tachycardia, hypotension, decreased pulmonary artery and central venous pressures, decreased urine output).
◆ Maintain I.V. therapy, and monitor effect of fluid bolus.
◆ Monitor electrolyte status and effects of electrolyte replacements.
◆ If the patient is awake and alert, rehydrate orally.
◆ Administer oxygen and monitor pulse oximetry.

◆ Ensure a patent airway and adequate circulation. Begin CPR.
◆ Monitor for respiratory distress (dyspnea, shortness of breath, decreasing oxygen saturations).
◆ Monitor for signs of cardiovascular collapse (hypotension, tachycardia, diaphoresis, diminished pulse).
◆ Administer oxygen and monitor the patient closely for its effects.
◆ Monitor the patient's neurologic status.
◆ Maintain patency of I.V. lines

◆ Monitor for signs of myocardial infarction, arrythmias, stroke, and peripheral vascular occlusion.
◆ Maintain patency of I.V. lines.
◆ Monitor intake and output.
◆ Administer antiarrhythmics and monitor the patient for their effects.
◆ Monitor the patient for changes in pulses and peripheral circulation.
◆ Administer oxygen and monitor pulse oximetry.
◆ Monitor effects of thrombolytics.

■ To avoid oxygen toxicity during recompression, advise the patient to alternate breathing oxygen for 5 minutes with breathing air for 5 minutes.

Diabetes mellitus

Diabetes mellitus is a metabolic disorder characterized by hyperglycemia (elevated serum glucose level) resulting from lack of insulin, lack of insulin effect, or both. Three general classifications are recognized:
■ type 1, absolute insulin insufficiency

(*Text continues on page 118.*)

DISORDERS AFFECTING
MANAGEMENT OF DIABETES MELLITUS

This chart highlights disorders that affect the management of diabetes mellitus.

DISORDER	SIGNS AND SYMPTOMS	DIAGNOSTIC TEST RESULTS
Coronary artery disease (complication)	◆ Angina or feeling of burning, squeezing, or tightness in the chest that may radiate to the left arm, neck jaw, or shoulder blade ◆ Nausea and vomiting ◆ Cool extremities and pallor ◆ Diaphoresis ◆ Xanthelasma (fat deposits on the eyelids)	◆ Electrocardiogram (ECG) may be normal between anginal episodes. During angina it may show ischemic changes (T-wave inversion, ST-segment depression, arrhythmias). ◆ Computed tomography may identify calcium deposits in coronary arteries. ◆ Stress testing may detect ST-segment changes during exercise or pharmacologic stress. ◆ Coronary angiography reveals location and degree of stenosis, obstruction, and collateral circulation. ◆ Intravascular ultrasound may define coronary anatomy and lumenal narrowing. ◆ Myocardial perfusion imaging detects ischemic areas as cold spots. ◆ Stress echocardiography shows abnormal wall motion in ischemic areas. ◆ Rest perfusion imaging rules out myocardial infarction.
Diabetic ketoacidosis (complication)	◆ Acetone breath ◆ Dehydration ◆ Weak and rapid pulse ◆ Kussmaul's respirations	◆ Blood glucose level is slightly above normal. ◆ Serum ketone level is elevated. ◆ Serum potassium is normal or elevated initially and then drops. ◆ Urine glucose is positive; urine acetone is high. ◆ Serum phosphorus, magnesium, and Chloride are decreased. ◆ Serum osmolality is slightly elevated, ranging from 300 to 350 mOsm/L. ◆ Hematocrit is slightly elevated. ◆ Arterial blood gas (ABG) analysis reveals metabolic acidosis. ◆ ECG shows arrhythmias.
Hyperosmolar hyperglycemic nonketotic syndrome (complication)	◆ Polyuria ◆ Thirst ◆ Neurologic abnormalities ◆ Stupor	◆ Blood glucose is markedly elevated above normal, usually greater than 800 mg/dl. ◆ Urine acetone is negative; serum ketones are negative. ◆ Urine glucose is positive. ◆ Serum osmolality is elevated, usually above 350 mOsm/L. ◆ Serum electrolyte levels reveal hypokalemia, hypophosphatemia, hypomagnesemia, and hypochloremia. ◆ Serum creatinine and blood urea nitrogen (BUN) are elevated. ◆ Hematocrit is slightly elevated.
Hypertension (complication)	◆ Usually asymptomatic ◆ Elevated blood pressure readings on at least two consecutive occasions ◆ Occipital headache ◆ Epistaxis	◆ Serial blood pressure measurements reveal elevations of 140/90 mm Hg or greater on two or more separate occasions. ◆ Urinalysis may show protein, casts, red blood cells, or white blood cells. ◆ BUN and serum creatinine are elevated. ◆ Complete blood count may reveal polycythemia or anemia.

Treatment and care

◆ During anginal attacks, monitor the patient's blood pressure and heart rate. Obtain an ECG during the episode and before administering nitroglycerin or other nitrates. Record duration of pain, amount of medication required to relieve it, and accompanying symptoms.

◆ Keep nitroglycerine available for immediate use. Instruct the patient to call immediately whenever he feels chest, arm, or neck pain.

◆ Before cardiac catheterization, explain the procedure and reinforce learning of the procedure.

◆ After catheterization, review recommended treatment. Check distal pulses, and monitor catheter site for bleeding. To counter diuretic effect of the dye, make sure the patient drinks plenty of fluids. Assess potassium levels.

◆ If the patient is scheduled for surgery, explain the procedure and reinforce learning.

◆ Administer nitrates, beta-adrenergic blockers, calcium channel blockers, antiplatelets, antilipemics, and antihypertensives.

◆ After surgery, monitor blood pressure, intake and output, breath sounds, chest tube drainage, and ECG. Monitor for arrhythmias. Give vigorous chest physiotherapy.

◆ Before discharge, stress the need to follow the prescribed drug regimen, exercise program, and diet.

◆ Assess level of consciousness (LOC) and maintain airway patency.

◆ Monitor vital signs at least every 15 minutes initially and then hourly as indicated; monitor hemodynamic status.

◆ Institute continuous cardiac monitoring and treat arrhythmias.

◆ Administer I.V. replacement therapy with normal saline to correct fluid deficit; dextrose may be added to prevent hypoglycemia.

◆ Administer regular insulin I.V. as ordered; monitor blood glucose levels and serum electrolyte levels frequently.

◆ Anticipate potassium replacement after insulin therapy is initiated; replace electrolytes as needed.

◆ If the patient is comatose, obtunded, or vomiting; insert a nasogastric (NG) tube to suction.

◆ Monitor the patient for signs of complications, such as infection, diabetic neuropathy, and hypoglycemia.

◆ Perform teaching regarding treatment regimen for diabetes; enlist the assistance of a diabetes educator and nutritionist as needed.

◆ Assess LOC and maintain a patent airway.

◆ Monitor vital signs at least every 15 minutes initially and then hourly as indicated; monitor hemodynamic status.

◆ Institute continuous cardiac monitoring and treat arrhythmias.

◆ Administer I.V. replacement therapy with isotonic or 0.45% saline to correct fluid deficit.

◆ Administer regular insulin I.V.; monitor blood glucose levels and serum electrolyte levels frequently.

◆ Replace electrolytes as necessary according to laboratory studies.

◆ If the patient is comatose, obtunded, or vomiting; insert an NG tube to suction.

◆ Assess peripheral circulation.

◆ Perform range-of-motion every 2 hours; use intermittent pneumatic sequential compression devices.

◆ Assess for hypoglycemia, diabetic neuropathy, or signs of infection.

◆ Consult a dietitian to plan a recommended diet; enlist assistance of a diabetes educator.

◆ Monitor blood pressure, the patient's response to antihypertensive medications, and laboratory studies.

◆ Encourage a reduced-sodium diet.

◆ Monitor for complications of hypertension, such as signs of stroke or myocardial infarction and renal disease.

◆ Administer thiazide diuretics, angiotensin-converting enzyme inhibitors, angiotensin receptor blockers, beta-adrenergic blockers, and calcium channel blockers.

(continued)

DISORDERS AFFECTING
MANAGEMENT OF DIABETES MELLITUS *(continued)*

DISORDER	SIGNS AND SYMPTOMS	DIAGNOSTIC TEST RESULTS
Hypertension *(continued)*	◆ Bruits ◆ Dizziness, confusion, fatigue ◆ Blurry vision ◆ Nocturia ◆ Edema	◆ Excretory urography may reveal renal atrophy. ◆ ECG may show left ventricular hypertrophy or ischemia. ◆ Chest X-rays may show cardiomegaly. ◆ Echocardiography may reveal left ventricular hypertrophy.
Hypoglycemia (complication)	◆ Decreased LOC ◆ Shakiness ◆ Sweating ◆ Numbness and tingling of extremities ◆ Hunger ◆ Irritability, anxiety	◆ Blood glucose level is less than normal.
Pneumonia (complication)	◆ Coughing, sputum production ◆ Pleuritic chest pain ◆ Shaking chills and fever ◆ Possible crackles	◆ Chest X-ray shows infiltrates. ◆ Sputum smear shows acute inflammatory cells. ◆ Positive blood cultures in patients with infiltrates suggest sepsis. ◆ Transtracheal aspirate of secretions or bronchoscopy are positive for organisms.
Retinopathy (complication)	◆ Progressive blindness or loss of vision	◆ Indirect ophthalmoscopy shows retinal changes, such as microaneurysms, retinal hemorrhages, edema, venous dilation exudates, and vitreous hemorrhage. ◆ Fluorescein angiography shows leakage of fluorescein from new blood vessels and differentiates between microaneurysms and true hemorrhages. ◆ History reveals long-standing diabetes and decreased vision.
Wound infection (complication)	◆ Wound that doesn't heal properly ◆ Foul discharge and inflammation at wound site ◆ Fever	◆ Culture confirms wound infection.

■ type 2, insulin resistance with varying degrees of insulin secretory defects
■ gestational diabetes, which emerges during pregnancy.

Onset of type 1 (insulin-dependent) diabetes usually occurs before age 30, although it may occur at any age. The patient is usually thin and requires exogenous insulin and dietary management to achieve control.

Conversely, type 2 (non-insulin-dependent) diabetes usually occurs in obese adults after age 40 and is treated with diet and exercise in combination with various oral antidiabetic drugs, although treatment may include insulin therapy. (See *Disorders affecting management of diabetes mellitus,* pages 116 to 119.)

- Monitor blood glucose level.
- Administer dextrose 50% I.V. if the patient is unable to eat or drink.
- Give the patient juice and carbohydrates (such as crackers) if the patient is awake and alert.
- Assess for the cause of hypoglycemia (such as extreme exercise, taking antidiabetic medication without eating, or illness).

- Maintain a patent airway and adequate oxygenation. Measure ABG levels.
- Teach the patient to deep breathe and cough effectively.
- Assist with endotracheal intubation or tracheostomy as necessary; suction to remove secretions.
- Obtain sputum specimens as directed and monitor for results; administer antibiotics as needed and record the patient's response to treatment.
- Maintain hydration and treat fever; fluid and electrolyte replacement may be necessary.
- Maintain adequate nutrition; supplemental oral feedings or parenteral nutrition may be needed; monitor intake and output.
- Dispose of secretions properly.
- Administer appropriate antibiotics.

- Carefully control blood glucose levels, and monitor levels closely.
- If the patient complains of sudden, unilateral vision loss, arrange for immediate ophthalmologic evaluation.
- Monitor blood pressure.
- Encourage the patient to comply with the prescribed regimen for treating diabetes.
- Assist with laser photocoagulation, which cauterizes the leaking blood vessels and eliminates the cause of the edema, as needed.

- Administer appropriate antibiotics and monitor the patient for their effects.
- Maintain hydration and treat fever; fluid and electrolyte replacement may be necessary.
- Maintain adequate nutrition; supplemental oral feedings or parenteral nutrition may be needed; monitor intake and output.
- Perform dressing changes, and look for signs of healing; debridement may be necessary.

ETIOLOGY

Evidence indicates that diabetes mellitus has diverse causes, including heredity, environment (infection, diet, toxins, stress), lifestyle changes in genetically susceptible persons, and pregnancy.

PATHOPHYSIOLOGY

In persons genetically susceptible to type 1 diabetes, a triggering event, possibly a viral infection, causes production of autoantibodies against the beta cells of the pancreas. The resultant destruction of the beta cells leads to a decline in and ultimate lack of insulin secretion. Insulin deficiency leads to hyperglycemia, enhanced lipolysis (decomposition of fat), and protein catabolism. These characteristics occur when more than 90% of the beta cells have been destroyed.

Type 2 diabetes mellitus is a chronic disease caused by one or more of the following factors: impaired insulin secretion, inappropriate hepatic glucose production, or peripheral insulin receptor insensitivity. Genetic factors are significant, and onset is accelerated by obesity and a sedentary lifestyle. Stress can also be a pivotal factor.

Gestational diabetes mellitus occurs when a woman not previously diagnosed with diabetes shows glucose intolerance during pregnancy. This may occur if placental hormones counteract insulin, causing insulin resistance. Gestational diabetes mellitus is a significant risk factor for the future occurrence of type 2 diabetes mellitus.

Cardiovascular system
■ Arterial thrombosis may develop due to persistent activated thrombogenic pathways and impaired fibrinolysis.

Gastrointestinal system
■ Autonomic neuropathy leads to abdominal discomfort and pain, causing gastroparesis and constipation.
■ Nausea, diarrhea, or constipation may develop due to dehydration, electrolyte imbalances, or autonomic neuropathy.

Metabolic system
■ Impaired or absent insulin function prevents normal metabolism of carbohydrates, fats, and proteins, leading to weight loss.
■ Muscle cramps, irritability, and emotional lability result from electrolyte imbalances.

Neurologic system
■ Low intracellular glucose levels may result in headaches, fatigue, lethargy, reduced energy levels, and impaired school and work performance.
■ Vision changes, such as blurring, occur due to glucose-induced swelling.
■ Numbness and tingling occur due to neural tissue damage.

Renal system
■ Polyuria and polydipsia occur because of high serum osmolality caused by high serum glucose levels.

ASSESSMENT
Type 1 diabetes usually presents rapidly, typically with polydipsia, polyuria, polyphagia, weakness, weight loss, dry skin, and ketoacidosis. Type 2 diabetes is typically slow and insidious in onset and is usually unaccompanied by symptoms.

Clinical findings
■ Asymptomatic (possibly) in type 1
■ Anorexia, nausea, vomiting
■ Headache
■ Fatigue
■ Lethargy
■ Visual changes
■ Numbness and tingling
■ Diarrhea or constipation
■ Abdominal pain
■ Slow healing of skin infections or wounds
■ Itchy skin
■ Recurrent monilial infections of the vagina or anus
■ Signs of dehydration (dry mucous membranes, poor skin turgor, hypovolemia, shock, decreased peripheral pulses)
■ Weight loss in type 1 with muscle wasting; possible weight gain in type 2
■ Skin ulcerations
■ Fruity breath odor

Diagnostic test results
In adult men and nonpregnant women, diabetes mellitus is diagnosed with two of the following criteria obtained more than 24 hours apart, using the same test twice or a combination of tests:
■ fasting plasma glucose level of more than 100 mg/dl on at least two occasions
■ blood glucose level of greater than or equal to 200 mg/dl 2 hours after ingesting 75 g of oral dextrose.

Diagnosis may also be based on:
■ diabetic retinopathy on ophthalmologic examination
■ other diagnostic and monitoring tests, including urinalysis for acetone and glycosylated hemoglobin (reflects glycemic control over the past 2 to 3 months).

COLLABORATIVE MANAGEMENT
The patient may be managed by an endocrinologist to help control blood glucose levels, rehydrate, and restore electrolyte and acid-base balance. Depending on the severity of

the symptoms, the patient may require a pulmonologist to assist with ventilatory support. Nutritional therapy is indicated to assist with dietary needs. A diabetes educator can be valuable in helping the patient learn about his disease and how to manage it. Social services may assist with identifying financial and community resources and with arranging follow-up care.

TREATMENT AND CARE

Effective treatment of all types of diabetes optimizes blood glucose control and decreases complications. Treatment for type 1 diabetes mellitus includes:

■ insulin replacement, meal planning, and exercise (current forms of insulin replacement include mixed-dose, split mixed-dose, and multiple daily injection regimens, and continuous subcutaneous insulin infusions)

■ pancreas transplantation (currently requires chronic immunosuppression).

Treatment of type 2 diabetes mellitus includes:

■ oral antidiabetic drugs to stimulate endogenous insulin production, increase insulin sensitivity at the cellular level, suppress hepatic gluconeogenesis, and delay GI absorption of carbohydrates (drug combinations may be used).

Treatment of both types of diabetes mellitus includes:

■ careful monitoring of blood glucose levels

■ individualized meal plan designed to meet nutritional needs, control blood glucose and lipid levels, and reach and maintain appropriate body weight (plan to be followed consistently with meals eaten at regular times)

■ weight reduction (obese patient with type 2 diabetes mellitus) or high-calorie allotment, depending on growth stage and activity level (type 1 diabetes mellitus).

Drug overdose

Drug overdose, also referred to as *drug poisoning,* most commonly involves overdose of prescription or over-the-counter medications.

ETIOLOGY

Overdose usually results from ingestion of a drug through inhalation, injection, or direct absorption through the skin and mucous membranes.

PATHOPHYSIOLOGY

The effects of drug overdose depend on:

■ type of substance ingested

■ amount of substance ingested

■ patient's tolerance to the toxin

■ number of toxins ingested

■ time between ingestion and treatment.

Changes produced by a drug overdose commonly result from an exaggeration of the drug's normal therapeutic and adverse effects. For example, when one or more drugs are ingested, the effects may be synergistic or antagonistic. Synergistic effects occur when a drug combination produces a response that is greater than the response that would occur if the drugs were taken alone. Antagonistic effects occur when the combined response of a drug combination is less than the response produced by either drug alone.

Some toxins, such as acetaminophen and ethylene glycol, have organ-specific toxic effects. (See *Understanding specific drug toxicities,* pages 122 and 123 and *Disorders affecting management of a drug overdose,* pages 124 and 125.)

Cardiovascular system

■ Hypotension and arrhythmias occur after ingestion of beta-adrenergic blockers and calcium channel blockers.

Nervous system

■ Depressed level of consciousness typically occurs after ingestion of sedatives and opioids.

Respiratory system

■ Hypoventilation typically occurs after ingestion of sedatives and opioids.

ASSESSMENT

Assessment of the patient experiencing a drug overdose must include a simultaneous history, assessment of airway, breathing, and circulation (ABCs), and initiation of life support (as indicated). The patient may be alert and able to respond to questions, or may be agitated, delirious, or obtunded and unre-

UNDERSTANDING SPECIFIC DRUG TOXICITIES

Acetaminophen

Acetaminophen, the active ingredient in many over-the-counter analgesics and antipyretics, is the most commonly reported pharmaceutical ingestion in adults and children. The drug is rapidly absorbed and metabolized in the liver. Normally, a small amount of acetaminophen (less than 5%) is metabolized to a toxic intermediate metabolite, N-acetyl-para-benzoquinoneimine (NAPQI), which is further metabolized by glutathione to nontoxic products.

NAPQI is a powerful oxidizing agent that leads to cell death by bonding to cellular proteins. After an acute single toxic dose (7.5 g in an adult), the glutathione is used up and can't regenerate fast enough to detoxify all of the intermediate metabolite. Consequently, NAPQI builds up, causing liver damage. Evidence of liver damage may not be apparent until 24 to 36 hours after ingestion.

Alcohols

All alcohols, including ethanol, ethylene glycol, methanol, and isopropanol, are rapidly absorbed from the GI tract and metabolized by the liver enzyme alcohol dehydrogenase. Isopropanol and methanol also are easily absorbed through the skin and mucous membranes and can result in toxicity. Ethylene glycol and methanol are the most toxic alcohols. Ethylene glycol commonly is found in antifreeze and cleaning solutions; methanol is found in windshield washer fluid and solvents. Both are minimally toxic before metabolism, but in addition to their inebriating effects, have specific organ toxicity once metabolized. Both alcohols are metabolized in the liver, and blood levels above 20 mg/dl are considered toxic for both.

Metabolism of ethylene glycol produces glycolaldehyde, glycolic acid, glyoxylic acid, and oxalic acid. Symptoms result from the direct effects of these toxins and progress through three stages. Symptoms in stage I (first 12 hours) include altered mental status, seizures, and severe anion-gap metabolic acidosis. Cardiac toxicity occurs in stage II (12 to 36 hours). Stage III, renal failure, the hallmark of ethylene glycol toxicity, occurs at 36 to 48 hours.

Metabolism of methanol produces formaldehyde and formic acid. Folic acid is required for further metabolism to nontoxic products. Symptoms of methanol toxicity appear 12 to 24 hours after ingestion and result primarily from the effects of formic acid. Formic acid damages the optic nerve. Hemorrhages also have been found in a portion of the basal ganglia called the *putamen*. Symptoms include severe anion-gap metabolic acidosis caused by acid production, hypotension, visual changes that can progress to blindness, coma, and sudden respiratory arrest.

---

sponsive. (See *Assessing drug overdose,* pages 126 and 127.)

The patient's history—whether it's from the patient or significant others—should reveal the substance involved, the form of exposure (ingestion, inhalation, injection, or skin contact), and when exposure occurred.

Clinical findings
■ Dilated pupils
■ Tremors or seizures
■ Possible coma or posturing neurologically
■ Rapid respirations, Kussmaul's respirations, or no respirations
■ Cardiac arrest
■ Diaphoretic, pink-tinged, or cyanotic skin
■ Dry mouth, diarrhea, nausea, vomiting, or hematemesis

Diagnostic test results
■ *Toxicologic studies* of the mouth, vomitus, urine, stool, blood, or the victim's hands or clothing confirm the diagnosis.
■ *Drug screens* identify the toxin and amount. If possible, have the family or patient bring the container of the ingested substance to the facility for a comparable study.
■ *Abdominal X-rays* may reveal iron pills or other radiopaque substances such as calcium, enteric-coated aspirin, and phenothiazine.
■ *Arterial blood gas levels* aid in ruling out hypoxia, hypercapnia, and metabolic acido-

Cocaine

Cocaine blocks the reuptake of norepinephrine, epinephrine, and dopamine, causing excesses at the postsynaptic receptor sites. This leads to central and peripheral adrenergic stimulation and to a generalized vasoconstriction that affects multiple organs. These effects may include hypertension, hyperthermia, tachycardia, excited delirium, and seizures. Hyperthermia can cause rhabdomyolysis and later renal failure. Direct effects on the heart include increased myocardial oxygen consumption, coronary artery spasm, ischemia, myocardial infarction, depressed myocardial contractility, acute heart failure, sudden death from arrhythmias, and dilated cardiomyopathy. Recent studies have shown that cocaine increases platelet aggregation and thrombus formation. I.V. drug users are also at risk for endocarditis.

Cyclic antidepressants

Cyclic antidepressants are responsible for almost half of all overdose-related adult admissions to critical care units and are the leading cause of overdose-related deaths in emergency departments. Cyclic drugs include the older tricyclics, such as amitriptyline and nortriptyline, and such newer agents as maprotiline (Ludiomil). These drugs are rapidly absorbed from the GI tract, although absorption may be delayed in large overdoses because of anticholinergic adverse effects. They're metabolized in the liver.

In an overdose, the enzymes responsible for metabolism become saturated, and some of the drug and its metabolites are secreted into the bile and gastric fluid to be reabsorbed later. Toxicity results from central and peripheral blockage of norepinephrine reuptake, anticholinergic effects, and quinidine-like effects on the heart. Central nervous system (CNS) effects may include initial agitation followed rapidly by lethargy, coma, and seizures. Anticholinergic effects include tachycardia, mydriasis, dry and flushed skin, hypoactive bowel sounds, and urine retention. Cardiovascular effects include hypotension, arrhythmias, and quinidine-like changes on the electrocardiogram with widening of the QRS complex.

Organophosphates and carbamates

Organophosphates and carbamates are commonly found in pesticides and account for 80% of pesticide-related hospital admissions. They are highly lipid-soluble and easily absorbed through skin and mucous membranes. The primary mechanism of toxicity is cholinesterase inhibition, which leads to excess acetylcholine at muscarinic, nicotinic, and CNS receptors. The effects of excessive acetylcholine include increased salivation and lacrimation, muscle fasciculations and weakness, constricted pupils, decreased level of consciousness, and seizures. Bradycardia is typically present, but tachycardia has also been reported.

sis as the cause of the patient's altered level of consciousness.

■ *Blood glucose level* aids in ruling out hypoglycemia as the cause of the patient's altered level of consciousness.

■ *Electrocardiography* reveals ischemia, arrhythmias, and widened QRS complexes associated with cyclic antidepressant therapy.

■ *Serum electrolyte levels* reveal high anion gap (associated with methanol, ethylene glycol, iron, and salicylate toxicity); low anion gap (associated with lithium toxicity); hyperkalemia (associated with ethylene glycol and methanol toxicity); hypokalemia (associated with loop diuretics and salicylate toxicity); and hypocalcemia (associated with ethylene glycol toxicity).

■ *Complete blood count* may reveal leukocytosis secondary to ethylene glycol toxicity.

■ *Coagulation studies* may reveal prolonged coagulation times suggesting warfarin toxicity.

COLLABORATIVE MANAGEMENT

Cardiac, renal, neurologic, and hepatic specialists may be consulted depending on the organs affected by the drug overdose. Respiratory therapy may be involved to assist with maintaining ventilation and perfusion. Renal specialists may be needed to assist with dialysis to remove the drug. Social services and psychological specialists may be needed to assist with coping mechanisms and provide therapy if it's determined that the ingestion

(*Text continues on page 128.*)

WATCHFUL EYE

DISORDERS AFFECTING MANAGEMENT OF A DRUG OVERDOSE

This chart highlights disorders that affect the management of a drug overdose.

DISORDER	SIGNS AND SYMPTOMS	DIAGNOSTIC TEST RESULTS
Arrhythmias (complication)	◆ May be asymptomatic ◆ Dizziness, hypotension, syncope ◆ Weakness ◆ Cool, clammy skin ◆ Altered level of consciousness ◆ Reduced urine output ◆ Shortness of breath ◆ Chest pain	◆ Electrocardiography (ECG) detects arrhythmias and ischemia and infarction that may result in arrhythmias. ◆ Laboratory testing may reveal electrolyte abnormalities, acid-base abnormalities, or drug toxicities that may cause arrhythmias. ◆ Holter monitoring, event monitoring, and loop recording can detect arrhythmias and effectiveness of drug therapy during a patient's daily activities. ◆ Exercise testing may detect exercise-induced arrhythmias. ◆ Electrophysiologic testing identifies the mechanism of an arrhythmia and the location of accessory pathways; it also assesses the effectiveness of antiarrhythmic drugs, radiofrequency ablation, and implanted cardioverter-defibrillators.
Liver failure (complication)	◆ Ascites, shortness of breath ◆ Right-upper-quadrant tenderness ◆ Jaundice ◆ Nausea and anorexia ◆ Fatigue and weight loss ◆ Pruritus ◆ Oliguria ◆ Splenomegaly ◆ Peripheral edema ◆ Varices ◆ Bleeding tendencies ◆ Petechia ◆ Amenorrhea ◆ Gynecomastia	◆ Liver function studies reveal elevated levels of aspartate aminotransferase, alanine aminotransferase, alkaline phosphatase, and bilirubin. ◆ Blood studies reveal anemia, impaired red blood cell production, elevated bleeding and clotting times, low blood glucose levels, and increased serum ammonia levels. ◆ Urine osmolarity is increased. ◆ Liver scan may show filling defects.
Renal failure (complication)	◆ Initially, oliguria ◆ Metabolic acidosis ◆ Nausea, vomiting ◆ Dry mucous membranes ◆ Headache ◆ Confusion ◆ Seizures ◆ Drowsiness ◆ Irritability ◆ Dry, pruretic skin ◆ Uremic breath odor ◆ Hypotension (early) ◆ Hypertension with arrhythmias (later) ◆ Systemic edema ◆ Pulmonary edema ◆ Kussmaul's respirations ◆ Tachycardia ◆ Bibasilar crackles ◆ Altered LOC	◆ Blood urea nitrogen, serum creatinine, and potassium levels are elevated. ◆ Bicarbonate level, hematocrit, hemoglobin, and pH are decreased. ◆ Urine studies show casts, cellular debris, decreased specific gravity; in glomerular diseases, proteinuria and urine osmolality close to serum osmolality are present; urine sodium level is less than 20 mEq/L if oliguria results from decreased perfusion, and more than 40 mEq/L if the cause is intrarenal. ◆ Creatinine clearance test measures glomerular filtration rate and reflects the number of remaining functioning nephrons. ◆ ECG shows tall, peaked T waves; widening QRS; and disappearing P waves if hyperkalemia is present. ◆ Ultrasonography, abdominal and kidney-ureter-bladder X-rays, excretory urography, renal scan, retrograde pyelography, computerized tomography, and nephrotomography reveal abnormalities of the urinary tract.

TREATMENT AND CARE

◆ When life-threatening arrhythmias develop, rapidly assess level of consciousness (LOC), respirations, and pulse rate.
◆ Initiate cardiopulmonary resuscitation if indicated.
◆ Evaluate cardiac output resulting from arrhythmias.
◆ If the patient develops heart block, prepare for cardiac pacing.
◆ Administer antiarrhythmic agents as ordered, and prepare to assist with medical procedures if indicated.
◆ Assess intake and output every hour; insert an indwelling urinary catheter, as indicated, to ensure accurate urine measurement.
◆ Document arrhythmias in a monitored patient and assess for possible causes and effects.
◆ If the patient's pulse is abnormally rapid, slow, or irregular, watch for signs of hypoperfusion, such as hypotension and diminished urine output.
◆ Monitor the patient for predisposing factors, such as fluid and electrolyte imbalance, or possible drug toxicity.

◆ Auscultate lung sounds for crackles, rhonchi, or stridor. Observe for signs of airway obstruction including labored breathing, severe hoarseness, and dyspnea.
◆ Administer supplemental humidified oxygen.
◆ Administer lactulose, potassium-sparing diuretics, and potassium supplements.
◆ Monitor oxygen saturation for evidence of hypoxemia with continous pulse oximetry and serial arterial blood gas (ABG) studies. Anticipate the need for endotracheal intubation and mechanical ventilation if patient's respiratory status deteriorates.
◆ Monitor ABGs for increasing partial pressure of arterial carbon dioxide and decreasing pH (respiratory acidosis).
◆ Administer I.V. fluid therapy. Obtain laboratory specimens to assess for drug, electrolytes, and glucose levels. Anticipate administering normal saline solution and vasopressors if the patient is hypotensive; administering dextrose 5% in water if the patient is hypoglycemic.
◆ For the patient who has a history of chronic alcohol abuse, use of dextrose solutions may precipitate Wernicke-Korsakoff syndrome, a thiamine deficiency with severe neurologic impairment.
◆ Place the patient in semi-Fowler's position to maximize chest expansion. Keep the patient as quiet and comfortable as possible to minimize oxygen demands.
◆ Monitor for encephalopathy; lactulose may provide palliative treatment.

◆ Administer hypertonic glucose, insulin, diuretics, and sodium bicarbonate.
◆ Measure intake and output, including body fluids, nasogastric output, and diarrhea. Weigh the patient daily.
◆ Measure hemoglobin and hematocrit; replace blood components.
◆ Monitor vital signs; check and report for signs of pericarditis (pleuritic chest pain, tachycardia, pericardial friction rub), inadequate renal perfusion (hypotension), and acidosis.
◆ Maintain proper electrolyte balance. Monitor potassium levels and monitor for hyperkalemia (malaise, anorexia, paresthesia or muscle weakness), and ECG changes.
◆ If patient receives hypertonic glucose and insulin infusions, monitor potassium and glucose levels. If giving sodium polystyrene sulfonate rectally, make sure patient doesn't retain it and become constipated to prevent bowel perforation.
◆ Maintain nutritional status with a high-calorie, low-protein, low-sodium, low-potassium diet and vitamin supplements.
◆ Monitor the patient carefully during peritoneal dialysis.
◆ If patient requires hemodialysis, monitor vascular access site carefully and assess patient and laboratory studies carefully.

ASSESSING DRUG OVERDOSE

DRUG	ASSESSMENT FINDINGS	DRUG	ASSESSMENT FINDINGS
Acetaminophen	◆ Plasma levels greater than 300 mcg/ml 4 hours after ingestion; 50 mcg/ml 12 hours after ingestion (suggestive of hepatoxicity) ◆ Nausea, vomiting, diaphoresis, and anorexia 12 to 24 hours after ingestion ◆ Cyanosis ◆ Anemia ◆ Jaundice ◆ Skin eruptions ◆ Fever ◆ Emesis ◆ Delirium ◆ Methemoglobinemia progressing to CNS depression, coma, vascular collapse, seizures, and death	Anticoagulants	◆ Hematuria ◆ Internal or external bleeding ◆ Skin necrosis
		Antihistamines	◆ Drowsiness ◆ Moderate anticholinergic symptoms (selected histamine-1 antagonists) ◆ Respiratory depression ◆ Seizures ◆ Coma
		Barbiturates	◆ Areflexia ◆ Confusion ◆ Pulmonary edema ◆ Respiratory depression ◆ Slurred speech ◆ Sustained nystagmus ◆ Somnolence ◆ Unsteady gait ◆ Coma
Amphetamines, cocaine	◆ Abdominal cramps ◆ Aggressiveness ◆ Arrhythmias ◆ Confusion ◆ Diarrhea ◆ Fatigue ◆ Hallucinations ◆ Hyperreflexia ◆ Nausea, vomiting ◆ Restlessness ◆ Seizures ◆ Tachypnea ◆ Tremor ◆ Coma ◆ Death	Benzodiazepines	◆ Bradycardia ◆ Confusion ◆ Dyspnea ◆ Hypoactive reflexes ◆ Hypotension ◆ Impaired coordination ◆ Labored breathing ◆ Slurred speech ◆ Somnolence
Anticholinergics	◆ Blurred vision ◆ Decreased or absent bowel sounds ◆ Dilated, nonreactive pupils ◆ Dry mucous membranes ◆ Dysphagia ◆ Flushed, hot, dry skin ◆ Hypertension ◆ Hyperthermia ◆ Increased respiratory rate ◆ Tachycardia ◆ Urine retention	Central nervous system (CNS) depressants	◆ Absent pupillary reflexes ◆ Apnea ◆ Dilated pupils ◆ Hypotension ◆ Hypothermia followed by fever ◆ Inadequate ventilation ◆ Loss of deep tendon reflexes ◆ Tonic muscle spasms ◆ Coma

Assessing drug overdose *(continued)*

Drug	Assessment findings	Drug	Assessment findings
Iron supplements	◆ GI irritation with epigastric pain, nausea, vomiting ◆ Diarrhea (initially green, then tarry, then progressing to melena) ◆ Hematemesis ◆ Metabolic acidosis ◆ Hepatic dysfunction ◆ Renal failure ◆ Bleeding diathesis ◆ Circulatory failure ◆ Coma ◆ Death	Salicylates	◆ Hyperpnea ◆ Metabolic acidosis ◆ Respiratory alkalosis ◆ Tachypnea
Nonsteroidal anti-inflammatory drugs	◆ Abdominal pain ◆ Apnea ◆ Cyanosis ◆ Dizziness ◆ Drowsiness ◆ Headache ◆ Nausea, vomiting ◆ Nystagmus ◆ Paresthesia ◆ Sweating	Tricyclic antidepressants	◆ CNS stimulation (first 12 hours after ingestion) – Agitation – Confusion – Constipation, ileus – Dry mucous membranes – Hallucinations – Hyperthermia – Irritation – Parkinsonism – Pupillary dilation – Seizures – Urine retention ◆ CNS depression – Cardiac irregularities – Cyanosis – Decreased or absent reflexes – Hypotension – Hypothermia – Sedation
Opioids	◆ Respiratory depression with or without CNS depression and miosis ◆ Hypotension ◆ Bradycardia ◆ Hypothermia ◆ Shock ◆ Cardiopulmonary arrest ◆ Circulatory collapse ◆ Pulmonary edema ◆ Seizures		
Phenothiazines	◆ Abnormal involuntary muscle movements ◆ Agitation ◆ Arrhythmias ◆ Autonomic nervous system dysfunction ◆ Deep, unarousable sleep ◆ Extrapyramidal symptoms ◆ Hypotension ◆ Hypothermia or hyperthermia ◆ Seizures		

was intentional. Social services may also assist with identifying financial and community resources and with arranging follow-up
care.

TREATMENT AND CARE

Initial treatment and care includes emergency resuscitation; support for the patient's
ABCs; prevention of further absorption of
the drug; administration of an antidote, if
available; enhancement of the drug's elimination; and prevention of complications.

■ Reduce drug absorption by administering
activated charcoal, inducing emesis, and gastric lavage. Gastric lavage is only recommended for patients who have ingested a potentially lethal amount of drug or toxin and
present within 1 hour of ingestion.

■ Administer methods used to enhance the
drug's elimination which may include
cathartics, such as sorbitol, magnesium citrate, or magnesium sulfate; repeated multiple doses of activated charcoal; whole bowel
irrigation with a solution such as a balanced electrolyte solution; forced diuresis;
and dialysis.

E–F

Electric shock

When an electric current passes through the body, the damage it does depends on the current's intensity (amperes, milliamperes, or microamperes), the resistance of the tissues through which it passes, the kind of current (AC, DC, or mixed), and the frequency and duration of current flow. Electric shock may cause ventricular fibrillation, respiratory paralysis, burns, and death. The prognosis depends on the site and extent of damage, the patient's health, and the speed and adequacy of treatment. In the United States, about 1,000 people die of electric shock each year.

ETIOLOGY

Electric shock usually follows accidental contact with exposed parts of electrical appliances or wiring, but it may also result from lightning or the flash of electric arcs from high-voltage power lines or machines. The increased use of electrical medical devices in hospitals, many of which are connected directly to the patient, has raised concerns about electrical safety and has led to the development of electrical safety standards. However, even well-designed equipment with reliable safety features can cause electric shock if mishandled.

PATHOPHYSIOLOGY

Electric current can cause injury in three ways: true electrical injury as the current passes through the body, arc or flash burns from current that doesn't pass through the body, and thermal surface burns caused by associated heat and flames.

Cardiovascular system
■ If it passes through the heart, even the smallest electric current may induce ventric-

ular fibrillation (or another arrhythmia) that progresses to fibrillation or myocardial infarction. (See *Disorders affecting management of electric shock,* pages 130 and 131.)

Integumentary system
■ Electric shock from a high-frequency current (which generates more heat in tissues than a low-frequency current) usually causes burns, local tissue coagulation, and necrosis.
■ Low-frequency currents can cause serious burns if the contact with the current is concentrated in a small area (for example, if a toddler bites into an electric cord).

Musculoskeletal system
■ Cell membrane resting potential is altered, causing depolarization in muscles. Muscle tetany can occur.
■ Contusions, fractures, and other injuries can result from violent muscle contractions, falls, or being thrown during the shock.

Neurologic system
■ Cell membrane resting potential is altered, causing depolarization in nerves. Numbness, tingling, or sensorimotor deficits can occur.

Renal system
■ Electrical current causes coagulation necrosis and tissue ischemia, which liberates myoglobin and hemoglobin.
■ Myoglobin and hemoglobin can precipitate in the renal tubules, causing tubular necrosis and renal shutdown.

Respiratory system
■ Respiratory paralysis occurs because of the electric current's direct effect on the respiratory nerve center, or because of prolonged contraction of respiratory muscles.
■ After momentary shock, hyperventilation may follow initial muscle contraction.

DISORDERS AFFECTING MANAGEMENT OF ELECTRIC SHOCK

This chart highlights disorders that affect the management of electric shock.

DISORDER	SIGNS AND SYMPTOMS	DIAGNOSTIC TEST RESULTS
Atrial fibrillation (complication)	◆ Irregularly irregular pulse rhythm with normal or abnormal heart rate ◆ Radial pulse rate slower than apical pulse rate ◆ Palpable peripheral pulse with stronger contractions ◆ Evidence of decreased cardiac output, such as hypotension and light-headedness, with new-onset atrial fibrillation and a rapid ventricular rate	◆ Electrocardiography (ECG) reveals no clear P waves, irregularly irregular ventricular response, and uneven baseline fibrillatory waves; wide variation in R-R intervals results in loss of atrial kick. Atrial fibrillation may be preceded by premature atrial contractions.
Heart failure (complication)	◆ Cough that produces pink, frothy sputum ◆ Cyanosis of the lips and nail beds ◆ Pale, cool, clammy skin ◆ Diaphoresis ◆ Jugular vein distention ◆ Ascites ◆ Pulsus alternans ◆ Tachycardia ◆ Hepatomegaly ◆ Decreased pulse pressure ◆ Third (S_3) and fourth (S_4) heart sounds ◆ Moist, basilar crackles ◆ Rhonchi ◆ Expiratory wheezing ◆ Decreased pulse oximetry ◆ Peripheral edema ◆ Decreased urinary output	◆ B-type natriuretic peptide immunoassay is elevated. ◆ Chest X-ray shows increased pulmonary vascular markings, interstitial edema, or pleural effusions and cardiomegaly. ◆ ECG reveals heart enlargement or ischemia, tachycardia, extrasystole, or atrial fibrillation. ◆ Pulmonary artery pressure, pulmonary artery wedge pressure, and left ventricular end-diastolic pressure are elevated in the presence of left-sided heart failure; right atrial or central venous pressure is elevated in right-sided heart failure.

ASSESSMENT

Assessment findings vary depending on the voltage exposure.

Clinical findings

- Burns
- Local tissue coagulation
- Entrance and exit wounds
- Cyanosis
- Apnea
- Decreased blood pressure
- Cold skin
- Unconsciousness
- Numbness or tingling or sensorimotor deficits
- Contusions
- Fractures
- No palpable pulse or heart sounds (if ventricular fibrillation occurs)
- Absent respirations
- Muscle contraction followed by unconsciousness and loss of reflex control (in severe electric shock)

Diagnostic test results

- *Electrocardiography* (ECG) reveals the cardiac arrhythmia (if present).
- *Urine studies* test positive for myoglobin.
- *X-rays* reveal fractures.

TREATMENT AND CARE

◆ Interventions aim to reduce the ventricular response rate to less than 100 beats/minute, establish anticoagulation, and restore and maintain a sinus rhythm.

◆ Treatment typically includes drug therapy (calcium channel blockers, beta-adrenergic blockers, antiarrhythmics, cardiac glycosides, anticoagulants) to control the ventricular response or a combination of electrical cardioversion and drug therapy. If drug therapy is used, monitor serum drug levels and observe the patient for evidence of toxicity.

◆ If the patient is hemodynamically unstable, synchronized electrical cardioversion should be performed right away. It's most successful if done within 48 hours after atrial fibrillation starts.

◆ A transesophageal echocardiogram may be obtained before cardioversion to rule out the presence of thrombi in the atria.

◆ Tell the patient to report changes in pulse rate, dizziness, feeling faint, chest pain, and signs of heart failure, such as dyspnea and peripheral edema.

◆ If the patient isn't on a cardiac monitor, be alert for an irregular pulse and differences in the radial and apical pulse rates.

◆ Monitor the patient's peripheral and apical pulses; watch for evidence of decreased cardiac output and heart failure.

◆ Limit fluid and sodium intake to decrease preload.

◆ Monitor the patient for signs of embolization (hematuria, pleuritic chest pain, left-upper-quadrant pain).

◆ Monitor oxygenation status, auscultate lung fields, and evaluate arterial blood gas studies.

◆ Monitor urine output.

◆ Administer supplemental oxygen and mechanical ventilation.

◆ Place the patient in Fowler's position.

◆ Administer diuretics, inotropic drugs, vasodilators, angiotensin-converting enzyme inhibitors, angiotensin-receptor blockers, cardiac glycosides, beta-adrenergic blockers, and electrolyte supplements.

◆ Initiate cardiac monitoring.

◆ Recurrent heart failure from valvular dysfunction may require surgery.

◆ A ventricular assist device may be needed.

◆ Maintain adequate cardiac output and monitor hemodynamic stability.

◆ Assess for deep vein thrombosis and apply antiembolism stockings.

■ *Arterial blood gas analysis* helps determine respiratory status.

■ *Electrolyte values* show electrolyte imbalances.

■ *Blood urea nitrogen* and *creatinine levels* show kidney damage.

COLLABORATIVE MANAGEMENT

Pulmonary and cardiovascular specialists may be needed, depending on the severity of the electrical current and degree of involvement.

TREATMENT AND CARE

■ Immediate emergency treatment consists of carefully separating the victim from the current source, quickly assessing vital functions, and performing emergency measures such as cardiopulmonary resuscitation (CPR) and defibrillation.

■ To separate the victim from the current source, immediately turn it off or unplug it. If this isn't possible, pull the victim free with a nonconductive device, such as a loop of dry cloth or rubber, a dry rope, or a leather belt with the metal buckle detached.

■ Continue until vital signs return or help arrives with a defibrillator and other advanced life-support equipment. Then monitor the patient's cardiac rhythm continuously and obtain a 12-lead ECG.

■ Because internal tissue destruction may be much greater than indicated by skin damage, administer I.V. lactated Ringer's solution to maintain urine output of 50 to 100 ml/hour.

■ Insert an indwelling urinary catheter and send the first specimen to the laboratory.

■ Measure intake and output hourly and watch for tea- or port wine-colored urine, which occurs when coagulation necrosis and tissue ischemia liberate myoglobin and hemoglobin.

■ Administer mannitol and furosemide to prevent renal shutdown.

■ Administer sodium bicarbonate to counteract acidosis caused by widespread tissue destruction and anaerobic metabolism.

■ Assess the patient's neurologic status frequently because central nervous system damage may result from ischemia or demyelination. Because a spinal cord injury may follow cord ischemia or a compression fracture, watch for sensorimotor deficits.

■ Check for neurovascular damage in the extremities by assessing peripheral pulses and capillary refill and by asking the patient if he feels numbness, tingling, or pain. Elevate injured extremities.

■ Apply a temporary sterile dressing, and admit the patient for surgical debridement and observation. Frequent debridement and use of topical and systemic antibiotics can help reduce the risk of infection.

■ Prepare the patient for grafting or, if his injuries are extreme, for amputation.

Emphysema

Emphysema is one of several diseases usually labeled collectively as chronic obstructive pulmonary disease (COPD). About 2 million Americans have emphysema, but the disease appears to be more prevalent in men than in women. Moreover, it's the most common cause of death from respiratory disease in the United States.

ETIOLOGY

Emphysema may be caused by a genetic deficiency of the enzyme alpha$_1$-antitrypsin (AAT), a major component of alpha$_1$-globulin, and by cigarette smoking.

AAT inhibits the activation of several proteolytic enzymes; deficiency of this enzyme is an autosomal recessive trait that predisposes an individual to develop emphysema because proteolysis in lung tissues isn't inhibited. Genetically, one in 3,000 neonates has the disease, and 1% to 3% of all cases of emphysema are due to AAT deficiency. Patients who develop emphysema before or during their early 40s and those who are nonsmokers are believed to have an AAT deficiency.

Cigarette smoking is thought to cause up to 20% of cases. Homozygous individuals have up to an 80% chance of developing lung disease; people who smoke have a greater chance of developing emphysema. Other causative factors are unknown.

PATHOPHYSIOLOGY

Recurrent inflammation associated with the release of proteolytic enzymes from lung cells causes destruction of the alveolar walls, resulting in a breakdown of elasticity and abnormal, irreversible enlargement of the air spaces distal to the terminal bronchioles. (See *What happens in emphysema.*)

In normal breathing, the air moves into and out of the lungs to meet metabolic needs. A change in airway size compromises the lungs' ability to circulate sufficient air.

The alveolar septa are initially destroyed, eliminating a portion of the capillary bed and increasing air volume in the acinus. This breakdown leaves the alveoli unable to recoil normally after expanding and results in bronchiolar collapse on expiration. The damaged or destroyed alveolar walls can't support the airways to keep them open. The amount of air that can be expired passively is diminished, thus trapping air in the lungs and leading to overdistension. Hyperinflation of the alveoli produces bullae (air spaces) adjacent to the pleura (blebs). Septal destruction also decreases airway calibration. Part of each inspiration is trapped because of increased residual volume and decreased calibration. Septal destruction may affect only the respiratory bronchioles and

WHAT HAPPENS IN EMPHYSEMA

In normal, healthy breathing, air moves in and out of the lungs to meet metabolic needs. Any change in airway size compromises the lungs' ability to circulate sufficient air.

In a patient with emphysema, recurrent pulmonary inflammation damages the alveolar walls and causes abnormal, irreversible enlargement of the air spaces. This breakdown leaves the alveoli unable to recoil normally after expanding and results in bronchiolar collapse on expiration. Air is trapped within the lungs.

Associated pulmonary capillary destruction usually allows a patient with severe emphysema to match ventilation to perfusion and thus avoid cyanosis.

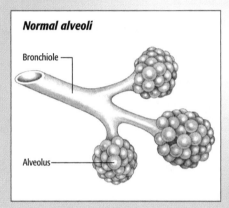

Normal alveoli

Bronchiole

Alveolus

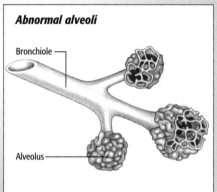

Abnormal alveoli

Bronchiole

Alveolus

alveolar ducts, leaving alveolar sacs intact (centriacinar emphysema), or it can involve the entire acinus (panacinar emphysema), with damage more random and involving the lower lobes of the lungs.

Cardiovascular system

■ Pulmonary hypertension causes cor pulmonale as the heart's workload increases and the right ventricle hypertrophies to force blood through the lungs. As this compensatory mechanism fails, the right ventricle dilates. (See *Disorders affecting management of emphysema,* pages 134 to 137.)

■ As blood viscosity increases due to prolonged hypoxia, pulmonary hypertension increases and heart failure can occur.

Hematologic system

■ Hypoxia causes the bone marrow to produce more red blood cells (RBCs) and blood viscosity increases, aggravating pulmonary hypertension.

ASSESSMENT

The patient's history may reveal that he's a long-time smoker. The patient may report shortness of breath and a chronic cough. The history may also reveal anorexia with resultant weight loss and a general feeling of malaise.

Clinical findings

■ Barrel chest
■ Pursed-lip breathing
■ Accessory muscle use
■ Peripheral cyanosis
■ Clubbed fingers and toes
■ Tachypnea
■ Decreased tactile fremitus and decreased chest expansion on palpation
■ Hyperresonance with percussion
■ Decreased breath sounds, crackles, and wheezing during inspiration, a prolonged expiratory phase with grunting respirations, and distant heart sounds on auscultation

(Text continues on page 136.)

DISORDERS AFFECTING
MANAGEMENT OF EMPHYSEMA

This chart highlights disorders that affect the management of emphysema.

DISORDER	SIGNS AND SYMPTOMS	DIAGNOSTIC TEST RESULTS
Cor pulmonale (complication)	◆ Progressive dyspnea worsening on exertion ◆ Tachypnea ◆ Orthopnea ◆ Edema ◆ Weakness ◆ Dependent edema ◆ Jugular vein distention ◆ Enlarged tender liver ◆ Tachycardia ◆ Hypotension ◆ Weak pulse	◆ Pulmonary artery pressures show increased right ventricular pressures. ◆ Echocardiography or angiography indicates right ventricular enlargement. ◆ Chest X-ray suggests right ventricular enlargement. ◆ Arterial blood gas (ABG) analysis shows partial pressure of arterial oxygen (Pao_2) of less than 70 mm Hg. ◆ Electrocardiography (ECG) may show various arrhythmias. ◆ Pulmonary function tests are consistent with underlying disorder.
Peptic ulcer disease (complication)	◆ Pallor ◆ Epigastric tenderness ◆ Hyperactive bowel sounds *Gastric ulcer* ◆ Recent weight loss or appetite loss ◆ Nausea or vomiting ◆ Pain triggered or worsened by eating *Duodenal ulcer* ◆ Pain relieved by eating; may occur 1½ hours to 3 hours after food intake ◆ Pain that awakens the patient from sleep ◆ Weight gain	◆ Barium swallow or upper GI and small-bowel series may reveal the presence of the ulcer. ◆ Upper GI endoscopy or esophagogastroduodenoscopy confirms the presence of an ulcer and permits cytologic studies and biopsy to rule out *Helicobacter pylori* or cancer. ◆ Upper GI tract X-rays reveal mucosal abnormalities. ◆ Laboratory analysis may disclose occult blood in stools. ◆ Immunoglobulin A anti-*H. pylori* test on a venous blood sample can be used to detect *H. pylori* antibodies. ◆ Serologic testing may disclose clinical signs of infection such as an elevated white blood cell (WBC) count. ◆ Gastric secretory studies show hyperchlorhydria. ◆ Carbon 13 urea breath test results reflect activity of *H. pylori*.
Respiratory failure (complication)	◆ Cyanosis of the oral mucosa, lips, and nail beds ◆ Yawning and use of accessory muscles ◆ Pursed-lip breathing ◆ Nasal flaring ◆ Ashen complexion ◆ Cold, clammy skin ◆ Rapid breathing ◆ Asymmetrical chest movement ◆ Decreased tactile fremitus over an obstructed bronchi or pleural effusion ◆ Increased tactile fremitus over consolidated lung tissue ◆ Hyperresonance ◆ Wheezes (in asthma) ◆ Diminished or absent breath sounds ◆ Rhonchi (in bronchitis) ◆ Crackles (in pulmonary edema)	◆ ABG analysis indicates respiratory failure by deteriorating values (typically Pao_2 less than 60 mm Hg and partial pressure of arterial carbon dioxide greater than 45 mm Hg) and a pH below 7.35. ◆ Chest X-ray identifies pulmonary diseases or conditions, such as emphysema, atelectasis, lesions, pneumothorax, infiltrates, and effusions. ◆ ECG can demonstrate arrhythmias; these are commonly found with cor pulmonale and myocardial hypoxia. ◆ Pulse oximetry reveals a decreasing arterial oxygen saturation; a mixed venous oxygen saturation level of less than 50% indicates impaired tissue oxygenation. ◆ WBC count helps detect an underlying infection as the cause. ◆ Abnormally low hemoglobin and hematocrit levels signal blood loss, indicating a decreased oxygen-carrying capacity.

TREATMENT AND CARE

◆ Provide meticulous respiratory care, including oxygen therapy, suctioning as needed, and deep-breathing and coughing exercises.
◆ Monitor ABG values and monitor for signs of respiratory failure (change in pulse rate, deep labored respiration's, and increased fatigue on exertion).
◆ Monitor fluid status carefully; limit fluid intake to 1,000 to 2,000 ml/day and provide a low sodium diet.
◆ Monitor serum potassium levels if patient is receiving diuretics; low serum potassium levels can potentiate arrhythmias.
◆ Administer digoxin, antibiotics, vasodilators, and oxygen.

◆ Support the patient emotionally and offer reassurance.
◆ Administer proton pump inhibitors, histamine-2-receptor agonists, gastric acid pump inhibitors, sedatives, anticholinergics (with duodenal ulcers), and prostaglandin analogs.
◆ Provide six small meals or small hourly meals as ordered. Advise the patient to eat slowly, chew thoroughly, and have small snacks between meals.
◆ Schedule the patient's care so that he can get plenty of rest.
◆ Teach the patient about peptic ulcer disease, and help him to recognize its signs and symptoms.
◆ Explain scheduled diagnostic tests and prescribed therapies.
◆ Review symptoms associated with complications, and urge him to notify the doctor if any of these occur.
◆ Emphasize the importance of complying with treatment, even after his symptoms are relieved.

◆ To reverse hypoxemia, administer oxygen at appropriate concentrations to maintain Pao_2 at a minimum pressure range of 50 to 60 mm Hg. The patient with chronic obstructive pulmonary disease usually requires only small amounts of supplemental oxygen. Watch for a positive response, such as improved breathing, color, and ABG values.
◆ Maintain a patent airway. If your patient retains carbon dioxide, encourage him to cough and breathe deeply with pursed lips. If he's alert, have him use an incentive spirometer.
◆ If the patient is intubated and lethargic, reposition him every 1 to 2 hours. Use postural drainage and chest physiotherapy to help clear secretions.
◆ Observe the patient closely for respiratory arrest. Auscultate chest sounds. Monitor ABG values, and report any changes immediately. Notify the physician of decreased oxygen saturation levels detected by pulse oximetry.
◆ Watch for treatment complications, especially oxygen toxicity and acute respiratory distress syndrome.
◆ Frequently monitor vital signs. Note and report an increasing pulse rate, increasing or decreasing respiratory rate, declining blood pressure, or febrile state.
◆ Monitor and record serum electrolyte levels carefully. Take appropriate steps to correct imbalances. Monitor fluid balance by recording the patient's intake and output and daily weight.
◆ Check the cardiac monitor for arrhythmias.
◆ Perform oral hygiene measures frequently.
◆ Position the patient for comfort and optimal gas exchange.
◆ Maintain the patient in a normothermic state to reduce the body's demand for oxygen. *(continued)*

DISORDERS AFFECTING MANAGEMENT OF EMPHYSEMA *(continued)*		
DISORDER	**SIGNS AND SYMPTOMS**	**DIAGNOSTIC TEST RESULTS**
Respiratory failure *(continued)*		◆ Serum electrolyte levels may reveal hypokalemia resulting from compensatory hyperventilation, the body's attempt to correct acidosis, or hypochloremia if the patient develops metabolic alkalosis. ◆ Blood cultures, sputum culture and Gram stain may identify pathogens.

Diagnostic test results

■ *Chest X-rays* in advanced disease may show a flattened diaphragm, reduced vascular markings at the lung periphery, overaeration of the lungs, a vertical heart, enlarged anteroposterior chest diameter, and large retrosternal air space.

■ *Pulmonary function tests* typically indicate increased residual volume and total lung capacity, reduced diffusing capacity, and increased inspiratory flow.

■ *Arterial blood gas analysis* usually shows reduced partial pressure of arterial oxygen and normal partial pressure of arterial carbon dioxide late in the disease.

■ *Electrocardiography* may reveal tall, symmetrical P waves in leads II, III, and aV_F; vertical QRS axis; and signs of right ventricular hypertrophy late in the disease.

■ *RBC count* usually demonstrates an increased hemoglobin level late in the disease when the patient has persistent severe hypoxia.

COLLABORATIVE MANAGEMENT

Pulmonary specialists will be consulted to manage respiratory treatments. Cardiologists may be utilized to manage cardiac complications that may arise. Nutritionists will be needed to ensure adequate nutritional status. Social services will be consulted if the patient requires long-term care at home.

TREATMENT AND CARE

■ Treatment of emphysema usually includes the use of bronchodilators, such as aminophylline to promote mucociliary clearance; antibiotics, to treat respiratory tract infection; and immunizations, to prevent influenza and pneumococcal pneumonia.

■ Other treatment measures include adequate hydration and (in selected patients) chest physiotherapy to mobilize secretions.

■ Some patients may require oxygen therapy (at low settings) to correct hypoxia. They may also require transtracheal catheterization to receive oxygen at home.

■ Counseling about avoiding smoking and air pollutants is essential.

Endocarditis

An infection of the endocardium (the innermost heart layer), heart valves, or cardiac prosthesis, endocarditis is usually fatal if left untreated; however, with proper treatment, about 70% of patients recover. The prognosis is worst when endocarditis causes severe valvular damage, leading to insufficiency and left-sided heart failure, or when it involves a prosthetic valve. Recurrent infection occurs in approximately 10% to 20% of patients.

Subacute infective endocarditis typically occurs in people with acquired valvular or congenital cardiac lesions. It can also follow dental, genitourinary, gynecologic, and GI procedures. The most common infecting organisms are *Streptococcus viridans,* which usually inhabits the upper respiratory tact, and *Enterococcus faecalis,* found in GI and perineal flora.

Preexisting conditions, including rheumatic valvular disease, congenital heart disease, mitral valve prolapse, degenerative heart disease, calcificic aortic stenosis (in elderly people), asymmetrical septal hyper-

◆ Schedule patient care activities to maximize the patient's energy level and provide needed rest.

trophy, Marfan syndrome, syphilitic aortic valve, I.V. drug abuse, and long-term hemodialysis with an arteriovenous shunt or fistula, can predispose a person to endocarditis. However, up to 40% of affected patients have no underlying heart disease.

ETIOLOGY
Endocarditis results from bacterial, viral, fungal, or rickettsial invasion. Four mechanisms are involved with the development of infective endocarditis:
■ a congenital or acquired defect in the heart valve or septum, with blood flowing from an area of high to low pressure through this narrowed opening, that allows an optimal area of growth for any organism
■ formation of a sterile platelet fibrin clot that leads to vegetation
■ bacteremia secondary to colonization at the site of vegetation
■ antibody agglutination promoting vegetation growth.

The most common causative organisms are group A nonhemolytic streptococci, staphylococci, and enterococci. However, almost any organism can cause endocarditis.

PATHOPHYSIOLOGY
Organisms enter the body through the mouth and GI tract, upper airway, skin, or external genitourinary tract and travel to the heart. In infective endocarditis, fibrin and platelets cluster on valve tissue and engulf circulating organisms. This produces friable verrucous vegetation. The vegetation may cover the valve surfaces, causing deformities and destruction of valvular tissue. It may also extend to the chordae tendineae, causing them to rupture and leading to valvular

insufficiency. (See *Disorders affecting management of endocarditis*, pages 138 to 141.)

Sometimes vegetation forms on the endocardium, usually in areas altered by rheumatic, congenital, or syphilitic heart disease. It may also form on normal surfaces. Vegetative growth on the heart valves, endocardial lining of a heart chamber, or endothelium of a blood vessel may embolize to the spleen, kidneys, central nervous system and lungs.

Cardiovascular system
■ Infective endocarditis can occur as a consequence of nonbacterial thrombotic endocarditis, which results from turbulence or trauma to the endothelial surface of the heart.
■ The bacteria invade the vegetative lesions, leading to infective endocarditis.
■ Atrial fibrillation can result as the cardiac muscle is destroyed (through progressive local tissue trauma and destruction).

Musculoskeletal system
■ Immune response to the infection and systemic infection can result in septic arthritis.

Renal system
■ Fragments of lesions in the valves and endocardium can form emboli and travel in the bloodstream to the renal system where they may form renal infarctions and abscesses, resulting in glomerulonephritis.

ASSESSMENT
Invasive procedures, such as temporary pacemaker or pulmonary or central venous catheter insertion, endoscopy, surgery, or dental work — especially in patients with a
(*Text continues on page 140.*)

DISORDERS AFFECTING
MANAGEMENT OF ENDOCARDITIS

This chart highlights disorders that affect the management of endocarditis.

DISORDER	SIGNS AND SYMPTOMS	DIAGNOSTIC TEST RESULTS
Atrial fibrillation (complication)	◆ Irregularly irregular pulse rhythm with normal or abnormal heart rate ◆ Radial pulse rate slower than apical pulse rate ◆ Palpable peripheral pulse with the stronger contractions ◆ Evidence of decreased cardiac output, such as hypotension and light-headedness, with new-onset atrial fibrillation and a rapid ventricular rate	◆ Electrocardiography (ECG) shows no clear P waves, irregularly irregular ventricular response, and uneven baseline fibrillatory waves; wide variation in R-R intervals results in loss of atrial kick. ◆ Atrial fibrillation may be preceded by premature atrial contractions.
Heart failure (complication)	◆ Cough that produces pink, frothy sputum ◆ Cyanosis of the lips and nail beds ◆ Pale, cool, clammy skin ◆ Diaphoresis ◆ Jugular vein distention ◆ Ascites ◆ Pulsus alternans ◆ Tachycardia ◆ Hepatomegaly ◆ Decreased pulse pressure ◆ Third (S_3) and fourth (S_4) heart sounds ◆ Moist, basilar crackles ◆ Rhonchi ◆ Expiratory wheezing ◆ Decreased pulse oximetry ◆ Peripheral edema ◆ Decreased urinary output	◆ Cardiac output is decreased. ◆ B-type natriuretic peptide immunoassay is elevated. ◆ Chest X-ray shows increased pulmonary vascular markings, interstitial edema, or pleural effusions and cardiomegaly. ◆ ECG reveals heart enlargement or ischemia, tachycardia, extrasystole, or atrial fibrillation. ◆ Pulmonary artery pressure, pulmonary artery wedge pressure (PAWP), and left ventricular end-diastolic pressure are elevated in the presence of left-sided heart failure; right atrial or central venous pressure is elevated in right-sided heart failure.
Septic arthritis (complication)	◆ Abrupt single swollen joint with pain on active or passive movement ◆ Low-grade fever	◆ Synovial fluid analysis may reveal an elevated leukocyte count. ◆ Gram stain of synovial fluid may reveal the infecting organism. ◆ X-rays reveal the inflamed synovial tissue and accompanying fluid in the joint as well as a symmetric soft-tissue swelling around the involved joint. ◆ Magnetic resonance imaging reveals inflammatory changes and fluid.
Valvular insufficiency (complication)	◆ Orthopnea ◆ Dyspnea ◆ Fatigue ◆ Angina	◆ Catheterization may show mitral insufficiency with increased left ventricular end-diastolic volume and pressure, and increased atrial pressure and PAWP.

TREATMENT AND CARE

◆ Interventions aim to reduce the ventricular response rate to less than 100 beats/minute, to establish anticoagulation, and to restore and maintain a sinus rhythm.
◆ Treatment typically includes drug therapy to control the ventricular response or a combination of electrical cardioversion and drug therapy.
◆ If the patient is hemodynamically unstable, synchronized electrical cardioversion should be performed right away.
◆ A transesophageal echocardiogram may be obtained before cardioversion to rule out the presence of thrombi in the atria.
◆ If drug therapy is used, monitor serum drug levels and observe the patient for evidence of toxicity.
◆ Tell the patient to report changes in pulse rate, dizziness, feeling faint, chest pain, and signs of heart failure, such as dyspnea and peripheral edema.
◆ If the patient isn't on a cardiac monitor, be alert for an irregular pulse and differences in the radial and apical pulse rates.
◆ Monitor the patient's peripheral and apical pulses; watch for evidence of decreased cardiac output and heart failure.

◆ Limit fluid and sodium intake to decrease preload.
◆ Monitor for signs of embolization (hematuria, pleuritic chest pain, left-upper-quadrant pain).
◆ Monitor oxygenation status, auscultate lung fields, and evaluate arterial blood gas (ABG) studies.
◆ Monitor urine output.
◆ Administer supplemental oxygen and mechanical ventilation.
◆ Place the patient in Fowler's position.
◆ Administer diuretics, inotropic drugs, vasodilators, angiotensin-converting enzyme inhibitors, angiotensin-receptor blockers, cardiac glycosides, beta-adrenergic blockers, and electrolyte supplements.
◆ Initiate cardiac monitoring.
◆ Recurrent heart failure from valvular dysfunction may require surgery.
◆ A ventricular assist device may be needed.
◆ Maintain adequate cardiac output and monitor hemodynamic stability.
◆ Assess for deep vein thrombosis and apply antiembolism stockings.

◆ Practice strict sterile technique for all procedures. Wash hands carefully before and after giving care. Dispose of soiled linens and dressings properly. Prevent contact between immunosuppressed patients and infected patients.
◆ Watch for signs of joint inflammation (heat, redness, swelling, pain, or drainage). Monitor vital signs and fever pattern. Remember that corticosteroids mask signs of infection.
◆ Check splints or traction regularly. Keep the joint in proper alignment, but avoid prolonged immobilization. Start passive range-of-motion exercises immediately, and progress to active exercises as soon as the patient can move the affected joint and put weight on it.
◆ Monitor pain levels and medicate accordingly, especially before exercise, remembering that the pain of septic arthritis is easy to underestimate. Administer analgesics and opioids for acute pain and heat or ice packs for moderate pain.
◆ Warn the patient before the first aspiration that it will be painful. Carefully evaluate the patient's condition after joint aspiration.

◆ Watch for signs of heart failure or pulmonary edema.
◆ Monitor for adverse effects of drug therapy.
◆ Teach the patient about diet restrictions, medications, and the importance of consistent follow-up care.
◆ Monitor vital signs, ABG studies, input and output, daily weight, blood chemistries, chest X-rays and pulmonary artery readings.

(continued)

DISORDERS AFFECTING
MANAGEMENT OF ENDOCARDITIS *(continued)*

DISORDER	SIGNS AND SYMPTOMS	DIAGNOSTIC TEST RESULTS
Valvular insufficiency *(continued)*	◆ Palpitations ◆ Peripheral edema ◆ Jugular vein distention ◆ Hepatomegaly ◆ Tachycardia ◆ Crackles ◆ Pulmonary edema ◆ Murmurs	◆ X-rays may show left atrial and ventricular enlargement and pulmonary venous congestion. ◆ Echocardiography shows abnormal valve leaflet motion and left atrial enlargement. ◆ ECG may show left atrial and ventricular hypertrophy, sinus tachycardia, and atrial fibrillation.
Valvular stenosis (complication)	◆ Dyspnea ◆ Orthopnea ◆ Palpitations ◆ Peripheral edema ◆ Jugular vein distention ◆ Ascites ◆ Crackles ◆ Cardiac arrhythmias ◆ Murmurs	◆ PAWP is increased. ◆ Severe pulmonary hypertension is present. ◆ X-rays may reveal left atrial and ventricular enlargement, enlarged pulmonary arteries, and mitral valve calcification. ◆ Echocardiography may show a thickened mitral valve. ◆ ECG may show left atrial hypertrophy, atrial fibrillation, right ventricular hypertrophy, and right axis deviation.

history of a preexisting valve disorder — greatly increase the risk of infective endocarditis. The patient may report a predisposing condition and complain of nonspecific symptoms, such as weakness, fatigue, weight loss, anorexia, arthralgia, night sweats, or an intermittent fever that may recur for weeks.

Clinical findings
■ Petechiae of the skin, especially common on the upper anterior trunk and the buccal, pharyngeal, or conjunctival mucosa
■ Splinter hemorrhages under the nails
■ Osler's nodes (tender, raised, subcutaneous lesions on the fingers or toes)
■ Roth's spots (hemorrhagic areas with white centers on the retina)
■ Janeway lesions (purplish macules on the palms or soles)
■ Clubbing of the fingers in the patient with long-standing disease
■ Loud and regurgitating murmur (except in those with early acute endocarditis and I.V. drug users with tricuspid valve infection), murmur that changes suddenly, or

new murmur that develops in the presence of fever
■ Splenomegaly (in long-standing disease)

Diagnostic test results
■ Three or more *blood cultures* taken during a 24- to 48-hour period identify the causative organism in up to 90% of patients; the remaining have negative blood cultures.
■ *White blood cell count* and *differential* are normal or elevated; histiocytes (macrophages) may be abnormal.
■ *Red blood cell studies* may reveal normocytic, normochromic anemia (in subacute infective endocarditis).
■ *Erythrocyte sedimentation rate* and *serum creatinine levels* are elevated.
■ *Serum studies* are positive for rheumatoid factor.
■ *Urinalysis* may reveal proteinuria and microscopic hematuria.
■ *Endocardiography* may identify valvular damage.
■ *Electrocardiography* may detect conduction defects due to spread of the infection.

TREATMENT AND CARE

♦ Therapies vary with the severity of symptoms.

♦ Watch for signs of heart failure or pulmonary edema.
♦ Monitor for adverse effects of drug therapy.
♦ Teach the patient about diet restrictions, medications, and the importance of consistent follow-up care.
♦ Monitor vital signs, ABG studies, input and output, daily weight, blood chemistries, chest X-rays and pulmonary artery readings.
♦ Therapies vary with the severity of symptoms.

■ *Arteriograms* or *computed tomography scanning* may identify possible embolization sites.

COLLABORATIVE MANAGEMENT

The acutely ill patient requires the attention of a cardiologist and a skilled team to stabilize and manage his condition. Specialists such as surgeons, nephrologists, and cardiac or stroke rehabilitation teams may be consulted if complications arise.

TREATMENT AND CARE

■ The goal of treatment is to eradicate all of the infecting organisms from the vegetation.
■ Therapy should start promptly and continue over several weeks.
■ Selection of an anti-infective drug is based on the infecting organism and sensitivity studies.
■ Although blood cultures are negative in 10% to 20% of the subacute cases, the physician may want to determine the probable infecting organism.
■ I.V. antibiotic therapy usually lasts about 4 to 6 weeks.

■ Supportive treatment includes bed rest, aspirin for fever and aches, and sufficient fluid intake.
■ Severe valvular damage, especially aortic regurgitation or infection of a cardiac prosthesis, may require corrective surgery if refractory heart failure develops, or if an infected prosthetic valve must be replaced.

Esophageal varices

Esophageal varices are dilated, torturous veins in the submucosa of the lower esophagus resulting from portal hypertension (elevated pressure in the portal vein). These varices can go undetected and result in sudden and massive bleeding. Care for the patient who has portal hypertension with esophageal varices focuses on monitoring for signs and symptoms of hemorrhage and subsequent hypotension, compromised oxygen supply, and altered level of consciousness.

DISORDER AFFECTING
MANAGEMENT OF ESOPHAGEAL VARICES

This chart highlights how aspiration pneumonitis affects the management of esophageal varices.

DISORDER	SIGNS AND SYMPTOMS	DIAGNOSTIC TEST RESULTS
Aspiration pneumonitis (complication)	◆ Fever ◆ Chills ◆ Sweats ◆ Pleuritic chest pain ◆ Cough ◆ Sputum production ◆ Hemoptysis ◆ Dyspnea ◆ Headache ◆ Fatigue ◆ Bronchial breath sounds over areas of consolidation ◆ Crackles ◆ Increased tactile fremitus ◆ Unequal chest wall expansion	◆ Chest X-rays reveal infiltrates, confirming the diagnosis. ◆ Sputum specimen for Gram stain and culture and sensitivity tests shows acute inflammatory cells. ◆ White blood cell count indicates leukocytosis in bacterial pneumonia and a normal or low count in viral or mycoplasmal pneumonia. ◆ Blood cultures reflect bacteremia and help to determine the causative organism. ◆ Arterial blood gas (ABG) levels vary depending on the severity of pneumonia and the underlying lung state. ◆ Bronchoscopy or transtracheal aspiration allows the collection of material for culture. Pleural fluid culture may also be obtained. ◆ Pulse oximetry may show a reduced level of arterial oxygen saturation.

Bleeding from esophageal varices accounts for approximately 10% of the cases of upper GI bleeding. If a patient experiences an episode of bleeding from esophageal varices, he has a 70% chance of experiencing additional bleeding episodes. Of these rebleeding episodes, one-third typically results in death. Comorbidity involving the renal, pulmonary, and cardiovascular systems adds to the mortality risk. If the patient experiences massive bleeding with a loss of approximately 40% of his blood volume, death can occur within 30 minutes.

ETIOLOGY

Portal hypertension occurs when blood flows meets increased resistance. The disorder is a common result of cirrhosis, but may also stem from mechanical obstruction and occlusion of the hepatic veins (Budd-Chiari syndrome).

PATHOPHYSIOLOGY

As pressure in the portal vein rises, blood backs up into the spleen and flows through collateral channels to the venous system, bypassing the liver. Consequently, portal hypertension produces splenomegaly; thrombocytopenia; dilated collateral veins in the esophagus (esophageal varices), abdomen, and rectum (hemorrhoids); and ascites.

Gastrointestinal system

■ The collateral circulation located in the submucosa of the lower esophagus and upper stomach results from communication between the portal vein and the gastric coronary vein.
■ Increased blood flow and higher pressure resulting from the opening of these collaterals cause the submucosa veins near the esophagogastric junction to become dilated and protrude into the lumen.

TREATMENT AND CARE

◆ Maintain a patent airway and adequate oxygenation. Measure the patient's ABG levels, especially if he's hypoxic. Administer supplemental oxygen if his partial pressure of arterial oxygen falls below 55 mm Hg. If he has an underlying chronic lung disease, give oxygen cautiously.

◆ In severe pneumonia that requires endotracheal (ET) intubation or a tracheostomy with or without mechanical ventilation, provide thorough respiratory care and suction often, using sterile technique, to remove secretions.

◆ Obtain sputum specimens as needed. Use suction if the patient can't produce a specimen. Collect the specimens in a sterile container, and deliver them promptly to the microbiology laboratory.

◆ Administer antibiotics and pain medication. Administer I.V. fluids and electrolyte replacement, if needed, for fever and dehydration.

◆ Provide a high-calorie, high-protein diet of soft foods to offset the calories the patient uses to fight the infection. If necessary, supplement oral feedings with nasogastric (NG) tube feedings or parenteral nutrition.

◆ To prevent aspiration during NG tube feedings, elevate the patient's head, check the tube position, and administer the feeding slowly. Don't give large volumes at one time because this can cause vomiting.

◆ If the patient has an ET tube, inflate the tube cuff before feeding. Keep his head elevated after feeding.

◆ Monitor the patient's fluid intake and output.

◆ To control the spread of infection, dispose of secretions properly. Tell the patient to sneeze and cough into a disposable tissue, and tape a waxed bag to the side of the bed for used tissues.

◆ Provide a quiet, calm environment, with frequent rest periods. Make sure the patient has diversionary activities appropriate to his age.

◆ Listen to the patient's fears and concerns, and remain with him during periods of severe stress and anxiety. Encourage him to identify actions and care measures that promote comfort and relaxation.

◆ Whenever possible, include the patient in decisions about his care.

◆ Include family members in all phases of the patient's care, and encourage them to visit.

Respiratory system

■ The patient is at risk for impaired gas exchange because of the possibility of aspiration pneumonitis. (See *Disorder affecting management of esophageal varices.*)

ASSESSMENT

In many patients, bleeding from esophageal varices is the first sign of portal hypertension. The bleeding may be painless. The patient history may reveal a history of excessive use of alcohol or previously diagnosed cirrhosis. In addition, the patient interview may reveal mechanical irritation, such as coarse or unchewed food, straining on defecation, or rigorous coughing preceding the bleeding episode.

Clinical findings

■ Massive hematemesis

■ Varied level of consciousness depending on the degree of bleeding
■ Tachycardia
■ Tachypnea
■ Hypotension
■ Weak peripheral pulses
■ Pale skin
■ Circumoral pallor
■ Dry mucous membranes
■ Poor skin turgor
■ Jaundice
■ Palpable splenomegaly
■ Diminished urine output

Diagnostic test results

■ *Endoscopy* identifies the ruptured varix as the bleeding site and excludes other potential sources in the upper GI tract.
■ *Complete blood count* reveals decreased hemoglobin levels, hematocrit, and red blood cell count; white blood cell and

platelet counts are decreased initially due to splenomegaly.

■ *Coagulation studies* reveal prolonged prothrombin time secondary to hepatocellular disease.

■ *Serum chemistry tests* may reveal elevated blood urea nitrogen, sodium, total bilirubin, and ammonia levels; decreased serum albumin due to liver damage; and elevated liver enzyme levels.

■ *Angiography* helps to identify patency of the portal vein and development of collateral vessels.

COLLABORATIVE MANAGEMENT

Respiratory therapy may be required to manage the patient's oxygenation, including the need for intubation and mechanical ventilation. A GI specialist may collaborate with a pulmonary specialist for ventilatory management especially if the patient requires endotracheal intubation and mechanical ventilation. Nutritional therapy may be needed after the patient's condition stabilizes to ensure adequate caloric intake in conjunction with any restrictions such as sodium or protein. If appropriate, social services may be consulted for assistance with rehabilitation programs if the patient has a substance abuse problem, support of the patient and his family, and for referrals to community support groups.

TREATMENT AND CARE

■ The goal of treatment is to stop the hemorrhage using direct tamponade with an inflatable balloon and injecting varices with a sclerosing agent through an endoscope tube.

■ Transjugular intrahepatic portosystemic shunting may be done to reduce portal pressure. This procedure creates a shunt within the liver between the systemic vascular system and portal system.

■ Surgical procedures may include portal systemic shunting, in which blood is diverted away from the obstructed portal system, or esophageal transaction and devascularization, in which the bleeding esophageal site is separated from the portal system.

■ Endoscopic variceal ligation or I.V. administration of vasopressin is used to reduce splenic blood flow and portal venous pressure.

■ Drug therapy may include propranolol to reduce portal pressure by blocking beta-adrenergic action and somastatin to produce selective vasodilation of the portal system, thereby reducing portal pressure.

DRUG ALERT *Vasopressin may cause adverse reactions such as hypothermia, myocardial and GI tract ischemia, and acute renal failure. Propranolol may cause decreased pulse and blood pressures, which may impair the patient's cardiovascular response to hemorrhage.*

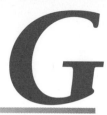

Gaucher's disease

Gaucher's disease is the most common lysosomal storage disease. It occurs in three forms: Type I (adult); Type II (infantile); and Type III (juvenile). Type II can be fatal within 9 months of onset, usually from pulmonary involvement. (See *Types of Gaucher's disease*.)

ETIOLOGY

Gaucher's disease results from an autosomal recessive inheritance. The faulty gene is located on the long arm (designated as "q") of chromosome 1 in region 21. This is commonly noted as *1q21*. More than 100 mutations of the gene have been identified. However, the mutation that appears is unrelated to the manifestations presented or the prognosis.

PATHOPHYSIOLOGY

The abnormal gene encoding leads to a deficiency in the enzyme glucocerebrosidase. Glucocerebrosidase plays a major role in phagocytosis, breaking down dead cells and cellular debris. This deficiency causes an abnormal accumulation of glucocerebrosides in reticuloendothelial cells.

Glucocerebrosidase deficiency leads to an accumulation of glucosylceramide in the storage compartments (lysosomes) of certain body cells. Glucosylceramide is an intermediate metabolite that forms from the breakdown of aging leukocytes. This metabolite, along with other fats and carbohydrates that aren't broken down, builds up in the monocytes and macrophages of the liver, spleen, bones, and bone marrow. These now enlarged cells are called *Gaucher cells* and are characteristic of the disease. Gaucher cells can affect any organ in the body. (See *Disor-*

ders affecting management of Gaucher's disease, pages 146 and 147.)

Hematologic system
■ Gaucher cells infiltrate the spleen, leading to splenomegaly and hypersplenism.
■ Hypersplenism results in over-filtering of circulating blood cells, possibly leading to anemia, leukopenia, and thrombocytopenia.
■ Fibrosis occurs, which affects red blood cell production, leading to anemia.

TYPES OF GAUCHER'S DISEASE

Gaucher's disease can be classified as one of three types. This classification is based on the age of onset and the degree of neurologic involvement.

Type I Gaucher's disease is the most common form of all lysosomal disorders. It occurs primarily in the Ashkenazi Jewish population. Although most cases are diagnosed in adulthood, some cases are diagnosed in infancy; others aren't diagnosed until age 70 or older. The disease initially presents as painless splenomegaly. Bone involvement may be so severe that the patient is confined to a wheelchair.

Type II Gaucher's disease is a rare form. Onset usually occurs by age 3 months. The disease initially presents as hepatosplenomegaly. Trismus, strabismus, and backward flexion of the neck develop within a few months. The disease involves rapid neurologic deterioration. Most patients die before age 1.

Type III is also rare and combines features of Type I and Type II disease. Splenomegaly and bone marrow damage occur along with neurologic manifestations. Onset occurs at an older age and progresses at a slower rate than with Type II disease.

DISORDERS AFFECTING MANAGEMENT OF GAUCHER'S DISEASE

This chart highlights disorders that affect the management of Gaucher's disease.

DISORDER	SIGNS AND SYMPTOMS	DIAGNOSTIC TEST RESULTS
Anemia (complication)	◆ Possibly asymptomatic early; signs and symptoms develop as anemia becomes more severe ◆ Dyspnea on exertion and fatigue ◆ Listlessness, inability to concentrate ◆ Pallor, irritability ◆ Tachycardia ◆ Brittle, thinning nails	◆ Total iron binding capacity is elevated and serum iron levels are decreased (early on). ◆ Bone marrow aspiration reveals reduced iron stores and reduced production of red blood cell (RBC) precursors. ◆ Complete blood count reveals decreased hemoglobin and hematocrit and low mean corpuscular hemoglobin. ◆ RBC indices reveal decreased cells that are microcytic and hypochromic.
Pathological fractures (complication)	◆ Increased pain with movement ◆ Inability to intentionally move body part ◆ Possible tingling sensation distal to fracture site ◆ Soft tissue edema ◆ Obvious deformity or shortening of limb ◆ Possible discoloration over fracture site ◆ Warmth, crepitus on palpation ◆ Numbness and coolness distal to site of fracture (indicative of possible nerve and vessel damage)	◆ Anteroposterior and lateral X-rays identify site of fracture, which displays as a break in the continuity of the bone. ◆ Computed tomography or magnetic resonance imaging indicates fracture site. ◆ Angiography reveals possible vascular injury due to fracture.

■ Blood cell production is compromised by infiltration of the Gaucher cells in the bone marrow.

Musculoskeletal system

■ Infiltration of osteocytes can lead to musculoskeletal abnormalities.

■ Remodeling of the distal femur and proximal tibia fails, producing a funnel-like, cylindrical-shaped bone instead of the typical flared shape.

■ Diffuse and localized bone loss occurs along with cortical thinning and loss of coarse cancellous bone. Bone loss is most severe in the axial skeleton.

■ Osteonecrosis occurs, most commonly affecting the femoral head or proximal humerus (although it may also affect the long bones), leading to pathologic fractures and bone pain.

Nervous system

■ Enzyme deficiency can result in Gaucher cells developing within the cells of the central nervous system.

■ Motor and sensory nerve dysfunction can occur leading to seizures, hypertonicity, spasticity, hyperreflexia, and cognitive dysfunction.

ASSESSMENT

Two key findings associated with Gaucher's disease are hepatosplenomegaly and bone lesions. Other findings may vary depending on the disease type.

Clinical findings

Findings with Type I disease may include:
■ pathologic fractures
■ collapsed hip joints
■ vertebral compression

TREATMENT AND CARE

◆ Assess for decreased perfusion to vital organs, including heart and lungs; monitor for dyspnea, chest pain, and dizziness.
◆ Administer oxygen therapy to prevent hypoxemia.
◆ Frequently monitor vital signs for changes.
◆ Administer iron replacement therapy.
◆ Prepare to administer blood component therapy, such as packed RBCs, if anemia is severe.
◆ Allow for frequent rest periods.

◆ Prepare for immobilization of fracture site with a splint, cast, or traction.
◆ Perform neurovascular assessment every 1 to 2 hours to detect changes in circulation or sensation.
◆ Administer analgesics for pain control.
◆ Increase fluid intake and maintain diet.
◆ Elevate the fractured extremity; for a fractured hip, keep the patient flat with the foot of the bed elevated 25 degrees and legs abducted.
◆ Provide active and passive range-of-motion exercises for unaffected limbs.
◆ Encourage coughing, deep breathing, and incentive spirometry.
◆ Assess vital signs frequently, watching for signs and symptoms of pulmonary or fat embolism, such as dypsnea, tachypnea, tachycardia, hemoptysis, chest pain, and crackles.

■ severe episodic pain in the legs, arms, and back
■ fever
■ abdominal distention (from hypotonicity of the large bowel)
■ respiratory problems (pneumonia or, rarely, cor pulmonale)
■ easy bruising and bleeding, anemia and, rarely, pancytopenia
■ yellow pallor and brown-yellow pigmentation on the face and legs (in older patients).
Findings in those with Type II disease may include:
■ motor dysfunction and spasticity
■ strabismus
■ muscle hypertonicity
■ retroflexion of the head
■ neck rigidity
■ dysphagia
■ laryngeal stridor
■ hyperreflexia
■ seizures
■ respiratory distress
■ easy bruising and bleeding.
Findings of Type III disease may include:
■ seizures
■ hypertonicity
■ strabismus
■ poor coordination and mental ability.

Diagnostic test results
■ *Direct assay of glucocerebrosidase activity,* which can be performed on venous blood, confirms the diagnosis.
■ *Bone marrow aspiration* shows Gaucher cells.
■ *Distal femur radiography* shows flask-shaped bone.

■ *Magnetic resonance imaging* of the skeleton, including femurs, shows infiltration of bone marrow and bone changes.

■ *Laboratory tests* reveal increased serum acid phosphatase level and decreased platelets and serum iron level.

■ *Electroencephalography* is abnormal after infancy in Type III disease.

COLLABORATIVE MANAGEMENT

Genetic counseling for patients with a family history of Gaucher's disease is important. (Clinical trials involving gene therapy have been performed; however, no new clinical trials are currently underway.) Additionally, prenatal testing can determine if a fetus has the syndrome. Other team members may include a nutritionist, to help the patient plan his meals to meet his dietary requirements; social services, to assist with continued care and follow-up and help with financial concerns and community support; and a spiritual counselor or pastoral care associate to help the family cope with the stress that a diagnosis may yield.

TREATMENT AND CARE

There's no cure for Gaucher's disease. Treatment is mainly supportive and may include:
■ enzyme replacement therapy
■ partial or total splenectomy to combat hypersplenism or mechanical obstruction due to splenomegaly
■ bone marrow transplantation
■ supplemental therapy including vitamins, supplemental iron or liver extract to prevent anemia caused by iron deficiency and to alleviate other hematologic problems, blood transfusions for anemia, and analgesics for bone pain.

Graft-versus-host disease

Graft-versus-host disease (GVHD) can occur when an immunologically impaired recipient receives a graft from an immunocompetent donor. The donor's lymphocytes recognize the recipient's cells as antigenically different and attempt to destroy them. Essentially, the transplant tries to reject the recipient rather than the recipient rejecting the transplant.

GVHD can be acute or chronic. Acute GVHD occurs within the first 100 days after a transplant. Chronic GVHD occurs after day 100 of a transplant and involves an autoimmune response that affects multiple organs. Older patients and those who have suffered previous acute GVHD face the greatest risk of chronic GVHD.

Less than one-half of recipients with histocompatibility identical to the donor develop GVHD. This incidence increases to greater than 60% when there is one antigen mismatch. Development of acute GVHD is a major contributing factor for mortality following bone marrow transplantation. Death with GVHD is commonly due to sepsis. Patients who develop chronic GVHD immediately following acute GVHD have the highest mortality rates.

ETIOLOGY

GVHD disease usually develops after a patient with impaired immune function — from congenital immunodeficiency, radiation treatment, or immunosuppressant therapy — receives a bone marrow transplant from an incompatible donor. It can also occur following solid organ transplants, most commonly liver transplants. Additionally, GVHD may result from the transfusion of a blood product containing viable lymphocytes. This means that patients may develop GVHD during the transfusion of whole blood or transplant of fetal thymus, liver, or bone marrow. The risk of GVHD disease transmission also exists during maternal-fetal blood transfusions and intrauterine transfusions.

PATHOPHYSIOLOGY

GVHD involves donor T-cells attacking and destroying host cells. Three criteria are necessary for the development of GVHD: immunologically competent cells in the graft; graft recognition of the host as foreign; and inability of the host to react to the graft. If donor and recipient cells aren't histocompatible, the foreign or graft cells may launch an attack against the host cells, which can't reject them. This process begins when graft cells become sensitized to the recipient's class II antigens. The exact mechanism by which this occurs remains unclear, although biopsy of active GVHD lesions usually reveals infiltration by mononuclear cells, eosinophils, and phagocytic and histiocytic cells.

Gastrointestinal system
■ Severe diarrhea, severe abdominal pain, GI bleeding, and malabsorption occur as cell loss from the bowel progresses.
■ Mild jaundice with elevated liver enzymes and possibly hepatic coma may result from liver damage. (See *Disorders affecting management of GVHD*, pages 150 and 151.)

Immune system
■ Infections (mostly bacterial and fungal) due to granulocytopenia are an issue immediately after transplantation. Later, interstitial pneumonitis predominates.
■ Because the patient is already immunocompromised from a graft or organ transplant, sepsis can occur.

Integumentary system
■ A pruritic maculopapular rash may develop on palms and soles 10 to 30 days after transplant, possibly progressing to generalized erythema with bullous formation and desquamation.

ASSESSMENT
Chronic GVHD is commonly manifested by skin changes that resemble scleroderma that can ultimately lead to ulcerations, joint contractures, and impaired esophageal motility.

Although graft survival typically hinges on early detection of transplant rejection, no single test or combination of tests proves definitive. Tests reveal only nonspecific evidence, which may easily be attributed to other causes, especially infection. Diagnosis commonly becomes a matter of exclusion and depends on careful evaluation of signs and symptoms along with results from specific organ function tests, standard laboratory studies, and tissue biopsy.

Clinical findings
■ Skin rash
■ Severe diarrhea
■ Jaundice
■ Abdominal cramps
■ GI bleeding

Diagnostic test results
■ *Tissue biopsy* usually reveals immunocompetent T cells along with the extent of lymphocytic infiltration and tissue damage.
■ *Repeat biopsies* detect early histologic changes characteristic of rejection, to determine the degree of change from previous biopsies, and to monitor the course and success of treatment.
■ *Liver function studies* reveal elevated levels of bilirubin, serum alkaline phosphatase, alanine aminotransferase, and aspartate aminotransferase.

COLLABORATIVE MANAGEMENT
Transplant specialists along with hematologic, dermatologic, and gastroenterologic specialists may be necessary to help guide treatment. Infection control personnel may be consulted to reduce the patient's risk for infection. Other specialists, including neurologists and nephrologists, may be consulted for assistance depending on the involvement of the patient's organs and prognosis. The patient and his family may also benefit from supportive counseling and a referral for social services.

TREATMENT AND CARE
■ Because patients may die of GVHD, initial interventions must focus on prevention. Most patients receive immunosuppressant therapy with methotrexate, with or without prednisone, antithymocyte globulin, cyclosporine, cyclophosphamide, or tacrolimus for the first 3 to 12 months after a transplant.
■ Other strategies to decrease the incidence of GVHD involve attempting to deplete donor marrow of T cells and radiating blood products before administration to prevent T-cell replication.

(*Text continues on page 152.*)

DISORDERS AFFECTING MANAGEMENT OF GVHD

This chart highlights disorders that affect the management of graft-versus-host disease (GVHD).

DISORDER	SIGNS AND SYMPTOMS	DIAGNOSTIC TEST RESULTS
Hypokalemia (complication)	◆ Abdominal cramps, nausea, and vomiting ◆ Muscle weakness ◆ Irritability, malaise, confusion ◆ Paresthesia and progression to paralysis ◆ Decreased cardiac output and possible cardiac arrest at any point ◆ Respiratory paralysis ◆ Metabolic alkalosis ◆ Characteristic electrocardiogram (ECG) changes ◆ Orthostatic hypotension ◆ Irregular heart rate ◆ Decreased bowel sounds ◆ Speech changes	◆ Serum potassium level is below 3.5 mEq/L. ◆ Bicarbonate (HCO_3^-) levels and pH are elevated. ◆ Serum glucose levels are slightly elevated. ◆ ECG changes show a flattened T wave, a depressed ST segment, and a characteristic U wave.
Septic shock (complication)	*Hyperdynamic phase* ◆ Pink and flushed skin ◆ Agitation ◆ Anxiety ◆ Irritability ◆ Shortened attention span ◆ Rapid and shallow respirations ◆ Urine output below normal ◆ Rapid, full, bounding pulse ◆ Warm, dry skin ◆ Normal or slightly elevated blood pressure *Hypodynamic phase* ◆ Pale and possibly cyanotic skin (peripheral areas may be mottled) ◆ Decreased level of consciousness (obtundation and coma may be present) ◆ Possible rapid, shallow respirations ◆ Urine output less than 25 ml/hour or absent ◆ Weak, thready, and rapid pulse or absent pulse; may be irregular if arrhythmias are present ◆ Cold, clammy skin ◆ Hypotension, usually with a systolic pressure below 90 mm Hg or 50 to 80 mm Hg below the patient's previous level ◆ Crackles or rhonchi if pulmonary congestion is present	◆ Blood cultures are positive for the offending organism. ◆ Complete blood count shows the presence or absence of anemia and leukopenia, severe or absent neutropenia, and (usually) the presence of thrombocytopenia. ◆ Blood urea nitrogen and creatinine levels are increased and creatinine clearance is decreased. ◆ Prothrombin time and partial thromboplastin time are abnormal. ◆ ECG shows ST-depression, inverted T waves, and arrhythmias resembling myocardial infarction. ◆ Serum lactate dehydrogenase levels are elevated with metabolic acidosis. ◆ Urine studies show increased specific gravity (more than 1.020) and osmolality and decreased sodium. ◆ Arterial blood gas analysis demonstrates elevated blood pH and partial pressure of arterial oxygen (Pao_2) and decreased partial pressure of arterial carbon dioxide ($Paco_2$) with respiratory alkalosis in early stages. As shock progresses, metabolic acidosis develops with hypoxemia indicated by decreased $Paco_2$, as well as decreasing Pao_2, HCO_3^-, and pH levels.

TREATMENT AND CARE

◆ Be prepared to administer I.V. potassium chloride with an infusion pump (never as a bolus) to prevent cardiac arrhythmias and cardiac arrest. Infusion rates are generally 10 mEq/hour, but should not exceed 40 to 60 mEq/hour.
◆ Provide continuous cardiac monitoring during I.V. potassium chloride infusions and report irregularities immediately, as well as toxic reactions.
◆ Assess the I.V. site for signs and symptoms of infiltration, phlebitis, or tissue necrosis. Advise the patient that I.V. potassium chloride administration can lead to burning at the infusion site.
◆ Monitor vital signs, ECG tracing, heart rate and rhythm, and respiratory status.
◆ Monitor serum potassium levels, intake and output, and signs of metabolic alkalosis.
◆ Provide a safe environment and assess the patient's risk for injury.
◆ Assess for constipation and gastric distention, but avoid the use of laxatives because of the potassium losses associated with these medications.
◆ Avoid crushing slow-released potassium supplements.
◆ After the potassium has returned to a normal level, the patient may need further dietary counseling and prescription of a sustained-release oral potassium supplement.
◆ A patient taking a diuretic should be changed to a potassium-sparing diuretic to prevent excessive loss of potassium in the urine.

◆ Remove I.V., intra-arterial, or urinary drainage catheters and send them to the laboratory to culture for the presence of the causative organism. New catheters can be reinserted in the intensive care unit.
◆ Start an I.V. infusion with normal saline solution or lactated Ringer's solution, using a large-bore (14G to 18G) catheter, which allows easier administration of later blood transfusions. (*Caution:* Don't start I.V. infusions in the legs of a shock patient who has suffered abdominal trauma because infused fluid may escape through the ruptured vessel into the abdomen.)
◆ Record the patient's blood pressure, pulse and respiratory rates, and peripheral pulses every 1 to 5 minutes until he's stabilized. Record hemodynamic pressure readings every 15 minutes. Monitor cardiac rhythm continuously. Systolic blood pressure less than 80 mm Hg usually results in inadequate coronary artery blood flow, cardiac ischemia, arrhythmias, and further complications of low cardiac output. When blood pressure drops below 80 mm Hg, increase the oxygen flow rate and notify the physician immediately.
◆ A progressive drop in blood pressure accompanied by a thready pulse generally signals inadequate cardiac output from reduced intravascular volume. Notify the physician and increase the infusion rate.
◆ Administer appropriate antimicrobial drugs I.V. to achieve effective blood levels rapidly.
◆ Measure hourly urine output. If output is less than 30 ml/hour in adults, increase the fluid infusion rate, but watch for signs of fluid overload, such as an increase in pulmonary artery wedge pressure. Notify the physician if urine output doesn't improve. A diuretic may be ordered to increase renal blood flow and urine output.
◆ Draw an arterial blood sample to measure blood gas levels. Administer oxygen by face mask or airway to ensure adequate tissue oxygenation. Adjust the oxygen flow rate to a higher or lower level, as blood gas measurements indicate.
◆ Provide emotional support to the patient and family members.
◆ Document the occurrence of a nosocomial infection and report it to the infection-control nurse. Investigating all hospital-acquired infections can help identify their sources and prevent future infections.

TYPES OF GUILLAIN-BARRÉ SYNDROME

Four variations of Guillain-Barré syndrome have been identified: ascending, descending, Miller-Fischer variant, and pure motor. These classifications reflect the degree of peripheral nerve involvement.

Ascending Guillain-Barré syndrome is the most common form. Weakness and numbness begin in the legs and progress upward to the trunk, arms, and cranial nerves. Motor deficits, which are symmetrical, range from paresis to quadriplegia. Sensory deficits involve mild numbness that's more severe in the toes. Reflexes are absent or diminished.

In descending Guillain-Barré syndrome, initial weakness of the cranial nerves, such as facial, glossopharyngeal, vagus, and hypoglossal nerves, progresses downward. Sensory deficits more commonly occur in the hands than in the feet. Reflexes are absent or diminished.

In Miller-Fisher variant Guillain-Barré syndrome, a rare form, ophthalmaplegia, areflexia, and pronounced ataxia occur, with no sensory loss.

In pure motor Guillain-Barré syndrome, a mild form, manifestations are similar to those of the ascending form, except that sensory deficits are absent.

Guillain-Barré syndrome

Guillain-Barré syndrome (also called *infectious polyneuritis, Landry-Guillain-Barré syndrome,* and *acute idiopathic polyneuritis*) is an acute, rapidly progressive, inflammatory polyneuropathy that primarily affects the motor component of the peripheral nerves. About 80% to 90% of patients have little or no residual disabilities from this syndrome. The prognosis is good when symptoms clear between 15 and 20 days after onset.

Guillain-Barré syndrome can occur at any age but is most common between ages 30 and 50; it affects both sexes equally. In the United States, it has an incidence of 0.6 to 2.4 cases per 100,000 people. Four types of Guillain-Barré syndrome have been identified. (See *Types of Guillain-Barré syndrome.*)

ETIOLOGY

Although the exact cause of Guillain-Barré syndrome is unknown, it's believed to be an autoimmune response to a viral infection. In most cases, the patient reports a recent history (usually within the previous 2 weeks) of an upper respiratory infection, viral pneumonia, or a GI infection. Rarely, the patient has received a vaccine before the onset of the syndrome.

PATHOPHYSIOLOGY

The major pathologic event is segmental demyelination of the peripheral nerves. This prevents normal transmission of electrical impulses along the sensorimotor nerve roots. Because this syndrome causes inflammation and degenerative changes in both the posterior (sensory) and anterior (motor) nerve roots, signs of sensory and motor losses occur simultaneously. (See *Understanding sensorimotor nerve degeneration.*)

Although the primary pathophysiologic mechanism involves the nervous system, the overall effects of the disorder can affect multiple systems. (See *Disorders affecting management of Guillain-Barré syndrome,* pages 154 and 155.)

Nervous system
- The proposed immunologic reaction causes segmental demyelination of the peripheral nerves, which prevents normal transmission of electrical impulses along the sensorimotor nerve roots.
- The myelin sheath, which covers the nerve axons and conducts electrical impulses along the nerve pathways, degenerates.
- With degeneration comes inflammation, swelling, and patchy demyelination.
- As myelin is destroyed, the nodes of Ranvier, located at the junctures of the myelin sheaths, widen. This widening delays and impairs impulse transmission along the dorsal and ventral nerve roots.
- Impairment of dorsal nerve roots affects sensory function leading to tingling and numbness.
- Impairment of ventral nerve roots affects motor function and leads to muscle weakness, immobility, and paralysis.

UNDERSTANDING SENSORIMOTOR
NERVE DEGENERATION

Guillain-Barré syndrome attacks the peripheral nerves so that they can't transmit messages to the brain correctly. Following is a synthesis of what goes wrong.

The myelin sheath degenerates for unknown reasons. This sheath covers the nerve axons and conducts electrical impulses along the nerve pathways. Degeneration brings inflammation, swelling, and patchy demyelination. As the disorder destroys myelin, the nodes of Ranvier (at the junction of the myelin sheaths) widen, which delays and impairs impulse transmission along the dorsal and anterior nerve roots.

Because the dorsal nerve roots handle sensory function, the patient may experience tingling and numbness. Similarly, because the anterior nerve roots are responsible for motor function, impairment causes varying weakness, immobility, and paralysis.

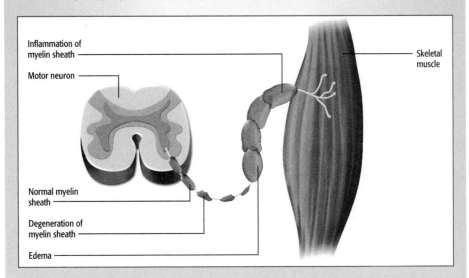

- Other neurologic problems include sensory loss, loss of position sense, and diminished or absent deep tendon reflexes.

Cardiovascular system
- Autonomic nervous system functioning may be affected, possibly leading to cardiac arrhythmias, tachycardia, bradycardia, hypertension, and postural hypotension.
- Vascular effects, primarily due to immobility from impaired motor function in conjunction with muscle weakness and paralysis, may lead to deep vein thrombosis.

Gastrointestinal system
- Swallowing may be impaired due to impaired cranial nerve function.
- Abdominal muscles are weakened because of nervous system dysfunction.

- Autonomic nervous system dysfunction can lead to decreased peristalsis, resulting in constipation. Bowel sphincter control may also be affected.

Integumentary system
- Immobility secondary to motor and sensory nerve dysfunction increases the risk of skin breakdown.

Musculoskeletal system
- Effects on the musculoskeletal system are directly related to the impaired motor function from ventral nerve root involvement.
- Impaired motor function leads to weakened muscles.
- Paralysis leads to a significant decrease in mobility. Joint pain and contractures may occur.

(*Text continues on page 156.*)

DISORDERS AFFECTING MANAGEMENT OF GUILLAIN-BARRÉ SYNDROME

This chart highlights disorders that affect the management of Guillain-Barré syndrome.

DISORDER	SIGNS AND SYMPTOMS	DIAGNOSTIC TEST RESULTS
Cardiac arrhythmias (complication)	◆ Palpitations ◆ Chest pain ◆ Dizziness ◆ Weakness, fatigue ◆ Irregular heart rhythm ◆ Hypotension ◆ Syncope ◆ Altered level of consciousness ◆ Diaphoresis ◆ Pallor ◆ Cold clammy skin	◆ 12-lead electrocardiography (ECG) identifies specific waveform changes associated with the arrhythmia. ◆ Laboratory testing reveals electrolyte abnormalities, hypoxemia, or acid-base abnormalities. ◆ Electrophysiologic testing identifies the mechanism of an arrhythmia and the location of accessory pathways.
Deep vein thrombosis (complication)	◆ Severe pain ◆ Fever ◆ Chills ◆ Malaise ◆ Swelling and cyanosis of the affected extremity ◆ Affected area possibly warm to the touch ◆ Positive Homans' sign (pain on dorsiflexion of the foot; false positives are common)	◆ Doppler ultrasonography identifies reduced blood flow to a specific area and any obstruction to venous flow, particularly in iliofemoral deep vein thrombophlebitis. ◆ Plethysmography shows decreased circulation distal to the affected area. ◆ Phlebography (also called *venography*), which usually confirms diagnosis, shows filling defects and diverted blood flow.
Respiratory failure (complication)	◆ Diminished chest movement ◆ Restlessness, irritability, confusion ◆ Decreasing level of consciousness ◆ Pallor, possible cyanosis ◆ Tachypnea, tachycardia (strong and rapid initially, but thready and irregular in later stages) ◆ Cold, clammy skin and frank diaphoresis, especially around the forehead and face ◆ Diminished breath sounds; possible adventitious breath sounds ◆ Possible cardiac arrhythmias	◆ Arterial blood gas (ABG) analysis shows a low partial pressure of arterial oxygen (usually less than 70 mm Hg), partial pressure of arterial carbon dioxide greater than 45 mm Hg, and a normal bicarbonate level, indicating early respiratory failure. ◆ Serial vital capacity is less than 800 mL. ◆ ECG may show arrhythmias. ◆ Pulse oximetry reveals a decreased oxygen saturation level. Mixed venous oxygen saturation levels less than 50% indicate impaired tissue oxygenation.

TREATMENT AND CARE

◆ Evaluate the patient's ECG regularly for arrhythmia and assess hemodynamic parameters as indicated. Document arrhythmias and notify the physician immediately.
◆ If the patient's pulse rate is abnormally rapid, slow, or irregular, watch for signs of hypoperfusion, such as hypotension and diminished urine output.
◆ Administer antiarrhythmics, and monitor for adverse effects.
◆ If a life-threatening arrhythmia develops, rapidly assess the patient's level of consciousness, pulse and respiratory rates, and hemodynamic parameters. Be alert for trends. Monitor EGG continuously. Be prepared to initiate cardiopulmonary resuscitation or cardioversion if indicated.
◆ Prepare for possible insertion of temporary pacemaker or implantable cardioverter-defibrillator if indicated.

◆ Administer anticoagulants, and monitor for adverse effects, such as bleeding, dark, tarry stools; coffee-ground vomitus, and ecchymoses.
◆ Assess pulses, skin color, and temperature of affected extremity and compare these findings with those of the unaffected extremity.
◆ Measure and record the circumference of the affected arm or leg daily. Compare this with the circumference of the other arm or leg.
◆ Maintain bed rest; use pillows for elevating the leg, placing them to support the entire length of the affected extremity and to prevent possible compression of the popliteal space.
◆ Perform range-of-motion exercises with unaffected extremities, and turn the patient every 2 hours.
◆ Apply warm soaks to improve circulation to the affected area and to relieve pain and inflammation. Give analgesics to relieve pain.
◆ Assess for signs of pulmonary emboli, such as crackles, dyspnea, hemoptysis, sudden changes in mental status, restlessness, and hypotension.

◆ Institute oxygen therapy immediately to optimize oxygenation of pulmonary blood.
◆ Prepare for endotracheal (ET) intubation and mechanical ventilation; anticipate the need for high-frequency or pressure ventilation to force airways open.
◆ Administer bronchodilators to open airways; corticosteroids to reduce inflammation; continuous I.V. solutions of positive inotropic agents to increase cardiac output; vasopressors to induce vasoconstriction to maintain blood pressure; and diuretics to reduce fluid overload and edema.
◆ Assess the patient's respiratory status at least every 2 hours, or more often as indicated. Observe for a positive response to oxygen therapy, such as improved breathing, color, and oximetry and ABG values.
◆ Position the patient for optimal breathing effort.
◆ Maintain a normothermic environment to reduce the patient's oxygen demand.
◆ Monitor vital signs, heart rhythm, and fluid intake and output.
◆ If intubated, auscultate the lungs to check for accidental intubation of the esophagus or the mainstem bronchus. Be alert for aspiration, broken teeth, nosebleeds, and vagal reflexes causing bradycardia, arrhythmias, and hypotension.
◆ Perform suctioning using strict aseptic technique when intubated.
◆ Monitor oximetry and capnography values to detect important indicators of changes in the patient's condition.
◆ Note the amount and quality of lung secretions and look for changes in the patient's status.
◆ Check cuff pressure on the ET tube to prevent erosion from an overinflated cuff.
◆ Implement measures to prevent nasal tissue necrosis. Position and maintain the nasotracheal tube midline in the nostrils and reposition daily. Tape the tube securely but use skin protection measures and nonirritating tape to prevent skin breakdown.
◆ Provide a means of communication for patients who are intubated and alert.

Respiratory system

- Paralysis of the internal and external intercostal muscles leads to a reduction in functional breathing.
- Vagus nerve paralysis causes a loss of the protective mechanisms that respond to brachial irritation and foreign bodies and a diminished or absent gag reflex.
- Immobility due to impaired motor function can lead to retained secretions, atelectasis, and pneumonia.

Urinary system

- Motor and sensory nerve dysfunction may lead to impaired bladder muscle tone and sphincter muscle function, possibly affecting urinary elimination.
- Autonomic nervous system dysfunction can lead to urine retention and loss of urinary sphincter control.

ASSESSMENT

The clinical course of Guillain-Barré syndrome has three phases. The *acute phase* begins when the first definitive symptom develops; it ends 1 to 3 weeks later, when no further deterioration is noted. The *plateau phase* lasts 1 to 2 weeks and is followed by the *recovery phase* (which is believed to coincide with remyelination and axonal process regrowth) extends over 4 to 6 months. However, patients with severe disease may take up to 2 to 3 years to recover (some patients never fully recover).

Most patients seek treatment when Guillain-Barré syndrome is in the acute stage. The patient's history typically reveals that he has experienced a minor febrile illness 1 to 4 weeks before his current symptoms. The patient may report feelings of tingling and numbness (paresthesia) in the legs. If the syndrome has progressed further, he may report that the tingling and numbness began in his legs and progressed to the arms, trunk and, finally, the face. The paresthesia usually precedes muscle weakness but tends to vanish quickly; in some patients, it may never occur. Some patients may also report stiffness and pain in the calves (such as a severe charley horse) and back.

RED FLAG *Guillain-Barré syndrome progresses rapidly. Symptoms may progress beyond the legs in 24 to 72 hours. Muscle weakness sometimes develops in the arms first (descending type), rather than in the legs (ascending type) — or in the arms and legs simultaneously. In milder forms of the syndrome, muscle weakness may affect only the cranial nerves or may not occur at all.*

Clinical findings

- Muscle weakness and sensory loss, usually in the legs and — if the syndrome has progressed — in the arms
- Difficulty talking, chewing, and swallowing
- Possible paralysis of the ocular, facial, and oropharyngeal muscles
- Possible loss of position sense and diminished or absent deep tendon reflexes
- Diplegia, possibly with ophthalmoplegia (ocular paralysis), from impaired motor nerve root transmission and involvement of cranial nerves III, IV and VI
- Dysphagia or dysarthria and, less commonly, weakness of the muscles supplied by cranial nerve XI (spinal accessory nerve)
- Hypotonia and areflexia from interruption of the reflex arc

Diagnostic test results

- *Cerebrospinal fluid (CSF)* analysis may show a normal white blood cell count, an elevated protein count, and, in severe disease, increased CSF pressure.
- *Electromyography* may demonstrate repeated firing of the same motor unit instead of widespread sectional stimulation.
- *Electrophysiologic testing* may reveal marked slowing of nerve conduction velocities.
- *Serum immunoglobulin levels* are elevated.

COLLABORATIVE MANAGEMENT

A neurologist is needed to evaluate the extent of nerve involvement. Pulmonary and respiratory specialists can help with clearing secretions and maintaining ventilation. The patient may require a physical therapist to help maintain joint range-of-motion, an occupational therapist to assist with activities of daily living, and a registered dietitian to maintain nutrition. Social services may be involved to assist with continued care and follow-up and help with financial concerns and community support. A spiritual counselor or pastoral care associate may also be called upon to help the patient and his family to cope.

TREATMENT AND CARE

■ Treatment is primarily supportive and may require endotracheal intubation or tracheotomy if the patient has difficulty clearing secretions.

■ Mechanical ventilation is necessary if the patient has respiratory difficulties.

■ Continuous electrocardiogram monitoring is necessary to identify cardiac arrhythmias.

■ Pharmacologic therapy may include propranolol to treat tachycardia and hypotension and atropine to treat bradycardia.

■ Marked hypotension may require volume replacement.

■ A trial dose (7 days) of prednisone may be given to reduce inflammatory response if the disease is relentlessly progressive; if prednisone produces no noticeable improvement, the drug is discontinued.

■ Plasmapheresis produces a temporary reduction in circulating antibodies. It's most effective when performed during the first few weeks of the disease. The patient may receive three to five plasma exchanges.

■ Immune globulin may be administered I.V. if plasmapheresis fails or isn't available.

■ Meticulous skin care prevents skin breakdown and contractures. Maintain a strict turning schedule, with skin inspection (especially sacrum, heels, and ankles) for breakdown, and repositioning every 2 hours. Use alternating pressure pads at points of contact.

■ Perform passive range-of-motion exercises within the patient's pain limits (proximal muscle group of the thighs, shoulders, and trunk are the most tender and cause the most pain on passive movement and turning), possibly using a Hubbard tank. When the patient's condition stabilizes, perform gentle stretching and active assistance exercises.

■ Administer analgesics to relieve muscle stiffness and spasm.

■ Test the patient's gag reflex and elevate the head of the bed before giving him anything to eat. If the gag reflex is absent, use nasogastric feedings until the reflex returns.

■ Frequently assess vital signs. As the patient regains strength and can tolerate a vertical position, monitor for postural hypotension.

■ Inspect the patient's legs for signs of thrombophlebitis (localized pain, tenderness, erythema, edema, positive Homans' sign). Use antiembolism stockings and possible prophylactic anticoagulants to prevent thrombophlebitis.

■ Provide mouth and eye care every 4 hours if the patient has facial paralysis; use isotonic eye drops and eye shields to protect the corneas.

■ Assess for urine retention: Measure and record intake and output every 8 hours; offer the bedpan every 3 to 4 hours; and encourage adequate fluid intake (2 qt/day [2 L/day]). If urine retention develops, use intermittent catheterization.

■ Increase the patient's fiber intake to prevent and relieve constipation. Administer daily or alternate-day suppositories (glycerin or bisacodyl) or enemas.

■ Offer diversional activities and emotional support.

H–K

Heart failure

Heart failure is a syndrome characterized by myocardial dysfunction that leads to impaired pump performance (diminished cardiac output) or to frank heart failure and abnormal circulatory congestion. Congestion of systemic venous circulation may result in peripheral edema or hepatomegaly; congestion of pulmonary circulation may cause pulmonary edema, an acute life-threatening emergency.

Although heart failure may be acute (as a direct result of myocardial infarction or infection), it's generally a chronic disorder associated with sodium and water retention by the kidneys. Advances in diagnostic and therapeutic techniques have greatly improved the outlook for patients with heart failure, but the prognosis still depends on the underlying cause and its response to treatment.

Chronic heart failure may worsen as a result of respiratory tract infections, pulmonary embolism, stress, increased sodium or water intake, or failure to adhere to the prescribed treatment regimen. Heart failure affects about two people out of every 100 between ages 27 and 74. It becomes more common with advancing age.

ETIOLOGY
Causes of heart failure can be divided into four general categories. (See *Causes of heart failure.*)

PATHOPHYSIOLOGY
Pump failure usually occurs in a damaged left ventricle (left-sided heart failure) but may occur in the right ventricle (right-sided heart failure) as a primary disorder or secondary to left-sided heart failure. Sometimes, left- and right-sided heart failure de-

velop simultaneously. (See *What happens in heart failure,* pages 160 and 161.)

Cardiovascular system
■ In left-sided heart failure, the pumping ability of the left ventricle fails and cardiac output falls. Blood backs up into the right atrium.
■ With right-sided heart failure, the right ventricle becomes stressed and hypertrophies, leading to increased conduction time and arrhythmias.

Gastrointestinal system
■ Congestion of the peripheral tissues leads to GI tract congestion and anorexia, GI distress, and weight loss.
■ Liver failure can occur as a result of blood backing up into the peripheral circulation and subsequent engorgement of organs. (See *Disorders affecting management of heart failure,* pages 162 and 163.)

Renal system
■ With right-sided heart failure, blood backs up into the right atrium and the peripheral circulation. The patient gains weight and develops peripheral edema and engorgement of the kidney and other organs.

Respiratory system
■ As blood backs up into the right atrium (because the hearts pumping ability has failed), blood backs into the lungs, causing pulmonary congestion.

ASSESSMENT
The patient will present with a disorder or condition that can predispose him to heart failure. He may complain of fatigue, dyspnea or paroxysmal nocturnal dyspnea, peripheral edema, insomnia, weakness, anorexia, nausea, and a sense of abdominal fullness (particularly in right-sided heart failure).

CAUSES OF HEART FAILURE

CAUSE	EXAMPLES
Abnormal cardiac muscle function	◆ Myocardial infarction ◆ Cardiomyopathy
Abnormal left ventricular volume	◆ Valvular insufficiency ◆ High-output states: – chronic anemia – ateriovenous fistula – thyrotoxicosis – pregnancy – septicemia – beriberi – infusion of large volume of intravenous fluids in a short time period
Abnormal left ventricular pressure	◆ Hypertension ◆ Pulmonary hypertension ◆ Chronic obstructive pulmonary disease ◆ Aortic or pulmonic valve stenosis
Abnormal left ventricular filling	◆ Mitral valve stenosis ◆ Tricuspid valve stenosis ◆ Atrial myxoma ◆ Constrictive pericarditis ◆ Atrial fibrillation ◆ Impaired ventricular relaxation: – hypertension – myocardial hibernation – myocardial stunning

Clinical findings

■ Cough that produces pink, frothy sputum
■ Cyanosis of the lips and nail beds
■ Pale, cool, clammy skin
■ Jugular vein distention
■ Diaphoresis
■ Ascites
■ Tachycardia
■ Pulsus alternans
■ Hepatomegaly and possibly hepatomegaly
■ Decreased pulse pressure
■ Third (S_3) and fourth (S_4) heart sounds
■ Moist, bibasilar crackles, rhonchi, and expiratory wheezing

Diagnostic test results

■ *B-type natriuretic peptide immunoassay* is elevated.

■ *Chest X-ray* shows increased pulmonary vascular markings, interstitial edema, or pleural effusions and cardiomegaly.
■ *Electrocardiography* reveals heart enlargement or ischemia, tachycardia, extrasystole, or atrial fibrillation.
■ *Pulmonary artery pressure, pulmonary artery wedge pressure,* and *left ventricular end-diastolic pressure* are elevated in the presence of left-sided heart failure; *right atrial* or *central venous pressure* is elevated in right-sided heart failure.
■ *Laboratory testing* may reveal abnormal liver function tests and elevated blood urea nitrogen and creatinine levels.
■ *Arterial blood gas levels* may reveal hypoxemia from impaired gas exchange and respiratory alkalosis secondary to patient's blowing off more carbon dioxide as respiratory rate rises in compensation.

WHAT HAPPENS IN HEART FAILURE

These step-by-step illustrations show what happens when myocardial damage leads to heart failure.

Left-sided heart failure

Increased workload and end-diastolic volume enlarge the left ventricle. Because of the lack of oxygen, however, the ventricle enlarges with stretched tissue rather than functional tissue. The patient may experience increased heart rate, pale and cool tingling in the extremities, decreased cardiac output, and arrhythmias.

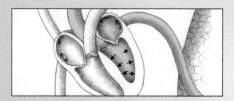

Diminished left ventricular function allows blood to pool in the ventricle and the atrium and eventually back up into the pulmonary veins and capillaries. The patient may experience dyspnea on exertion, confusion, dizziness, postural hypotension, decreased peripheral pulses and pulse pressure, cyanosis, and an S_3 gallop.

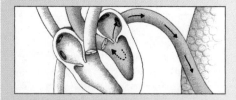

As the pulmonary circulation becomes engorged, rising capillary pressure pushes sodium (Na) and water (H_2O) into the interstitial space, causing pulmonary edema. Note coughing, subclavian retractions, crackles, tachypnea, elevated pulmonary artery pressure, diminished pulmonary compliance, and increased partial pressure of carbon dioxide.

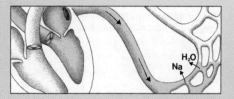

When the patient lies down, fluid in the extremities moves into systemic circulation. Because the left ventricle can't handle the increased venous return, fluid pools in the pulmonary circulation, worsening pulmonary edema. You may note decreased breath sounds, dullness on percussion, crackles, and orthopnea.

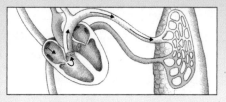

The right ventricle may now become stressed because it's pumping against greater pulmonary vascular resistance and left ventricular pressure. When this occurs, the patient's symptoms worsen.

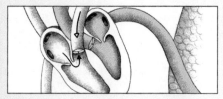

Right-sided heart failure

The stressed right ventricle hypertrophies with the formation of stretched tissue. Increasing conduction time and deviation of the heart from its normal axis can cause arrhythmias. If the patient doesn't already have left-sided heart failure, he may experience increased heart rate, cool skin, cyanosis, decreased cardiac output, palpitations, and dyspnea.

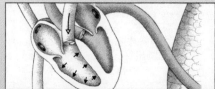

■ *Echocardiography* may reveal left ventricular hypertrophy, dilation, and abnormal contractility.

■ *Radionuclide ventriculography* may reveal an ejection fraction less than 40%; in diastolic dysfunction, the ejection fraction may be normal.

COLLABORATIVE MANAGEMENT

Multidisciplinary care is needed to determine the underlying cause and precipitating factors and may include the expertise of a respiratory therapist, a dietician and a physical therapist. Surgery may be indicated for the patient with coronary artery disease or one experiencing severe limitations or recurrent hospitalizations despite maximal medical treatment. Social services may be necessary to help the patient's transition to his home setting after the acute situation is resolved.

TREATMENT AND CARE

The aim of treatment is to improve pump function and may involve:

■ correction of the underlying cause, if known

■ angiotensin-converting enzyme inhibitors for patients with left ventricle dysfunction to reduce production of angiotensin II (resulting in preload and afterload reduction)

■ digoxin for patients with heart failure due to left ventricular systolic dysfunction to increase myocardial contractility, improve cardiac output, reduce the volume of the ventricle, and decrease ventricular stretch

■ diuretics to reduce fluid volume overload, venous return, and preload

■ beta-adrenergic blockers in patients with mild to moderate heart failure caused by left ventricular systolic dysfunction to prevent remodeling

■ diuretics, nitrates, morphine, and oxygen to treat pulmonary edema

■ lifestyle modifications (to reduce symptoms of heart failure) such as weight loss (if obese); limited sodium (to 3 g/day) and alcohol intake; reduced fat intake; smoking cessation; reduced stress; and development of a moderate exercise program.

■ coronary artery bypass surgery or angioplasty for heart failure due to coronary artery disease

(*Text continues on page 164.*)

Blood pools in the right ventricle and right atrium. The backed-up blood causes pressure and congestion in the vena cava and systemic circulation. The patient has elevated central venous pressure, jugular vein distention, and hepatojugular reflux.

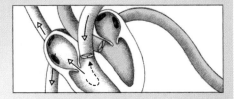

Backed-up blood also distends the visceral veins, especially the hepatic vein. As the liver and spleen become engorged, their function is impaired. The patient may develop anorexia, nausea, abdominal pain, palpable liver and spleen, weakness, and dyspnea secondary to abdominal distention.

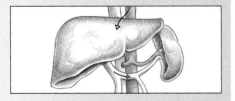

Increasing capillary pressure forces excess fluid from the capillaries into the interstitial space. This causes tissue edema, especially in the lower extremities and abdomen. The patient may experience weight gain, pitting edema, and nocturia.

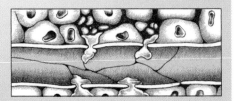

DISORDERS AFFECTING
MANAGEMENT OF HEART FAILURE

This chart highlights disorders that affect the management of heart failure.

DISORDER	SIGNS AND SYMPTOMS	DIAGNOSTIC TEST RESULTS
Pulmonary edema (complication)	◆ Restlessness and anxiety ◆ Rapid, labored breathing ◆ Intense, productive cough ◆ Frothy, bloody sputum ◆ Mental status changes ◆ Jugular vein distention ◆ Wheezing ◆ Crackles ◆ Third heart sound (S_3) ◆ Tachycardia ◆ Hypotension ◆ Thready pulse ◆ Peripheral edema ◆ Hepatomegaly	◆ Arterial blood gas (ABG) analysis shows hypoxemia, hypercapnia, or acidosis. ◆ Chest X-ray shows diffuse haziness of the lung fields, cardiomegaly, and pleural effusion. ◆ Pulse oximetry may reveal decreased oxygenation of the blood. ◆ Pulmonary artery catheterization may reveal increased pulmonary artery wedge pressures. ◆ Electrocardiogram (ECG) may show valvular disease and left ventricular hypokinesis or akinesis.
Renal failure (complication)	◆ Oliguria (initially) ◆ Azotemia ◆ Electrolyte imbalance ◆ Metabolic acidosis ◆ Anorexia, nausea, and vomiting ◆ Diarrhea or constipation ◆ Dry mucous membranes ◆ Headache ◆ Confusion ◆ Seizures ◆ Drowsiness ◆ Irritability ◆ Coma ◆ Dry skin ◆ Pruritus ◆ Pallor ◆ Purpura ◆ Uremic frost ◆ Hypotension (early) ◆ Hypertension with arrhythmias (later) ◆ Fluid overload ◆ Heart failure ◆ Systemic edema ◆ Anemia ◆ Altered clotting mechanisms ◆ Pulmonary edema ◆ Kussmaul's respirations	◆ Blood urea nitrogen, serum creatinine, and potassium levels are elevated. ◆ Bicarbonate level, hematocrit, hemoglobin, and pH are decreased. ◆ Urine studies show casts, cellular debris, decreased specific gravity; in glomerular diseases proteinuria and urine osmolality close to serum osmolality; urine sodium level is less than 20 mEq/L if oliguria results from decreased perfusion, and more than 40 mEq/L if the cause is intrarenal. ◆ Creatinine clearance tests reveal the number of remaining functioning nephrons. ◆ ECG shows tall, peaked T waves; widening QRS; and disappearing P waves if hyperkalemia is present. ◆ Ultrasonography, abdominal and kidney-ureter-bladder X-rays, excretory urography, renal scan, retrograde pyelography, computed tomography, nephrotomography reveal abnormalities of the urinary tract.

TREATMENT AND CARE

- Identify and attempt to correct or manage the underlying disease.
- Closely monitor for changes in the patient's respiratory status.
- Institute energy conservation strategies; plan activities as dictated by respiratory ability.
- Provide supplemental oxygen and mechanical ventilation.
- Implement fluid and sodium restriction.
- Monitor intake and output.
- Implement cardiac monitoring.
- Administer antiarrhythmics, diuretics, preload and afterload reducing agents, bronchodilators, and vasopressors.
- Maintain adequate cardiac output.
- Weigh the patient daily.
- Monitor pulse oximetry, ABG, and hemodynamic values.

- Measure input and output, including body fluids, nasogastric output, and diarrhea. Weigh the patient daily.
- Measure hemoglobin and hematocrit and replace blood components.
- Monitor vital signs; check and report for signs of pericarditis (pleuritic chest pain, tachycardia, pericardial friction rub), inadequate renal perfusion (hypotension), and acidosis.
- Maintain proper electrolyte balance. Monitor potassium levels and monitor the patient for hyperkalemia (malaise, anorexia, paresthesia or muscle weakness) and ECG changes.
- Administer diuretics.
- If the patient receives hypertonic glucose and insulin infusions, monitor potassium and glucose levels. If giving sodium polystyrene sulfonate rectally, make sure the patient doesn't retain it and become constipated (to prevent bowel perforation).
- Maintain nutritional status with a high-calorie, low-protein, low-sodium, and low-potassium diet and vitamin supplements.
- Monitor the patient carefully during peritoneal dialysis.
- If the patient requires hemodialysis, monitor the venous access site carefully, and assess the patient and laboratory work carefully.

- cardiac transplantation in patients receiving aggressive medical treatment but still experiencing limitations or repeated hospitalizations
- other surgery or invasive procedures for patients with severe limitations or repeated hospitalizations, despite maximal medical therapy.

Hepatitis

Viral hepatitis is a fairly common systemic disease. It's marked by hepatic cell destruction, necrosis, and autolysis, leading to anorexia, jaundice, and hepatomegaly. In most patients, hepatic cells eventually regenerate with little or no residual damage, allowing recovery. However, old age and serious underlying disorders make complications more likely. The prognosis is poor if edema and hepatic encephalopathy develop.

More than 70,000 cases of hepatitis are reported annually in the United States. Six types of viral hepatitis are recognized, and a seventh is suspected.

ETIOLOGY

The six major forms of viral hepatitis — A, B, C, D, E, and G — result from infection with the causative viruses.

Type A hepatitis is highly contagious and is usually transmitted by the fecal-oral route, commonly within institutions or families. It may also be transmitted parenterally. Hepatitis A usually results from ingestion of contaminated food, milk, or water. Outbreaks of this type are commonly traced to ingestion of seafood from polluted water.

Type B hepatitis, once thought to be transmitted only by the direct exchange of contaminated blood, is now known to be transmitted also by contact with contaminated human secretions and stools. As a result, nurses, physicians, laboratory technicians, and dentists are frequently exposed to type B hepatitis, typically as a result of wearing defective gloves. Transmission of this type also occurs during intimate sexual contact and through perinatal transmission.

Type C hepatitis is a blood-borne illness transmitted primarily by sharing of needles by I.V. drug users and through blood transfusions. This causes 80% of post-transfusion hepatitis. Although it seldom causes an acute disease, 90% of infected persons develop chronic infection. This type was formerly labeled *non-A, non-B hepatitis.*

Type D hepatitis is found only in patients with an acute or a chronic episode of hepatitis B. Type D infection requires the presence of the hepatitis B surface antigen; the type D virus depends on the double-shelled type B virus to replicate. For this reason, type D infection can't outlast a type B infection.

Type E hepatitis is transmitted enterically and is commonly waterborne. Because this virus is inconsistently shed in stools, detection is difficult. Outbreaks of type E hepatitis have occurred in developing countries.

Type G hepatitis is a newly identified virus. It's thought to be blood-borne, with transmission similar to that of type C hepatitis.

Hepatitis may also be caused by bacteria, toxins, and autoimmune destruction of the liver. Toxic hepatitis results from hepatic injury secondary to exposure to various agents — predominantly drugs, alcohol, industrial toxins, and certain plants. Drugs known to be hepatotoxins include acetaminophen, diazepam, erythromycin, antitubercular medications, anticonvulsants, 6-mercaptopurine, and antifungals. Other hepatotoxic agents include carbon tetrachloride, toluene, and mushrooms.

Autoimmune hepatitis is associated with high serum globulin levels and autoantibodies. The exact cause of this form is unknown. Diagnosis can be difficult because symptoms are usually vague. Autoimmune hepatitis commonly progresses to cirrhosis.

PATHOPHYSIOLOGY

Hepatic damage is usually similar in all types of viral hepatitis; however, varying degrees of cell injury and necrosis can occur.

On entering the body, the virus causes hepatocyte injury and cell death, either by directly killing the cells or by activating inflammatory and immune reactions. The inflammatory and immune reactions will, in turn, injure or destroy hepatocytes by lysing the infected or neighboring cells. Later, direct antibody attack against viral antigens causes further destruction of the infected cells. Edema and swelling of the interstitium lead to collapse of capillaries and decreased blood flow, tissue hypoxia, and scarring and fibrosis.

Neurologic system

■ Hepatic encephalopathy develops when the liver can no longer detoxify the blood. Liver dysfunction and collateral vessels that shunt blood around the liver to the systemic circulation permit toxins absorbed from the GI tract to circulate freely to the brain. The normal liver transforms ammonia (a by-product of protein metabolism) to urea, which the kidneys then excrete. When the liver fails, ammonia blood levels rise and circulate to the brain, causing encephalopathic damage.

■ Short-chain fatty acids, serotonin, tryptophan, and false neurotransmitters may accumulate in the blood and contribute to hepatic encephalopathy. (See *Recognizing asterixis*. See also *Disorders affecting management of hepatitis*, pages 166 to 169.)

Renal system

■ Accumulation of vasoactive substances or a compensatory response to portal hypertension and the pooling of blood in the splenic circulation may lead to decreased glomerular filatration, oliguria, and hepatorenal syndrome (renal failure concurrent with liver disease; the kidneys appear normal but abruptly cease functioning).

■ Hepatorenal syndrome causes expanded blood volume, accumulation of hydrogen ions, and electrolyte disturbances.

ASSESSMENT

Assessment findings are similar for the different types of hepatitis.

Clinical findings

Typically, signs and symptoms progress in several stages.

Prodromal (preicteric) stage

■ Fatigue and anorexia (possibly with mild weight loss)
■ Generalized malaise
■ Depression
■ Headache
■ Weakness
■ Arthralgia

RECOGNIZING ASTERIXIS

With asterixis, the patient's wrists and fingers are observed to "flap" because there is a brief, rapid relaxation of dorsiflexion of the wrist.

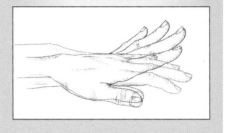

■ Myalgia
■ Photophobia
■ Nausea with vomiting
■ Changes in senses of taste and smell
■ Temperature of 100° to 102° F (37.8° to 38.9° C)
■ Dark-colored urine and clay-colored stools (usually 1 to 5 days before the onset of the clinical jaundice stage)

Clinical jaundice stage

■ Pruritus
■ Abdominal pain or tenderness
■ Indigestion
■ Anorexia (early; appetite may return)
■ Jaundiced sclerae, mucous membranes, and skin (hepatitis occasionally occurs without jaundice)
■ Rashes, erythematous patches, or urticaria (especially if the patient has type B or C hepatitis)
■ Enlarged and tender liver on palpation
■ Splenomegaly and cervical adenopathy (in some cases)
■ Asterixis

Diagnostic test results

■ A *hepatitis profile* identifies antibodies specific to the causative virus, establishing the type of hepatitis.
■ *Serum aspartate aminotransferase* and *serum alanine aminotransferase* levels are increased in the prodromal stage of acute viral hepatitis.

(*Text continues on page 168.*)

DISORDERS AFFECTING
MANAGEMENT OF HEPATITIS

This chart highlights disorders that affect the management of hepatitis.

DISORDER	SIGNS AND SYMPTOMS	DIAGNOSTIC TEST RESULTS
Hepatic encephalopathy (complication)	◆ Jaundice ◆ Nausea and anorexia ◆ Abdominal pain or tenderness ◆ Fatigue and weight loss ◆ Pruritus ◆ Oliguria ◆ Splenomegaly ◆ Ascites ◆ Peripheral edema ◆ Esophageal varices ◆ Bleeding tendencies ◆ Petechiae *Prodromal stage (Grade I)* ◆ Personality changes such as agitation, belligerence, disorientation, and forgetfulness ◆ Fatigue ◆ Drowsiness ◆ Slurred or slow speech ◆ Slight tremor *Impending stage (Grade II)* ◆ Confusion ◆ Disoriented to time, place, and person ◆ Asterixis (liver flap, flapping tremor) *Stuporous stage (Grade III)* ◆ Marked mental confusion ◆ Drowsiness ◆ Stupor ◆ Hyperventilation ◆ Muscle twitching ◆ Asterixis *Comatose stage (Grade IV)* ◆ Fetor hepaticus (musty odor of breath and urine) ◆ Seizures ◆ Hyperactive reflexes ◆ Coma	◆ Liver function tests reveal elevated levels of aspartate aminotransferase, alanine aminotransferase, alkaline phosphatase, and bilirubin. ◆ Blood studies reveal anemia, impaired red blood cell production, elevated bleeding and clotting times, low platelet levels, low blood glucose levels, low albumin, decreased blood urea nitrogen (BUN), and increased serum ammonia levels. ◆ Serum electrolyte studies commonly reveal hyponatremia and hypokalemia in patients with ascites. ◆ Urinalysis reveals increased urobilinogen, bilirubin, and osmolarity. ◆ Electroencephalogram is typically abnormal with hepatic encephalopathy, but the changes are nonspecific.
Renal failure (complication)	◆ Altered urinary elimination (oliguria or anuria) ◆ Irritability, drowsiness, or confusion ◆ Altered level of consciousness ◆ Dry, pruritic skin ◆ Infection related to an altered immune status ◆ Hematuria, petechiae, and ecchymosis related to bleeding abnormalities	◆ Blood studies show elevated BUN, serum creatinine, and potassium levels. Bicarbonate level, hematocrit, hemoglobin, and acid pH are decreased. ◆ Urine studies show casts, cellular debris, and decreased specific gravity.

TREATMENT AND CARE

◆ Frequently assess and record the patient's level of consciousness. Continually orient him to place and time. Remember to keep a daily record of the patient's handwriting to monitor the progression of neurologic involvement.
◆ Promote rest, comfort, and a quiet atmosphere.
◆ Monitor intake, output, and fluid and electrolyte balance. Check the patient's weight, and measure abdominal girth daily. Watch for and immediately report signs of anemia (decreased hemoglobin), alkalosis (increased serum bicarbonate), GI bleeding (melena, hematemesis), and infection. Monitor the patient's serum ammonia level.
◆ Administer lactulose, neomycin, potassium supplements, and salt-poor albumin. Monitor the patient for the desired effects, and watch for adverse reactions.
◆ Provide a low-protein diet, with carbohydrates supplying most of the calories. Provide good mouth care. Provide parenteral nutrition to the semicomatose or comatose patient.
◆ Use appropriate safety measures to protect the patient from injury. Avoid physical restraints, if possible.
◆ Provide emotional support for the patient's family during the terminal stage of encephalopathy.

◆ Measure and record intake and output of all fluids.
◆ Follow standard precautions.
◆ Weigh the patient and measure his abdominal girth daily.
◆ Assess hematocrit and hemoglobin levels and replace blood components.
◆ Monitor vital signs. Watch for and report signs of pericarditis (pleuritic chest pain, tachycardia, and pericardial friction rub), inadequate renal perfusion (hypotension), and acidosis.

(continued)

DISORDERS AFFECTING
MANAGEMENT OF HEPATITIS *(continued)*

DISORDER	SIGNS AND SYMPTOMS	DIAGNOSTIC TEST RESULTS
Renal failure *(continued)*	◆ Fatigue, dyspnea, and malaise related to anemia ◆ Anorexia, nausea, and vomiting ◆ Edema related to fluid retention ◆ Tachycardia ◆ Bibasilar crackles ◆ Uremic breath odor ◆ Hypertension or hypotension depending on the stage of acute renal failure ◆ Dry mucous membranes	*In glomerular disease* ◆ Urine studies show proteinuria and a urine osmolality close to the serum osmolality. ◆ A creatinine clearance test reveals the number of functioning nephrons and measures the glomerular filtration rate. ◆ An electrocardiogram shows tall, peaked T waves; widening QRS complex; and disappearing P waves if hyperkalemia is present. ◆ Ultrasonography, abdominal and kidney-ureter-bladder X-rays, excretory urography, renal scan, retrograde pyelography, computerized tomography, and nephrotomography reveal abnormalities of the urinary tract.

■ *Serum alkaline phosphatase levels* are slightly increased.

■ *Serum bilirubin levels* are elevated. Levels may continue to be high late in the disease, especially if the patient has severe disease.

■ *Prothrombin time* is prolonged (more than 3 seconds longer than normal indicates severe liver damage).

■ *White blood cell counts* commonly reveal transient neutropenia and lymphopenia followed by lymphocytosis.

■ *Liver biopsy* is performed if chronic hepatitis is suspected. (This study is performed for acute hepatitis only if the diagnosis is questionable.)

■ *Serum toxicology* identifies a hepatotoxic agent.

■ *Laboratory studies* reveal the presence of antinuclear antibodies and antimitochondrial antibodies in autoimmune hepatitis.

COLLABORATIVE MANAGEMENT

Depending on the severity of the disease and the organ involvement, neurologists and nephrologists may be consulted. The patient and his family may benefit from supportive counseling and a referral for social services.

TREATMENT AND CARE

■ Persons believed to have been exposed to hepatitis A and the household contacts of patients with confirmed cases should be treated with standard immunoglobulin.

■ Travelers planning visits to areas known to harbor such viruses should receive hepatitis A vaccine.

■ Hepatitis B globulin is given to individuals exposed to blood or body secretions of infected individuals.

■ Hepatitis B vaccine should be given to people at risk for exposure. This group includes neonates of infected mothers, sexual contacts of infected individuals, hemodialysis patients, health care workers, and male homosexuals.

■ There's no vaccine against hepatitis C, but it has been treated with alfa interferon.

■ In the early stages of the disease, the patient is advised to rest and combat anorexia by eating small, high-calorie, high-protein meals. (Protein intake should be reduced if signs of precoma, such as lethargy, confusion, and mental changes, develop.) Large meals are usually better tolerated in the morning because many patients experience nausea late in the day.

◆ Maintain proper electrolyte balance. Strictly monitor potassium levels. Watch for symptoms of hyperkalemia. Avoid administering medications that contain potassium.

◆ If the patient receives hypertonic glucose and insulin infusions, monitor potassium and glucose levels. If you give sodium polystyrene sulfonate rectally, make sure the patient doesn't retain it and become constipated. This can lead to bowel perforation.

◆ Provide a diet high in calories and low in protein, sodium, and potassium, with vitamin supplements.

◆ Encourage frequent coughing and deep breathing; perform passive range-of-motion exercises.

◆ Provide mouth care frequently to lubricate dry mucous membranes.

◆ Test all stools for occult blood.

◆ Provide meticulous perineal care.

◆ Use appropriate safety measures, such as side rails and restraints.

◆ Anticipate the need for peritoneal dialysis or hemodialysis.

◆ Administer medications after hemodialysis is completed. Many medications are removed from the blood during treatment.

◆ Administer diuretics.

■ In acute viral hepatitis, hospitalization is usually required only for those patients with severe symptoms or complications.

■ Parenteral nutrition may be required if the patient has persistent vomiting and is unable to maintain oral intake.

■ Antiemetics (trimethobenzamide or benzquinamide) may be administered 30 minutes before meals to relieve nausea and prevent vomiting; phenothiazines have a cholestatic effect and should be avoided.

■ For severe pruritus, the resin cholestyramine, which sequesters bile salts, may be administered.

DRUG ALERT *Most medications are metabolized in the liver; therefore, only essential drugs should be administered to the patient with hepatitis.*

■ For toxic hepatitis, the hepatotoxic agent is identified, and an antidote (if available) is administered. Acetylcysteine (Mucomyst) is administered for acetaminophen toxicity. Gastric lavage may also be used. Corticosteroids are used to manage autoimmune hepatitis.

■ Patients require education on how to prevent exposure to known hepatotoxins such as dry cleaning fluids and excessive amounts of acetaminophen.

■ Patients receiving drugs known to have hepatotoxic potential should have liver functions tests monitored.

Hepatic failure

Hepatic failure is the possible end result of any liver disease, and prognosis is generally poor. The only cure for hepatic failure is a liver transplant.

ETIOLOGY

Hepatic failure can be caused by nonviral hepatitis, viral hepatitis, cirrhosis, or liver cancer.

PATHOPHYSIOLOGY

When the liver fails, a complex syndrome involving impairment of many organs and body functions ensues. (See *Disorders affecting management of hepatic failure*, pages 170 and 171.)

Neurologic system

■ Hepatic encephalopathy develops when the liver can no longer detoxify the blood.

(*Text continues on page 172.*)

DISORDERS AFFECTING
MANAGEMENT OF HEPATIC FAILURE

This chart highlights disorders that affect the management of hepatic failure.

DISORDER	SIGNS AND SYMPTOMS	DIAGNOSTIC TEST RESULTS
GI hemorrhage (complication)	◆ Anxiety ◆ Agitation ◆ Confusion ◆ Tachycardia ◆ Hypotension ◆ Oliguria ◆ Diaphoresis ◆ Pallor ◆ Cool, clammy skin ◆ Hematochezia ◆ Hematemesis ◆ Melena	◆ Upper GI endoscopy reveals the source of bleeding, such as an ulcer, esophageal varice, or Mallory-Weiss tear. ◆ Colonoscopy reveals the source of bleeding, such as polyps. ◆ Complete blood count reveals a decrease in hemoglobin level and hematocrit (usually 6 to 8 hours after the initial symptoms) and the amount of blood lost (hematocrit may be normal initially, but then drops dramatically), increased reticulocyte and platelet levels, and decreased red blood cell count. ◆ Arterial blood gas (ABG) studies reveal low pH and bicarbonate levels, indicating lactic acidosis from massive hemorrhage and possible hypoxemia. ◆ A 12-lead electrocardiogram (ECG) may reveal evidence of cardiac ischemia secondary to hypoperfusion. ◆ Abdominal X-ray may indicate air under the diaphragm, suggesting ulcer perforation. ◆ Angiography may aid in visualizing the site of bleeding.
Renal failure (complication)	◆ Initially oliguria ◆ Electrolyte imbalance ◆ Metabolic acidosis ◆ Nausea, vomiting ◆ Dry mucous membranes ◆ Headache ◆ Confusion ◆ Seizures ◆ Drowsiness ◆ Irritability ◆ Dry, pruretic skin ◆ Uremic breath odor ◆ Hypotension (early) ◆ Hypertension with arrhythmias (later) ◆ Systemic edema ◆ Pulmonary edema ◆ Kussmaul's respirations ◆ Tachycardia ◆ Bibasilar crackles ◆ Altered level of consciousness	◆ Blood urean nitrogen, serum creatinine, and potassium levels are elevated. ◆ Bicarbonate level, hematocrit, hemoglobin, and pH are decreased. ◆ Urine studies show casts, cellular debris, decreased specific gravity; in glomerular diseases proteinuria and urine osmolality close to serum osmolality; urine sodium level less than 20 mEq/L if oliguria results from decreased perfusion, and more than 40 mEq/L if the cause is intrarenal. ◆ Creatinine clearance tests reveal the number of remaining functioning nephrons. ◆ ECG shows tall, peaked T waves; widening QRS; and disappearing P waves if hyperkalemia is present. ◆ Ultrasonography, abdominal and kidney-ureter-bladder X-rays, excretory urography, renal scan, retrograde pyelography, computerized tomography, and nephrotomography reveal abnormalities of the urinary tract.

TREATMENT AND CARE

◆ Assess the patient for the amount of blood lost and begin fluid resuscitation.
◆ Obtain a type and cross match for blood component therapy.
◆ Ensure a patent airway and assess breathing and circulation. Monitor cardiac and respiratory status closely, at least every 15 minutes – or more depending on the patient's condition.
◆ Administer supplemental oxygen. Monitor oxygen saturation and serial ABG levels for evidence of hypoxemia. Anticipate endotracheal intubation and mechanical ventilation should the patient's respiratory status deteriorate. Keep the patient in semi-Fowler's position to maximize chest expansion. Keep the patient as quiet and as comfortable as possible to minimize oxygen demands.
◆ Monitor vital signs continuously for changes indicating hypovolemic shock. Observe skin color and check capillary refill. Notify the physician if capillary refill is greater than 2 seconds.
◆ Assist with insertion of central venous or pulmonary artery catheter to evaluate hemodynamic status. Monitor hemodynamic parameters including central venous pressure, pulmonary artery wedge pressure, cardiac output, and cardiac index every 15 minutes to evaluate the patient's status and response to treatment.
◆ Assess level of consciousness approximately every 30 minutes until the patient stabilizes, and then every 2 to 4 hours as indicated by the patient's status.
◆ Obtain serial hemoglobin and hematocrit; notify the physician of hematocrit below the prescribed parameter.
◆ Monitor intake and output closely, including all losses from the GI tract. Insert an indwelling urinary catheter and assess urine output hourly. Check stools and gastric drainage for occult blood.
◆ Provide emotional support and reassurance appropriately in the wake of massive GI bleeding.
◆ Administer histamine-2-receptor agonists and other agents, such as sucralfate, misoprostol, and omeprazole (a protein-pump inhibitor).
◆ Prepare the patient for endoscopic or surgical repair of bleeding sites.
◆ Assist with gastric intubation and gastric pH monitoring.

◆ Measure intake and output including body fluids, nasogastric output, and diarrhea; weigh the patient daily.
◆ Measure hemoglobin and hematocrit and replace blood components as ordered.
◆ Monitor vital signs.
◆ Check for and report signs of pericarditis (pleuritic chest pain, tachycardia, pericardial friction rub), inadequate renal perfusion (hypotension), and acidosis.
◆ Maintain proper electrolyte balance. Monitor for hyperkalemia (malaise, anorexia, paresthesia or muscle weakness) and ECG changes.
◆ If the patient receives hypertonic glucose and insulin infusions, monitor potassium and glucose levels. If giving sodium polystyrene sulfonate rectally, make sure the patient doesn't retain it and become constipated; doing so prevents bowel perforation.
◆ Maintain the patient's nutritional status with a high-calorie, low-protein, low-sodium, low-potassium diet and vitamin supplements.
◆ Monitor the patient carefully during peritoneal dialysis.
◆ If the patient requires hemodialysis, monitor the venous access site carefully; assess the patient and laboratory work carefully.
◆ Administer diuretics.

Liver dysfunction and collateral vessels that shunt blood around the liver to the systemic circulation permit toxins absorbed from the GI tract to circulate freely to the brain. Ammonia is a by-product of protein metabolism. The normal liver transforms ammonia (by-product of protein metabolism) to urea, which the kidneys excrete. When the liver fails, ammonia blood levels rise and circulate to the brain.

■ Short-chain fatty acids, serotonin, tryptophan, and false neurotransmitters may accumulate in the blood and contribute to hepatic encephalopathy.

Renal system

■ Accumulation of vasoactive substances or a compensatory response to portal hypertension and the pooling of blood in the splenic circulation may lead to decreased glomerular filatration, oliguria, and hepatorenal syndrome (renal failure concurrent with liver disease; the kidneys appear normal but abruptly cease functioning).

■ Hepatorenal syndrome causes expanded blood volume, accumulation of hydrogen ions, and electrolyte disturbances.

ASSESSMENT

Hepatic encephalopathy is a key assessment finding associated with hepatic failure. The clinical features of hepatic encephalopathy vary depending on the severity of the neurologic involvement. The disorder usually progresses through four stages (or grades). The patient's symptoms can fluctuate from one stage to another.

In the *prodromal stage*, or Grade I, early symptoms are typically overlooked because they're so subtle. The patient's history may reveal slight personality changes, such as agitation, belligerence, disorientation, or forgetfulness. The patient may also have trouble concentrating or thinking clearly. He may report feeling fatigued or drowsy, or may have slurred speech.

In the *impending stage,* or Grade II, the patient undergoes continuing mental changes. He may be confused and disorientated as to time, place, and person. As encephalopathy progresses, the patient's ability to write becomes more difficult, and his writing tends to be illegible.

In the *stuporous stage,* or Grade III, the patient shows marked mental confusion.

The patient can still be aroused, however, and is commonly noisy and abusive (when aroused).

In the *comatose stage,* or Grade IV, the patient can't be aroused and is obtunded with no asterixis. Seizures may occur, although they're uncommon. Eventually, this stage progresses to coma and death.

Clinical findings

■ Jaundice
■ Nausea and anorexia
■ Abdominal pain or tenderness
■ Fatigue and weight loss
■ Pruritus
■ Oliguria
■ Splenomegaly
■ Ascites
■ Peripheral edema
■ Esophageal varices
■ Bleeding tendencies
■ Petechiae

Prodromal stage (Grade I) hepatic encephalopathy

■ Slurred speech
■ Slight tremor

Impending stage (Grade II) hepatic encephalopathy

■ Asterixis (liver flap, flapping tremor)
■ Lethargy
■ Aberrant behavior
■ Apraxia

Stuporous stage (Grade III) hepatic encephalopathy

■ Marked mental confusion
■ Drowsiness
■ Stupor
■ Hyperventilation
■ Muscle twitching
■ Asterixis

Comatose stage (Grade IV) hepatic encephalopathy

■ Fetor hepaticus (musty odor of breath and urine)
■ Seizures
■ Hyperactive reflexes
■ Coma

Diagnostic test results

■ *Liver function tests* reveal elevated levels of aspartate aminotransferase, alanine aminotransferase, alkaline phosphatase, and bilirubin.

■ *Blood studies* reveal anemia, impaired red blood cell production, elevated bleeding and clotting times, low platelet levels, low blood glucose levels, low albumin, decreased blood urea nitrogen, and increased serum ammonia levels.

■ *Serum electrolyte studies* commonly reveal hyponatremia and hypokalemia in patients with ascites.

■ *Urinalysis* reveals increased urobilinogen, bilirubin, and osmolarity.

■ *Electroencephalogram* is typically abnormal with hepatic encephalopathy, but the changes are nonspecific.

COLLABORATIVE MANAGEMENT

A respiratory therapist may be consulted for airway and ventilation maintenance, especially if the patient is experiencing problems such as impaired gag reflex, aspiration, or difficulty with respiration due to ascites. Nutritional therapy is critical in providing high-calorie, protein-restricted, and possibly moderately sodium-restricted diet. Enteral or parenteral nutritional therapy may also be necessary. Physical therapy may be involved to assist with measures to maintain joint function while the patient is maintained on strict bedrest. Various specialists, including neurologists and nephrologists, may be consulted for assistance depending on the involvement of the patient's organs and prognosis. The patient and his family may also benefit from supportive counseling and a referral for social services.

TREATMENT AND CARE

■ The goal of therapy is to eliminate the underlying cause of the disorder and to lower serum ammonia levels to stop progression of encephalopathy.

■ Treatments to eliminate ammonia from the GI tract include sorbitol-induced catharsis to produce osmotic diarrhea, continuous aspiration of blood from the stomach, reduction of dietary protein intake, and administration of lactulose to reduce serum ammonia levels.

■ Lactulose syrup may be administered orally. In acute hepatic coma, lactulose may be administered by retention enema. Lactulose therapy requires careful monitoring of fluid and electrolyte balance.

■ Although it's now considered a second-line treatment because of potential toxicity, neomycin may be administered to suppress bacterial flora (preventing them from converting amino acids into ammonia). Neomycin is administered orally or by retention enema.

■ Potassium supplements (80 to 120 mEq/day given by mouth or I.V.) to correct alkalosis (from increased ammonia levels) may be administered, especially if the patient is taking diuretics.

■ Salt-poor albumin may be used to maintain fluid and electrolyte balance, replace depleted albumin levels, and restore plasma.

■ Liver transplantation may be indicated.

Hypercalcemia

Hypercalcemia occurs when the serum calcium level rises above 10.1 mg/dl, the ionized serum calcium level rises above 5.1 mg/dl, and the rate of calcium entry into extracellular fluid exceeds the rate of calcium excretion by the kidneys.

ETIOLOGY

Hypercalcemia is usually caused by an increase in calcium absorption from bone related to hyperparathyroidism and cancer. Other causes include an increase in calcium absorption in the GI tract or a decrease in the excretion by the kidneys. These mechanisms can occur in isolation or in combination.

Hyperthyroidism can lead to an increase in calcium release as more calcium is reabsorbed from bone. Multiple fractures or prolonged immobilization can also cause an increase in calcium release from bone.

Certain medications such as antacids containing calcium, oral or I.V. calcium supplements, lithium, thiazide diuretics, vitamin A, and vitamin D can lead to hypercalcemia. Milk-alkali syndrome, a condition in which calcium and alkali are combined, also increases calcium levels.

PATHOPHYSIOLOGY

Hyperparathyroidism, the most common cause of hypercalcemia, occurs when the body excretes more parathyroid hormone

DISORDERS AFFECTING MANAGEMENT OF HYPERCALCEMIA

This chart highlights disorders that affect the management of hypercalcemia.

DISORDER	SIGNS AND SYMPTOMS	DIAGNOSTIC TEST RESULTS
Hypertension (complication)	◆ Headache ◆ Dizziness ◆ Fatigue ◆ Bounding pulse ◆ Pulsating abdominal mass ◆ Elevated blood pressure ◆ Bruits over the abdominal aorta	◆ Urinalysis may show proteinuria, red blood cells or white blood cells, or possibly glucose. ◆ Serum potassium levels are less than 3.5 mEq/L. ◆ Blood urea nitrogen is normal or elevated to more than 20 mg/dL. ◆ Serum creatinine levels normal or elevated to more than 1.5 mg/dL.
Renal calculi (complication)	◆ Severe pain that travels from the costovertebral angle to the flank and then to the suprapubic region and external genitalia ◆ Nausea and vomiting ◆ Fever ◆ Chills ◆ Hematuria ◆ Abdominal distention	◆ Kidney-ureter-bladder (KUB) radiography reveals most renal calculi. ◆ Excretory urography helps confirm the diagnosis and determine the size and location of calculi. ◆ Kidney ultrasonography is used to detect obstructive changes, such as unilateral or bilateral hydronephrosis and radiolucent calculi not seen on the KUB radiography. ◆ Urine culture of a midstream specimen may indicate pyuria, a sign of urinary tract infection. ◆ A 24-hour urine collection reveals the presence of calcium oxalate, phosphorus, and uric acid excretion. Three separate collections, along with blood samples, are needed for accurate testing. ◆ Calculus analysis shows mineral content. ◆ Serial blood calcium and phosphorus levels indicate hyperparathyroidism and show an increased calcium level in proportion to normal serum protein levels. ◆ Blood protein levels determine the level of free calcium unbound to protein.

(PTH) than normal, greatly increasing the effects of this hormone on the body. Calcium reabsorption from the bones, kidneys, and intestines also increases.

Cancer, the second most common cause of hypercalcemia, causes bone destruction as malignant cells invade the bones and trigger the release of a substance similar to PTH. This hormone secretion causes an increase in serum calcium levels. The kidneys can become overwhelmed and unable to excrete the excess calcium, which leads to elevated calcium levels. Patients with squamous cell carcinoma of the lung, myeloma, or breast cancer are especially prone to hypercalcemia.

Hypophosphatemia and acidosis increase calcium ionization and are associated with hypercalcemia.

Cardiovascular system

■ The heart muscle and cardiac conduction system are affected by hypercalcemia, which may lead to arrhythmias such as bradycardia and subsequent cardiac arrest.

■ Effects of excess calcium on the heart muscle may lead to hypertension. (See *Disorders affecting management of hypercalcemia*.)

Gastrointestinal system

■ GI symptoms such as anorexia, nausea, and vomiting may be the first symptoms the patient experiences.

TREATMENT AND CARE

- ◆ Monitor blood pressure for stability.
- ◆ Help the patient identify risk factors and modify his lifestyle. Encourage dietary changes.
- ◆ Advise patient to follow medication regimen in order to control blood pressure.
- ◆ Help the patient identify stress factors and establish effective coping mechanisms.
- ◆ Administer thiazide diuretics, angiotensin-converting enzyme inhibitors, angiotensin receptor blockers, and calcium channel blockers.

- ◆ To aid diagnosis, maintain a 24- to 48-hour record of urine pH using nitrazine pH paper. Strain all urine through gauze or a tea strainer, and save all solid material recovered for analysis.
- ◆ To facilitate spontaneous passage of calculi, encourage the patient to walk, if possible. Also, encourage fluids to maintain a urine output of 3.2 to 4.2 qt (3 to 4 L)/day (urine should be very dilute and colorless).
- ◆ If the patient can't drink the required amount of fluid, give supplemental I.V. fluids.
- ◆ Record intake and output and daily weight to assess fluid status and renal function.
- ◆ Medicate the patient for pain when he's passing a calculus.
- ◆ To help acidify urine, offer fruit juices, especially cranberry juice.

If the patient had calculi surgically removed
- ◆ Anticipate that the patient will have an indwelling catheter or a nephrostomy tube.
- ◆ Unless one of his kidneys was removed, expect bloody drainage from the catheter.
- ◆ Check dressings regularly for bloody drainage, and know how much drainage to expect.
- ◆ Immediately report excessive drainage or a rising pulse rate (symptoms of hemorrhage).
- ◆ Use sterile technique when changing dressings or providing catheter care.
- ◆ Administer antibiotics for infection.
- ◆ If lithotripsy is planned, expect to discontinue anticoagulants, aspirin, vitamin E, and platelet inhibitors for three days before the procedure.

■ Excess calcium affects the smooth muscle leading to decreased GI motility resulting in decreased bowel sounds, constipation, abdominal pain, and possibly a paralytic ileus.

Musculoskeletal system
■ As calcium levels increase, the patient may experience the onset of muscle weakness, hyporeflexia, and decreased muscle tone.
■ Pathological fractures and bone pain may result from the excess levels of calcium.

Neurologic system
■ Excess calcium levels can affect the nerve cells and the nervous system, leading to drowsiness, lethargy, headaches, depression or apathy, irritability, and confusion. (See *How hypercalcemia develops,* page 176.)

Renal system
■ The kidneys work overtime to remove excess calcium, which may lead to renal problems such as polyuria, dehydration, and renal failure.
■ Kidney stones and other calcifications may develop.

ASSESSMENT
Signs and symptoms of hypercalcemia are intensified if the condition develops acutely and if calcium levels are greater than 15 mg/dl.

HOW HYPERCALCEMIA DEVELOPS

Calcium resorption from bone increases.

▼

Calcium enters extracellular fluid at an increased rate.

▼

Calcium movement into extracellular fluid exceeds the rate of calcium excretion by the kidneys.

▼

Excess calcium enters the cells.

▼

Excess intracellular calcium decreases cell membrane excitability.

▼

Reduced membrane excitability affects skeletal and cardiac muscles and the nervous system.

▼

Patient may display fatigue, confusion, and decreased level of consciousness.

Clinical findings

- Abdominal pain and constipation
- Anorexia
- Behavioral changes, including confusion
- Bone pain
- Extreme thirst
- Lethargy
- Muscle weakness
- Nausea
- Polyuria
- Vomiting
- Constipation
- Bradycardia
- Decreased deep tendon reflexes
- Hypertension
- Flank pain

Diagnostic test results

- *Serum calcium level* is above 10.1 mg/dl.
- *Ionized calcium level* is above 5.1 mg/dl.
- *X-rays* reveal pathological fractures.
- *Electrocardiography* may reveal a shortened QT interval and shortened ST segment.

COLLABORATIVE MANAGEMENT

Nephrologists and cardiologists may be consulted depending on the patient's symptoms and organs involved. A nutritionist may be called in to help devise a low-calcium diet. If the patient is on bedrest, physical therapy may be indicated to provide passive range-of-motion exercises to prevent complications from immobility. The patient and family may also benefit from supportive counseling and a referral to social services.

TREATMENT AND CARE

- If hypercalcemia produces no symptoms, treatment may consist of managing the underlying cause.
- Hydration increases the excretion of calcium from the body through the process of diuresis. Normal saline solution is typically used for hydration in the presence of hypercalcemia because the sodium in the solution inhibits renal tubular reabsorption of calcium.
- Loop diuretics promote calcium excretion.
- Hemodialysis or peritoneal dialysis may be instituted if the hypercalcemia is life-threatening.
- Administration of corticosteroids I.V. and then orally may inhibit bone resorption of

calcium and decrease calcium absorption from the GI tract.

■ Etidronate disodium is commonly used to treat hypercalcemia; it inhibits the action of osteoclasts in bone and reduces resorption. The effects of etidronate disodium take 2 to 3 days.

■ When hypercalcemia results from cancer, mithramycin, a chemotherapeutic drug, is used to decrease bone resorption of calcium.

■ Monitor vital signs, cardiac rhythm, intake and output volumes, response to I.V. therapy and loop diuretics, and laboratory values.

■ Encourage mobility when possible to decrease the bone release of calcium. Perform passive range-of-motion exercises if mobility isn't possible.

■ Provide a safe environment and use caution when repositioning the patient to prevent pathological fractures.

■ Encourage a low-calcium diet and consult the dietitian as appropriate for teaching and diet evaluation.

■ Discontinue all medications that contain calcium or increase calcium levels or absorption.

Hyperchloremia

Hyperchloremia is an excess of chloride in extracellular fluid and occurs when serum chloride levels exceed 106 mEq/L. In patients between ages 60 and 90, the normal serum chloride level ranges from 98 to 107 mEq/L; in patients ages 90 and older, normal serum chloride levels range from 98 to 111 mEq/L. Hyperchloremia is commonly associated with acid-base imbalances and rarely occurs alone.

ETIOLOGY

Chloride regulation and sodium regulation are closely related. Hyperchloremia is often associated with hypernatremia. Chloride and bicarbonate (HCO_3^-) have an inverse relationship, so an excess of chloride may be associated with a decrease in HCO_3^-. Excess serum chloride may also result from increased intake of chloride or retention of chloride by the kidney. Increased chloride absorption by the bowel can occur in pa-

tients who have anastomoses joining the ureter and intestines. Conditions such as dehydration, renal tubular acidosis, renal failure, respiratory alkalosis, salicylate toxicity, hyperparathyroidism, hyperaldosteronism, and hypernatremia alter fluid, electrolyte, and acid-base balances and can lead to hyperchloremia.

Several drugs can contribute to hyperchloremia such as ammonium chloride, acetazolamide, phenylbutazone, sodium polystyrene sulfonate, and excessive amounts of salicylates and triamterene.

PATHOPHYSIOLOGY

Increased intake of chloride in the form of sodium chloride can lead to hyperchloremia, especially if water is lost from the body at the same time. Water loss elevates the chloride level even more. Increased renal retention of chloride also elevates levels.

Hyperchloremia increases the risk of metabolic acidosis. A normal anion gap in a patient with metabolic acidosis indicates that the acidosis is most likely caused by a loss of HCO_3^- ions by the kidneys or the GI tract. This situation leads to a corresponding increase in chloride ions. Acidosis can also result from an accumulation of chloride ions in the form of acidifying salts. A corresponding decrease in HCO_3^- ions occurs at the same time.

In patients with hyperchloremia caused by medications, ion exchange resins that contain sodium can cause chloride to be exchanged for potassium in the bowel. When chloride follows the sodium into the blood stream, serum chloride levels rise. Chloride retention in the body can also be related to medications.

Cardiovascular system

■ As the pH drops, central nervous system (CNS) depression affects myocardial function and leads to decreased cardiac output and hypotension.

■ Arrhythmias may result from hyperchloremia as a result of untreated acidosis.

■ Hypertension may also occur as a result of fluid overload. (See *Disorders affecting management of hyperchloremia*, pages 178 and 179.)

WATCHFUL EYE

DISORDERS AFFECTING
MANAGEMENT OF HYPERCHLOREMIA

This chart highlights disorders that affect the management of hyperchloremia.

DISORDER	SIGNS AND SYMPTOMS	DIAGNOSTIC TEST RESULTS
Hyperkalemia (complication)	*Mild hyperkalemia* ♦ Diarrhea ♦ Intestinal cramping ♦ Neuromuscular irritability ♦ Restlessness ♦ Tingling lips and fingers *Severe hyperkalemia* ♦ Loss of muscle tone ♦ Muscle weakness ♦ Paralysis	♦ Electrocardiography reveals regular rhythm; rate within normal limits; P wave that has a low amplitude (mild hyperkalemia), that's wide and flattened (moderate hyperkalemia), or indiscernible (severe hyperkalemia); PR interval that's normal or prolonged or not measurable if P wave can't be detected; a widened QRS complex; tall, peaked T wave; shortened QT interval; intraventricular conduction disturbances; and ST-segment elevation (in severe hyperkalemia).
Hypertension (complication)	♦ Headache ♦ Dizziness ♦ Fatigue ♦ Bounding pulse ♦ Pulsating abdominal mass ♦ Elevated blood pressure ♦ Bruits over the abdominal aorta	♦ Urinalysis may show proteinuria, red blood cells or white blood cells, or possibly glucose. ♦ Serum potassium levels are less than 3.5 mEq/L. ♦ Blood urea nitrogen is normal or elevated to more than 20 mg/dL. ♦ Serum creatinine levels normal or elevated to more than 1.5 mg/dL.

Endocrine and metabolic systems

■ A decrease in the serum HCO_3^- level leads to an increase in the chloride level.(See *How hyperchloremia develops,* page 180.)
■ The patient with diabetes experiencing metabolic acidosis may experience catabolism of fats and excretion of acetone through the lungs, leading to a fruity breath odor.

Gastrointestinal system

■ Urinary diversion into the sigmoid colon or ileal segment leads to hyperchloremic acidosis and is associated with HCO_3^- secretion into the colon in exchange for the reabsorption of urinary chloride.

Integumentary system

■ Initially, the skin is warm and dry due to peripheral vasodilation, but as shock develops the skin becomes cool and clammy.

Musculoskeletal system

■ Metabolic acidosis may lead to diminish muscle tone and deep tendon reflexes.

Neurologic system

■ Metabolic acidosis can produce lethargy, weakness and diminished thought processes related to CNS depression from the decreased pH level.
■ Headache may result from cerebral vessel dilation.

Renal system

■ Renal tubular acidosis is characterized by either HCO_3^- loss in the urine or the inability to generate new HCO_3^-.
■ Renal HCO_3^- wasting can result from the use of carbonic anhydrase inhibitors.

Respiratory system

■ As acids build in the bloodstream, the lungs compensate by increasing the depth and rate of respirations (Kussmaul's respirations).

ASSESSMENT

The signs and symptoms associated with hyperchloremia are generally related to meta-

TREATMENT AND CARE

◆ Identify the underlying cause.
◆ Administer I.V. calcium gluconate to decrease neuromuscular irritability, I.V. insulin to facilitate entry of potassium into cells, and I.V. sodium bicarbonate to correct metabolic acidosis.
◆ Administer oral or rectal cation exchange resins (sodium polystyrene sulfonate) that exchange sodium for potassium in the intestine.
◆ Dialysis may be needed with renal failure or severe hyperkalemia.
◆ Monitor serum potassium levels closely.
◆ Identify and manage arrhythmias.

◆ Monitor blood pressure for stability
◆ Help the patient identify risk factors and modify his lifestyle. Encourage dietary changes.
◆ Advise the patient to follow medication regimen in order to control blood pressure.
◆ Help the patient identify stress factors and establish effective coping mechanisms.
◆ Administer thiazide diuretics, angiotensin-converting enzyme inhibitors, angiotensin-receptor blockers, and calcium channel blockers.

bolic acidosis; hyperchloremia rarely produces signs and symptoms on its own.

Clinical findings
- Dull headache
- Anorexia
- Decreased level of consciousness that may progress to seizures and coma
- Lethargy
- Muscle weakness
- Nausea and vomiting
- Dyspnea
- Diminished muscle tone
- Decreased deep tendon reflexes
- Hypervolemia
- Hypertension related to fluid overload
- Hypotension related to CNS involvement
- Tachycardia
- Hyperkalemic signs including abdominal cramping, diarrhea, muscle weakness and electrocardiogram changes

Diagnostic test results
- *Serum chloride level* is above 106 mEq/L.
- *Serum sodium level* is greater than 145 mEq/L.
- *Serum pH level* is less than 7.35, *serum HCO_3^- level* is less than 22 mEq/L, and a normal anion gap (8 to 14 mEq/L) all indicate metabolic acidosis.

COLLABORATIVE MANAGEMENT
Nephrologists, cardiologists, and respiratory therapists may be consulted depending on the patient's symptoms, the organ system involved, and complications that may develop. Nutritional therapy may be necessary to devise a sodium- and chloride-free diet. The patient and family may also benefit from supportive counseling and a referral to social services.

TREATMENT AND CARE
- Treatments for hyperchloremia include correcting the underlying cause and restoring fluid, electrolyte, and acid-base balance.
- Dehydrated patients may need fluids to dilute the chloride and increase renal excretion of the chloride ions.

UP CLOSE

HOW HYPERCHLOREMIA DEVELOPS

Chloride intake, absorption, or retention increases.

▼

Water loss may worsen chloride accumulation in extracellular fluid.

▼

Sodium bicarbonate level falls, and sodium level increases.

▼

Patient develops signs and symptoms of metabolic acidosis.

■ A diuretic may be ordered to eliminate chloride, but be aware that other electrolytes will also be lost.

■ In the presence of normal liver function, the patient may receive an infusion of lactated Ringer's solution to convert lactate to HCO_3^- in the liver. This leads to an increase in the base HCO_3^- level and corrects acidosis.

■ If the hyperchloremia is severe, I.V. sodium bicarbonate may be administered to correct the acidosis because HCO_3^- and chloride compete for sodium and can lead to renal excretion of the chloride ions. Assess for overcompensation when administering I.V. sodium bicarbonate that will be manifested as metabolic alkalosis.

■ Continually monitor vital signs, intake and output, cardiac rhythm, CNS involvement, and laboratory results.

■ Provide a safe environment if the patient is confused or at risk for injury.

■ Provide information on the disorder, symptoms, and treatment plan to the patient and his family members.

Hypermagnesemia

Hypermagnesemia occurs when the body's serum magnesium level rises above 2.5 mEq/L. Although hypermagnesemia is less common than hypomagnesemia, it does oc-

cur more often than is diagnosed. Most causes of hypermagnesemia are iatrogenic.

ETIOLOGY

Hypermagnesemia is most likely to occur in patients with renal insufficiency. Magnesium is primarily excreted by the kidneys, and decreased renal function results in retention of magnesium. Elderly patients are at increased risk for hypermagnesemia because they have age-related reduced renal function and tend to consume magnesium-containing products such as antacids or mineral supplements. Older patients may also have GI disorders such as gastritis and colitis that alter the GI mucosal barrier and lead to increased magnesium absorption. Additionally, hypocalcemia may accompany hypermagnesemia because a low calcium level suppresses parathyroid hormone production.

Patients with Addison's disease, adrenocortical insufficiency, dehydration, hypothyroidism and untreated diabetic ketoacidosis are also at risk for hypermagnesemia. Other causes for excessive magnesium intake include:

■ magnesium sulfate administration during pregnancy or to control seizures

■ overuse of medications containing magnesium, such as antacids and laxatives

■ hemodialysis with a magnesium-rich dialysate solution

■ total parenteral solutions containing large concentrations of magnesium

DISORDER AFFECTING
MANAGEMENT OF HYPERMAGNESEMIA

This chart highlights how complete heart block affects the management of hypermagnesemia.

DISORDER	SIGNS AND SYMPTOMS	DIAGNOSTIC TEST RESULTS	TREATMENT AND CARE
Complete heart block (complication)	◆ Changes in level of consciousness ◆ Changes in mental status ◆ Chest pain ◆ Diaphoresis ◆ Dyspnea ◆ Hypotension ◆ Light-headedness ◆ Pallor ◆ Severe fatigue ◆ Slow peripheral pulse rate	◆ Serum magnesium is 10 mEq/L. ◆ Electrocardiogram shows ventricular depolarization typically initiated by junctional escape pacemaker (at a rate of 40 to 60 beats/minute); a normal-looking QRS complex, if the block is at the atrioventricular node level; or an intrinsic rate less than 40 beats/minute because of unstable ventricular escape pacemaker located distal to site of block and a wide, bizarre QRS complex.	◆ If the patient has serious signs and symptoms, immediate treatment includes maintaining transcutaneous pacing (most effective) and administering I.V. atropine, dopamine, epinephrine, or a combination of these drugs (for short-term use in emergencies). ◆ If the patient has no symptoms, maintain temporary transvenous pacing until the need for a permanent pacemaker is determined. Make sure patient has a patent I.V. line, administer oxygen, assess for correctable causes of arrhythmia (such as drugs and myocardial ischemia), minimize the patient's activity level, and maintain bed rest.

■ fetal absorption after administration to the mother to manage pregnancy-induced hypertension or preterm labor.

PATHOPHYSIOLOGY

Hypermagnesemia may go undiagnosed because magnesium isn't measured as often as other electrolytes.

Cardiovascular system
■ Cardiovascular effects of hypermagnesemia are related to its calcium channel blocker effect on the cardiac conduction system and the smooth muscle of blood vessels.
■ Bradycardia, atrioventricular block, and asystole may occur. (See *Disorder affecting management of hypermagnesemia.*)
■ Arrhythmias may lead to decreased cardiac output.(See *How hypermagnesemia develops,* page 182.)
■ A high serum magnesium level may cause vasodilation, which lowers the blood

pressure and leads to the patient feeling flushed or warm all over his body.
■ Hypotension related to vasodilation occurs early.

Respiratory system
■ Weakening of the respiratory muscles may lead to slow, shallow, and depressed respirations and may progress to respiratory arrest and the need for mechanical ventilation.

Neuromuscular system
■ Excessive magnesium depresses the central nervous system (CNS). The patient may appear lethargic or drowsy and experience a change in level of consciousness or advance to the level of a coma.
■ CNS depression depresses muscle and nerve activities, leading to hypoactive deep tendon reflexes that, without treatment, progress to a loss of the patellar reflex.

UP CLOSE

HOW HYPERMAGNESEMIA DEVELOPS

> Magnesium excretion decreases, or magnesium intake increases.
>
> ▼
>
> High magnesium level suppresses acetylcholine release at myoneural junctions.
>
> ▼
>
> Reduced acetylcholine blocks neuromuscular transmission and reduces cell excitability.
>
> ▼
>
> The neuromuscular system and central nervous system become depressed.
>
> ▼
>
> Level of consciousness decreases and respiratory distress occurs.
>
> ▼
>
> Arrhythmias and other cardiac complications may develop.

ASSESSMENT

Assessment of the patient at risk for hypermagnesemia is key because of the infrequent use of magnesium monitoring.

Clinical findings

- Nausea and vomiting
- Hypocalcemia
- Muscle weakness, drowsiness, lethargy and flaccidity
- Decreased cardiac output and possible cardiac arrest
- Sense of feeling warm due to vasodilation
- Bradycardia
- Hypotension
- Flushed appearance
- Respiratory depression that may advance to respiratory failure without treatment
- Decreased or absent deep tendon reflexes
- Coma

Diagnostic test results

- *Serum magnesium* level is above 2.5 mEq/L.
- *Electrocardiography* shows a prolonged PR interval, widened QRS complex, a shortened QT interval, and a tall T wave.

COLLABORATIVE MANAGEMENT

Collaborative management and consultation depends on the severity of the hypermagnesemia and the complications that develop. A respiratory therapist and a pulmonologist may be needed if the patient requires mechanical ventilation. A nephrologist will be consulted if the patient requires dialysis. A cardiologist will be consulted if the patient develops cardiac arrhythmias. A nutritionist is also necessary to provide the patient with a diet low in magnesium.

TREATMENT AND CARE

- Treatment and management of hypermagnesemia focuses on lowering the magnesium level and treating or eliminating the cause.
- Increase fluid intake—either orally or I.V.—to increase urine output, thus clear magnesium from the body.
- If the patient doesn't respond to increased fluid intake, a loop diuretic may be ordered to promote magnesium excretion.
- In severe cases of hypermagnesemia, expect to administer calcium gluconate, a magnesium antagonist.
- Some patients with severe hypermagnesemia develop respiratory depression and require mechanical ventilation.

TESTING THE PATELLAR REFLEX

One way to gauge your patient's magnesium status is to test her patellar reflex, one of the deep tendon reflexes that the serum magnesium level affects. To test the reflex, strike the patellar tendon just below the patella with the patient sitting or lying in a supine position, as shown. Look for leg extension or contraction of the quadriceps muscle in the front of the thigh.

If the patellar reflex is absent, notify the physician immediately. This finding may mean your patient's serum magnesium level is 7 mEq/L or higher.

Sitting
Have the patient sit on the side of the bed with her legs dangling freely, as shown here. Then test the reflex.

Supine position
Flex the patient's knee at a 45-degree angle, and place your non-dominant hand behind it for support. Then test the reflex.

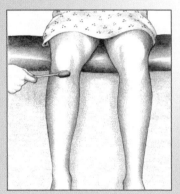 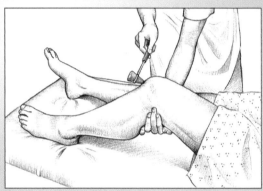

■ Patients with renal failure require hemodialysis using a magnesium-free dialysate to clear the magnesium from the body because impaired kidneys aren't capable.

■ If the patient isn't responding to treatment, evaluate his blood urea nitrogen and creatinine levels to determine renal function. If renal function is impaired, dialysis will likely be initiated.

■ Provide continuous cardiac monitoring for arrhythmias or rhythm changes.

■ Expect to monitor the patient's intake and output, vital signs, laboratory tests, deep tendon reflexes, mental status, muscle strength, risk for injury, and respiratory status (See *Testing the patellar reflex.*)

■ Evaluate the patient's medications for those containing magnesium and decrease or terminate the doses.

■ Restrict the patient's dietary intake of magnesium.

Hypernatremia

Hypernatremia occurs when the serum sodium level is greater than 145 mEq/L. In non-hospitalized patients, this disorder is primarily seen in elderly patients; however, hospital-acquired hypernatremia occurs in patients of all ages. Hypernatremia occurs in approximately 1% of all hospitalized patients and occurs in males and females equally. Mortality range from 40% to more than 60%, which is partly influenced by the severity of the hypernatremia.

Hypernatremia may occur in any patient with a diminished mental status related to impairment in the ability to perceive and respond to thirst. In the elderly, age is associated with lowered osmotic stimulation of thirst and the decreased ability of the kid-

DISORDER AFFECTING
MANAGEMENT OF HYPERNATREMIA

This chart highlights how hypertension affects the management of hypernatremia

DISORDER	SIGNS AND SYMPTOMS	DIAGNOSTIC TEST RESULTS	TREATMENT AND CARE
Hypertension (complication)	◆ Headache ◆ Dizziness ◆ Fatigue ◆ Bounding pulse ◆ Pulsating abdominal mass ◆ Elevated blood pressure ◆ Bruits over the abdominal aorta	◆ Urinalysis may show proteinuria, red blood cells or white blood cells, or possibly glucose. ◆ Serum potassium levels are less than 3.5 mEq/L. ◆ Blood urea nitrogen is normal or elevated to more than 20 mg/dL. ◆ Serum creatinine levels are normal or elevated to more than 1.5 mg/dL.	◆ Monitor blood pressure for stability. ◆ Help the patient identify risk factors and modify his lifestyle. Encourage dietary changes. ◆ Advise the patient to follow his medication regimen to control blood pressure. ◆ Help the patient identify stress factors and establish effective coping mechanisms.

neys to conserve water in times of need. Infants, who are unable to ask for water, are also at increased risk for hypernatremia.

ETIOLOGY

Causes of hypernatremia include a gain of sodium in excess of water, or a loss of water in excess of sodium. Conditions that increase insensible water loss, such as fever, hyperventilation, pulmonary infections, tracheostomy, exposure to hot temperatures, or massive burns, may result in hypernatremia. Watery diarrhea is a major cause of hypernatremia in children. Loss of hypotonic fluid in the stool of patients with end-stage liver disease treated with lactulose may also result in severe hypernatremia.

Excessive administration of parenteral sodium solutions or a high sodium intake from food or medications can elevate sodium levels. For example, antacids with sodium bicarbonate, specific antibiotics, salt tablets, I.V. sodium bicarbonate, I.V. sodium chloride preparations, and sodium polystyrene sulfonate can cause hypernatremia. Ingestion of sea water, which has a sodium concentration of 450 to 500 mEq/L, also increases sodium levels.

Diabetes insipidus, a disorder of water balance that's associated with the lack of antidiuretic hormone (ADH) or with kidney resistance to the affects of ADH, can lead to hypernatremia. Hypernatremia occurs if water losses aren't sufficiently replaced orally or intravenously. Excess adrenocortical hormones, as occurs in Cushing's syndrome, can lead to hypernatremia.

Respiratory hyperventilation leads to excessive water loss and places the patient at risk for hypernatremia.

PATHOPHYSIOLOGY

The body usually protects itself against hypernatremia by increasing the release of ADH and stimulating the thirst mechanism. When serum sodium increases, water retention and increased consumption of water lower sodium concentrations. Thus, the failure of these responses can lead to hypernatremia.

Urine specific gravity increases with hypernatremia as the kidneys attempt to conserve water that's lost through the GI tract, skin, or lungs. If the physiological defect involves water loss from the kidneys, the urine specific gravity is very low.

Cardiovascular system

■ Fluid shifts out of the cells into the extracellular fluid and results in hypertension and

UP CLOSE

HOW HYPERNATREMIA DEVELOPS

Sodium intake or water loss becomes excessive.

▼

Serum osmolality increases.

▼

Fluid moves by osmosis from inside cells to outside cells to balance intracellular and extracellular fluid levels.

Cells become dehydrated, causing neurologic impairment; extracellular volume in vessels increases, causing hypervolemia.

peripheral edema. (See *Disorder affecting management of hypernatremia.*)

Gastrointestinal system
■ High serum osmolality due to increased solute concentrations in the blood stimulates the hypothalamus and initiates the thirst mechanism. (See *How hypernatremia develops.*)
■ Diarrhea leads to water loss (major cause of hypernatremia in children).

Metabolic and endocrine systems
■ ADH is secreted by the posterior pituitary gland as the body strives to maintain a normal serum sodium level. ADH causes water to be retained and results in lowering the sodium levels.
■ Excessive water loss can occur when the patient experiences fever or heatstroke.

Neuromuscular system
■ Fluid shifting from the cells leads to cellular dehydration and significantly affects the central nervous system (CNS), leading to agitation, confusion, restlessness, lethargy, stupor, seizures, and — without treatment — coma.

Renal system
■ Renal impairment may lead to oliguria.

Respiratory system
■ Dyspnea, respiratory arrest, and death may result from a dramatic rise in osmotic pressure.

ASSESSMENT
Sodium imbalance has profound physiological effects and can induce severe CNS, cardiovascular, and GI abnormalities. Laboratory studies are necessary to determine cause.

Clinical findings
■ Agitation, restlessness, confusion
■ Flushed skin, low-grade fever
■ Dyspnea or respiratory hyperventilation
■ Irritability and high-pitched crying in infants
■ Bounding pulse, dyspnea, pulmonary edema, and hypertension resulting from hypervolemia
■ Dry mucous membranes, oliguria, and orthostatic hypotension from hypovolemia
■ Nerve involvement, possibly leading to twitching, seizures, or coma
■ Muscle weakness, muscle irritability, or convulsions
■ Rough, dry, swollen tongue

Diagnostic test results
■ *Serum magnesium level* is above 145 mEq/L.
■ *Serum osmolality* is greater than 295 mOsm/kg

■ *Urine specific gravity* is greater than 1.030, unless the water loss occurs from the kidneys (as in diabetes insipidus) where urine specific gravity is decreased.

COLLABORATIVE MANAGEMENT

Collaborative management and consultation depends on the severity of the hypernatremia and the complications that develop. A neurologist will need to be consulted if the patient develops seizures or coma. Additionally, a nutritionist can devise a sodium-restricted diet for the patient.

TREATMENT AND CARE

■ Treatment depends on the cause of the imbalance. If water loss is the cause, water needs to be replaced; if sodium excess is the cause, sodium needs to be removed.
■ Hypernatremia-correction should be gradual to prevent the onset of cerebral edema, seizures, permanent neurologic damage, and death (unless the hypernatremia is severe). In most cases, the correction of hypernatremia in adults and children should extend over a period of 48 hours.
■ Serum electrolyte levels should be monitored every 2 hours while the sodium level is being corrected.
■ Administer I.V. salt-free solution, such as dextrose in water, followed by an infusion of half-normal saline to prevent hyponatremia.
■ All drugs that promote hypernatremia or sodium retention should be discontinued.
■ The patient should consume a sodium-restricted diet.
■ Monitor vital signs, fluid intake and output, risk for injury, seizures and mental status changes, and signs of cerebral edema during fluid replacement therapy.

Hyperparathyroidism

Hyperparathyroidism results from excessive secretion of parathyroid hormone (PTH) from one or more of the four parathyroid glands. PTH promotes bone resorption, and hypersecretion leads to hypercalcemia and hypophosphatemia. Renal and GI absorption of calcium increases. The condition is two to three times more common in women than in men.

ETIOLOGY

Hyperparathyroidism may be primary or secondary. In primary hyperparathyroidism one or more parathyroid glands enlarge (commonly caused by a single adenoma) and increase PTH secretion and serum calcium levels, but this gland enlargement and hypersecretion may be a component of multiple endocrine neoplasia (all four glands are usually involved).

In secondary hyperparathyroidism, a hypocalcemia-producing abnormality outside the parathyroids causes excessive compensatory production of PTH. Causes include rickets, vitamin D deficiency, chronic renal failure, and osteomalacia (inadequate mineralization of bone) caused by phenytoin.

PATHOPHYSIOLOGY

Overproduction of PTH by a tumor or hyperplastic tissue increases intestinal calcium absorption, reduces renal calcium clearance, and increases bone calcium release. Response to this excess varies with each patient for an unknown reason.

Hypophosphatemia results when excessive PTH inhibits renal tubular phosphate reabsorption. The hypophosphatemia aggravates hypercalcemia by increasing the sensitivity of the bone to PTH.

Cardiovascular system

■ Cardiac arrhythmias, vascular damage, hypertension, and heart failure can occur because of increased levels of calcium.

Endocrine system

■ Calcium microthrombi can travel to the pancreas causing pancreatitis.

Musculoskeletal system

■ Untreated hyperparathyroidism damages the skeleton and kidneys from hypercalcemia.
■ Bone and articular problems, such as chondrocalcinosis, osteoporosis, subperiosteal resorption, occasional severe osteopenia, erosions of the juxta-articular surface, subchondral fractures, traumatic synovitis, and pseudogout, may occur. (See *Disorders*

affecting management of hyperparathyroidism, pages 188 and 189.)

Neurologic system
■ Central nervous system changes can result from parathyroid poisoning and may progress to coma.

Renal system
■ Renal complications that result from hypercalcemia include nephrolithiasis; hypercalciuria; renal calculi, colic, and insufficiency.
■ Renal failure can occur as a result of parathyroid poisoning and elevated calcium levels.

Respiratory system
■ Calcium microthrombi can travel to the lungs causing pulmonary emboli and respiratory distress.

ASSESSMENT
Primary hyperparathyroidism is usually diagnosed based on elevated calcium levels found on laboratory test results in asymptomatic patients. Secondary hyperparathyroidism may produce the same features of calcium imbalance with skeletal deformities of the long bones (such as rickets) as well as symptoms of the underlying disease.

Clinical findings
■ Polyuria, nephrocalcinosis, nocturia, polydipsia, dehydration, uremia symptoms, renal colic pain, nephrolithiasis, and renal insufficiency
■ Vague aches and pains, arthralgias, and localized swellings
■ Chronic lower back pain and easy fracturing caused by bone degeneration; bone tenderness; chondrocalcinosis (decreased bone mass); osteopenia and osteoporosis, especially on the vertebrae; erosions of the adjoining joint surface; subchondral fractures; traumatic synovitis; and pseudogout (skeletal and articular systems)
■ Pancreatitis causing constant, severe epigastric pain that radiates to the back; peptic ulcers, causing abdominal pain, anorexia, nausea, and vomiting (GI system)
■ Muscle weakness and atrophy, particularly in the legs (neuromuscular system)

■ Psychomotor and personality disturbances, emotional lability, depression, slow mentation (mental activity), poor memory, drowsiness, ataxia, overt psychosis, stupor and, possibly, coma
■ Pruritus caused by ectopic calcifications in the skin
■ Skin necrosis, cataracts, calcium microthrombi to lungs and pancreas, anemia, and subcutaneous calcification (other systems)

Diagnostic test results
■ *Urine or serum studies* reveal increased alkaline phosphatase, osteocalcin, tartrate-resistant acid phosphatase, PTH, calcium, and chloride levles; increased basal acid secretion; decreased serum phosphorus levels; and possible increased creatinine and serum amylase levels in primary disease and normal or slightly serum calcium, variable serum phosphorus, and increased serum PTH levels.
■ *X-rays* show diffuse bone demineralization, bone cysts, outer cortical bone absorption, and subperiosteal erosion of the phalanges and distal clavicles in primary disease.
■ *X-ray spectrophotometry* shows increased bone turnover in primary disease.
■ *Esophagography, thyroid scan, parathyroid thermography, ultrasonography, thyroid angiography, computed tomography scan,* and *magnetic resonance imaging* may show location of parathyroid lesions.

COLLABORATIVE MANAGEMENT
An endocrinologist, cardiologist, and pulmonologist may be called in to treat pseudogout, cardiac arrhythmias, and complications involving pulmonary emboli, respectively.

TREATMENT AND CARE
■ Treatment for secondary hyperparathyroidism must correct the underlying cause of parathyroid hypertrophy, which includes vitamin D therapy or aluminum hydroxide for hyperphosphatemia in the patient with renal disease.
■ In the patient with chronic secondary hyperparathyroidism, the enlarged glands may not revert to normal size and function even after calcium levels have been controlled; if so, they should be surgically removed.

(Text continues on page 190.)

WATCHFUL EYE

DISORDERS AFFECTING
MANAGEMENT OF HYPERPARATHYROIDISM

This chart highlights disorders that affect the management of hyperparathyroidism.

DISORDER	SIGNS AND SYMPTOMS	DIAGNOSTIC TEST RESULTS
Pancreatitis (complication)	◆ Midepigastric abdominal pain, which can radiate to the back ◆ Mottled skin ◆ Tachycardia ◆ Low-grade fever ◆ Cold, sweaty extremities ◆ Restlessness ◆ Extreme malaise (in chronic pancreatitis)	◆ Serum amylase levels are dramatically elevated – in many cases over 500 U/L. ◆ Urine and pleural fluid analysis amylase are dramatically elevated in ascites. ◆ Serum lipase levels are increased. ◆ Serum calcium levels are decreased (hypocalcemia). ◆ White blood cell counts range from 8,000 to 20,000/ul, with increased polymorphonuclear leukocytes. ◆ Glucose levels are elevated – as high as 500 to 900 mg/dl. ◆ Abdominal X-rays or computed tomography (CT) scans show dilation of the small or large bowel or calcification of the pancreas. ◆ An ultrasound or CT scan reveals an increased pancreatic diameter and helps distinguish acute cholecystitis from acute pancreatitis.
Pseudogout (complication)	◆ Pain in the great toe ◆ Swollen, red or purple joint with limited movement ◆ Tophi, especially in the outer ears, hands, and feet ◆ Warmth over the joint and extreme tenderness ◆ Fever ◆ Hypertension	◆ Joint aspiration and synovial biopsy detect calcium pyrophosphate crystals. ◆ X-rays show calcium deposits in the fibrocartilage and linear markings along the bone ends. ◆ Blood tests may detect an underlying endocrine or metabolic disorder.
Renal calculi (complication)	◆ Severe pain that travels from the costovertebral angle to the flank and then to the suprapubic region and external genitalia ◆ Nausea ◆ Vomiting ◆ Fever ◆ Chills ◆ Hematuria ◆ Abdominal distention	◆ Kidney-ureter-bladder (KUB) radiography reveals renal calculi. ◆ Excretory urography determines the size and location of calculi. ◆ Kidney ultrasonography detects obstructive changes, such as unilateral or bilateral hydronephrosis and radiolucent calculi not seen on the KUB radiography. ◆ Urine culture of a midstream specimen may indicate pyuria. ◆ A 24-hour urine collection may detect the presence of calcium oxalate, phosphorus, and uric acid excretion. Three separate collections, along with blood samples, are needed for accurate testing. ◆ Calculus analysis shows mineral content. ◆ Serum blood calcium and phosphorus levels show an increased calcium level in proportion to normal serum protein levels. ◆ Blood protein levels determine the level of free calcium unbound to protein.

TREATMENT AND CARE

◆ Monitor the patient's vital signs and pulmonary artery pressure or central venous pressure closely. Give plasma or albumin to maintain blood pressure. Record fluid intake and output, check urine output hourly, and monitor electrolyte levels. Assess for crackles, rhonchi, or decreased breath sounds.

◆ For bowel decompression, maintain constant nasogastric suctioning, and give nothing by mouth.

◆ Watch for signs and symptoms of calcium deficiency (tetany, cramps, carpopedal spasm, and seizures). If you suspect hypocalcemia, keep airway and suction apparatus handy and pad side rails.

◆ Administer analgesics to relieve the patient's pain and anxiety. Remember that anticholinergics reduce salivary and sweat gland secretions. Warn the patient that he may experience dry mouth and facial flushing. *Caution:* Narrow-angle glaucoma contraindicates the use of atropine or its derivatives.

◆ Monitor glucose levels.

◆ Watch for complications of total parenteral nutrition, such as sepsis, hypokalemia, overhydration, and metabolic acidosis. Watch for fever, cardiac irregularities, changes in arterial blood gas measurements, and deep respirations. Use strict aseptic technique when caring for the catheter insertion site.

◆ Urge the patient to perform as much self-care as his immobility and pain allow.

◆ Encourage bed rest, but use a bed cradle to keep bed linens off of sensitive, inflamed joints.

◆ Carefully evaluate the patient's condition after joint aspiration.

◆ Give pain medication (especially during acute attacks), and monitor the patient's response.

◆ Apply cold packs to inflamed joints to ease discomfort and reduce swelling.

◆ To promote sleep, administer pain medication.

◆ Help the patient identify techniques and activities that promote rest and relaxation.

◆ Administer anti-inflammatory medication and other drugs, and watch for adverse reactions. Be alert for GI disturbances in the patient taking colchicine.

◆ When encouraging fluids, record intake and output accurately. Be sure to monitor serum uric acid levels regularly. Administer sodium bicarbonate or other agents to alkalinize the patient's urine.

◆ Provide a nutritious but purine-poor diet.

◆ Watch for acute gout attacks 24 to 96 hours after surgery. Administering colchicine before and after surgery may help prevent gout attacks.

◆ Maintain a 24- to 48-hour record of urine pH using nitrazine pH paper. Strain urine and save solid material for analysis.

◆ To facilitate spontaneous passage of calculi, encourage patient mobility and fluids.

◆ If the patient can't drink the required amount of fluid, give supplemental I.V. fluids.

◆ Record intake and output and daily weight to assess fluid status and renal function.

◆ Medicate the patient for pain when he's passing a calculus.

◆ To help acidify urine, offer fruit juices, especially cranberry juice.

If the patient had calculi surgically removed

◆ Anticipate that the patient will have an indwelling catheter or a nephrostomy tube.

◆ Unless one of his kidneys was removed, expect bloody drainage from the catheter.

◆ Check dressings regularly for bloody drainage, and know how much drainage to expect. Immediately report excessive drainage or a rising pulse rate (symptoms of hemorrhage).

◆ Use sterile technique when changing dressings or providing catheter care.

◆ Watch for signs of infection, such as a rising fever or chills, and give antibiotics.

If lithotripsy is planned

◆ Expect to discontinue anticoagulants, aspirin, vitamin E, and platelet inhibitors for 3 days before the procedure.

Hyperphosphatemia

Hyperphosphatemia occurs when the serum phosphorus levels exceed 4.5 mg/dl (or 2.6 mEq/L). It usually reflects the kidneys' inability to excrete excess phosphorus. The condition commonly occurs along with an increased release of phosphorus from damaged cells. Severe hyperphosphatemia occurs when the serum phosphorus levels reach 6 mg/dl or higher.

ETIOLOGY

Three basic mechanisms can lead to hyperphosphatemia: reduced renal phosphate excretion, shifting of phosphorus from the intracellular space into the extracellular fluid, and increased phosphate intake or absorption. For example, hyperphosphatemia can result from such conditions as hypocalcemia, hypervitaminosis D, hypoparathyroidism, and renal failure, and from the overuse of laxatives with phosphates or phosphate enemas.

DRUG ALERT *Certain agents, such as oral phosphorus supplements, parenteral phosphorus supplements, and vitamin D supplements, can be associated with hyperphosphatemia.*

Infants who are fed cow's milk–based formula are predisposed to hyperphosphatemia because this kind of formula contains more phosphorus than breast milk does.

Phosphorus shifting to extracellular fluid may be caused by acid-base imbalances, chemotherapy, sepsis, hypothermia, muscle necrosis, and rhabdomyolysis. Impaired phosphorus excretion can also be related to any renal disorder that causes the glomerular filtration rate to fall below 30 ml/minute. Additionally, patients with slowed GI motility or defects of the bowel mucosa are at an increased risk for hyperphosphatemia.

PATHOPHYSIOLOGY

The pathophysiologic processes involved in hyperphosphatemia can vary depending on the cause of the condition. For example, large quantities of phosphates may be released into the circulation when chemotherapy is administered for a neoplastic condi-

tion. The increased levels are the result of cell destruction and release of intracellular phosphates (tumor lysis).

Conditions that lead to tissue necrosis, such as rhabdomyolysis, cause a shift of phosphorus from the cellular space into the extracellular fluid because muscle tissue contains the bulk of soft tissue phosphate. Blood transfusions can also be a source of exogenous phosphorus because of the leakage from the blood cells during storage.

Cardiovascular system

- Arrhythmias, palpitations, and an irregular heart rate may be related to hypocalcemia of calcium-phosphate calcification.

Endocrine and metabolic systems

- Hyperphosphatemia in renal failure results in acidosis; because acidosis favors increased calcium ionization, patients are less prone to develop hypocalcemia.

Integumentary system

- Calcium-phosphate calcification can lead to soft-tissue calcification causing dry, itchy skin with papular eruptions.
- Calcification of ocular vessels can lead to conjunctivitis and corneal haziness that progresses to impaired vision.

Neuromuscular system

- Associated hypocalcemia can lead to signs of tetany such as tingling (paresthesia) of the tips of the fingers and around the mouth. These sensations may increase in severity and spread along the limbs and to the face, resulting in numbness, muscle spasms, and pain.
- Hyperreflexia, mental status changes, muscle weakness, or seizures may develop because of hypocalcemia.

Renal system

- Oliguria related to acute or chronic renal failure may develop.
- Precipitation of calcium phosphate can lead to progressive renal impairment.

Respiratory system

- The patient may experience respiratory compromise related to lung tissue calcification.

■ Hyperphosphatemia commonly leads to respiratory acidosis. (See *Disorders affecting management of hyperphosphatemia,* pages 192 to 195.)

ASSESSMENT

The clinical signs and symptoms of hyperphosphatemia are primarily those associated with hypocalcemia because hyperphosphatemia results when elevated serum phosphate combines with ionized calcium. Insoluble calcium phosphate is formed when the calcium-phosphate product exceeds 75. The calcium-phosphate product is obtained by multiplying the serum calcium level with the serum phosphate level.

Clinical findings
■ Paresthesia, especially in the fingertips and around the mouth
■ Conjunctivitis or impaired vision
■ Anorexia
■ Impaired mental status and seizures
■ Muscle weakness, cramps, and spasms
■ Nausea and vomiting
■ Dry, itchy skin
■ Arrhythmias and irregular heart rate
■ Chvostek's sign or Trousseau's sign
■ Hyperreflexia
■ Papular eruptions
■ Decreased urine output
■ Corneal haziness

Diagnostic test results
■ *Serum phosphorus level* is 4.6 to 6 mg/dl in moderate hyperphosphatemia; more than 6 mg/dl in severe hyperphosphatemia.
■ *Serum calcium level* is below 8.9 mg/dl.
■ *Red blood cell 2, 3-DPG levels* may be increased.
■ *Electrocardiography* shows such changes as prolonged QT intervals and ST segments.
■ *X-rays* reveal skeletal changes caused by osteodystrophy in chronic hyperphosphatemia.
■ *Blood urea nitrogen and creatinine levels* are increased, reflecting worsening renal function.

COLLABORATIVE MANAGEMENT

Because hyperphosphatemia can affect multiple body systems, a multidisciplinary approach to care is needed. A renal specialist or nephrologist can help evaluate, treat, and manage the patient's kidney function. Respiratory and cardiology specialists may be consulted, depending on the patient's history and complications he may develop. Nutritional therapy may be involved to help institute necessary restrictions or supplementations. Physical and occupational therapy may help with energy conservation and rehabilitation, depending on the patient's condition and length of stay. If a prolonged hospital stay is expected and the patient requires long-term care or home care, social services may be consulted early on in the patient's care. The patient may also benefit from psychological or spiritual counseling if he's acutely ill or will require continued care upon discharge.

TREATMENT AND CARE
■ When possible, treatment is directed at the underlying disorder.
■ If the imbalance is related to excess phosphate intake, eliminate the source of phosphorus; dietary restriction may be needed.
■ A patient with renal failure may be placed on phosphate-binding medications. These medications bind phosphorus from dietary sources in the gut, which leads to elimination of the phosphorus in the patient's stools. Patients on phosphate binders should take this medication with meals to allow for the binding of phosphorus in the GI tract.
■ In acute hyperphosphatemia, I.V. infusions of saline may promote renal phosphorus excretion if the patient has normal renal function.
■ It may be necessary to administer hypertonic dextrose in conjunction with regular insulin to temporarily move the phosphorus into the cells.
■ Hemodialysis or peritoneal dialysis may be indicated if the hyperphosphatemia is related to renal failure.
■ Monitor for signs and symptoms of hypocalcemia, calcium phosphate calcification, and cardiac arrhythmias.
■ Monitor vital signs, intake and output, electrolyte levels, and renal studies.
■ Provide safety measures, and monitor for mental status changes and seizures.
■ Encourage the patient to avoid foods high in phosphorus, such as beans, bran,

(Text continues on page 194.)

WATCHFUL EYE

DISORDERS AFFECTING
MANAGEMENT OF HYPERPHOSPHATEMIA

This chart highlights disorders that affect the management of hyperphosphatemia.

DISORDER	SIGNS AND SYMPTOMS	DIAGNOSTIC TEST RESULTS
Heart failure (complication)	◆ Cough that produces pink, frothy sputum ◆ Cyanosis of the lips and nail beds ◆ Pale, cool, clammy skin ◆ Diaphoresis ◆ Jugular vein distention ◆ Ascites ◆ Pulsus alternans ◆ Tachycardia ◆ Hepatomegaly ◆ Decreased pulse pressure ◆ Third and fourth heart sounds ◆ Moist, basilar crackles ◆ Rhonchi ◆ Expiratory wheezing ◆ Decreased pulse oximetry ◆ Peripheral edema ◆ Decreased urinary output	◆ B-type natriuretic peptide immunoassay is elevated. ◆ Chest X-ray shows increased pulmonary vascular markings, interstitial edema, or pleural effusions and cardiomegaly. ◆ Electrocardiography (ECG) reveals heart enlargement or ischemia, tachycardia, extrasystole, or atrial fibrillation. ◆ Pulmonary artery pressure, pulmonary artery wedge pressure, and left ventricular end-diastolic pressure are elevated in the presence of left-sided heart failure; right atrial or central venous pressure is elevated in right-sided heart failure.
Hypocalcemia (complication)	◆ Anxiety, confusion, irritability ◆ Seizures ◆ Paresthesia of the toes, fingers, or face, especially around the mouth ◆ Twitching ◆ Muscle cramps ◆ Tremors ◆ Laryngospasm ◆ Bronchospasm ◆ Positive Trousseau's or Chvostek's signs ◆ Brittle nails ◆ Dry skin and hair ◆ Diarrhea ◆ Hyperactive deep tendon reflexes ◆ Decreased cardiac output ◆ Arrhythmias (prolonged ST segment, lengthened QT interval [risk of torsades de pointes] or decreased myocardial contractility, leading to angina, bradycardia, hypotension, and heart failure)	◆ Total serum calcium level is less than 8.5 mg/dl. ◆ Ionized calcium level is below 4.5 mg/dl. ◆ Albumin level is low. ◆ ECG reveals a prolonged ST segment and lengthened QT interval.
Respiratory acidosis (complication)	◆ Apprehension ◆ Confusion ◆ Decreased deep tendon reflexes ◆ Diaphoresis ◆ Dyspnea with rapid, shallow respirations ◆ Headache ◆ Nausea or vomiting ◆ Restlessness	◆ Arterial blood gas (ABG) analysis reveals pH below 7.35 and partial pressure of arterial carbon dioxide above 45 mm Hg. ◆ HCO_3^- level varies depending on how long the acidosis has been present. In the patient with acute respiratory acidosis, HCO_3^- level may be normal; in the patient with chronic respiratory acidosis, it may be above 26 mEq/L.

TREATMENT AND CARE

◆ Administer supplemental oxygen and mechanical ventilation, if needed.
◆ Place the patient in Fowler's position.
◆ Administer diuretics, inotropic drugs, vasodilators, angiotensin-converting enzyme inhibitors, angiotensin receptor blockers, cardiac glycosides, beta-adrenergic blockers, and electrolyte supplements.
◆ Initiate cardiac monitoring.
◆ Recurrent heart failure from valvular dysfunction may require surgery.
◆ A ventricular assist device may be needed.
◆ Maintain adequate cardiac output and monitor hemodynamic stability.
◆ Assess for deep vein thrombosis and apply antiembolism stockings.

◆ Monitor vital signs and assess the patient frequently.
◆ Monitor respiratory status, including rate, depth, and rhythm.
◆ Watch for stridor, dyspnea, and crowing.
◆ If the patient shows overt signs of hypocalcemia, keep a tracheotomy tray and a handheld resuscitation bag at the bedside in case laryngospasm occurs.
◆ Place your patient on a cardiac monitor, and evaluate him for changes in heart rate and rhythm, such as ventricular tachycardia or heart block.
◆ Check the patient for Chvostek's sign or Trousseau's sign.
◆ Monitor the patient receiving I.V. calcium for arrhythmias, especially if he's also taking digoxin. Calcium and digoxin have similar effects on the heart.
◆ Administer I.V. calcium replacement therapy carefully. Ensure the patency of the I.V. line because infiltration can cause tissue necrosis and sloughing.
◆ Administer oral replacements. Give calcium supplements 1 to 1½ hours after meals. If GI upset occurs, give the supplement with milk.
◆ Monitor pertinent laboratory test results, including calcium levels, albumin levels, and other electrolyte levels. Check the ionized calcium level after every 4 units of blood transfused.
◆ Encourage the older patient to take a calcium supplement and to exercise as much as he can tolerate to prevent calcium loss from bones.
◆ Take seizure precautions such as padding bedside rails.
◆ Reorient the confused patient. Provide a calm, quiet environment.

◆ Maintain a patent airway. Provide adequate humidification to ensure moist secretions.
◆ Monitor vital signs and assess cardiac rhythm. Respiratory acidosis can cause tachycardia, alterations in respiratory rate and rhythm, hypotension, and arrhythmias.
◆ Continue to assess respiratory patterns. Immediately report changes. Prepare for mechanical ventilation, if indicated.
◆ Monitor the patient's neurologic status and report significant changes.
◆ Monitor the patient's cardiac function because respiratory acidosis may progress to shock and cardiac arrest.
◆ Report variations in ABG values, pulse oximetry, or serum electrolyte levels.
◆ Administer antibiotics or bronchodilators.

(continued)

DISORDERS AFFECTING MANAGEMENT OF HYPERPHOSPHATEMIA *(continued)*		
DISORDER	**SIGNS AND SYMPTOMS**	**DIAGNOSTIC TEST RESULTS**
Respiratory acidosis *(continued)*	◆ Tachycardia ◆ Tremors ◆ Warm, flushed skin	◆ Serum electrolyte levels reveal a potassium level greater than 5 mEq/L. In acidosis, potassium leaves the cell, so expect the serum level to be elevated.

cheese, chocolate, dairy products, dark-colored sodas, lentils, nuts, peanut butter, and seeds.

Hyperpituitarism

Hyperpituitarism is a chronic, progressive disease marked by hormonal dysfunction and skeletal overgrowth. Although the prognosis depends on the causative factor, the disease usually reduces life expectancy if left untreated.

Hyperpituitarism appears in two forms: acromegaly and gigantism. Acromegaly occurs after epiphyseal closure, causing bone thickening and transverse growth and visceromegaly. This rare form of hyperpituitarism occurs equally among men and women, usually between the ages of 30 and 50.

Gigantism begins before epiphyseal closure and causes proportional overgrowth of all body tissues. As the disease progresses, loss of other trophic hormones, such as thyroid-stimulating hormone, luteinizing hormone, follicle-stimulating hormone, and corticotropin, may cause dysfunction of the target organs.

ETIOLOGY

In most patients, the source of excessive growth hormone (GH) or human growth hormone (HGH) secretion is a GH-producing adenoma of the anterior pituitary gland, usually macroadenoma (eosinophilic or mixed cell). The cause of the tumor is unclear. Occasionally, however, hyperpituitarism occurs in more than one family member, suggesting a genetic cause.

PATHOPHYSIOLOGY

A GH-secreting tumor creates an unpredictable GH secretion pattern, which replaces the usual peaks that occur 1 to 4 hours after the onset of sleep. Elevated GH and somatomedin levels stimulate tissue growth. Prolonged effects of excess GH secretion can affect other body systems.

Cardiovascular system

■ Excess GH causes enlargement of internal organs, which can result in cardiovascular disease, arteriosclerosis, hypertension, left-sided heart failure, and acromegalic cardiomyopathy with arrhythmias. (See *Disorders affecting management of hyperpituitarism,* pages 196 and 197.)

Endocrine system

■ Gigantism and acromegaly can cause signs of glucose intolerance and clinically apparent diabetes mellitus because of the insulin-antagonistic character of GH.

Musculoskeletal system

■ Excessive GH secretion may lead to arthritis, carpal tunnel syndrome, osteoporosis, and kyphosis.
■ In acromegaly, the excess GH increases bone density and width and the proliferation of connective and soft tissues.

- Administer oxygen. Generally, lower concentrations of oxygen are given to patients with chronic obstructive pulmonary disease because the medulla of these patients is accustomed to high carbon dioxide levels.
- Perform tracheal suctioning, incentive spirometry, postural drainage, and coughing and deep breathing as indicated.
- Make sure the patient takes in enough oral and I.V fluids, and maintain accurate intake and output records.
- Provide reassurance to the patient and family.
- Keep in mind that sedatives can decrease his respiratory rate.
- Institute safety measures as needed to protect a confused patient.

■ In pituitary gigantism — because the epiphyseal plates aren't closed — the excess GH stimulates linear growth.

Neurologic system
■ Acromegaly may result in blindness and severe neurologic disturbances due to compression of surrounding tissues by the tumor.
■ Bilateral temporal hemianopsia is common because of optic chiasm compression.

ASSESSMENT
The patient may complain of diaphoresis, oily skin, fatigue, heat intolerance, weight gain, headaches, decreased vision, decreased libido, impotence, oligomenorrhea, infertility, joint pain (possibly from osteoarthritis), hypertrichosis, and sleep disturbances (related to obstructive sleep apnea from an enlarged tongue [macroglossia]).

Clinical findings
■ Enlarged jaw, thickened tongue, enlarged and weakened hands, coarsened facial features, oily or leathery skin, and a prominent supraorbital ridge
■ Deep, hollow-sounding voice caused by laryngeal hypertrophy
■ Enlarged paranasal sinuses
■ Irritability, hostility, and other psychological disturbances
■ Cartilaginous and connective tissue overgrowth, causing a characteristic hulking appearance and thickened ears and nose
■ Prognathism (projection of the jaw) that may interfere with chewing

■ Thick fingers with tips that appear "tufted" (may appear as arrowheads on X-ray)
■ Multinodular goiter
■ Mild hirsutism in women

Diagnostic test results
■ *GH radioimmunoassay* shows increased plasma GH levels. However, because GH isn't secreted at a steady rate, a random sampling may be misleading. This test also shows increased levels of insulin-like growth factor (IGF) I. IGF-I (somatomedin-C) levels are a better screening option.
■ *Glucose suppression test* offers more reliable information. Glucose normally suppresses GH secretion; therefore, a glucose infusion that fails to suppress the hormone level to below the accepted norm of 2 ng/ml strongly suggests hyperpituitarism when combined with characteristic clinical features.
■ *Skull X-ray, computed tomography scan,* or *magnetic resonance imaging* may help locate the pituitary tumor.
■ *Bone X-rays* show a thickening of the cranium (especially of frontal, occipital, and parietal bones) and of the long bones as well as osteoarthritis in the spine.

COLLABORATIVE MANAGEMENT
Hypertension affects multiple body systems; thus, a multidisciplinary approach to care is necessary. A cardiologist may be called in to treat cardiovascular complications that can occur such as heart failure. An endocrinologist may be needed to prescribe treatment for developing diabetes and for glucose con-

DISORDERS AFFECTING
MANAGEMENT OF HYPERPITUITARISM

This chart highlights disorders that affect the management of hyperpituitarism.

DISORDER	SIGNS AND SYMPTOMS	DIAGNOSTIC TEST RESULTS
Diabetes mellitus (complication)	◆ Weight loss despite voracious hunger ◆ Weakness ◆ Vision changes ◆ Frequent skin and urinary tract infections ◆ Dry, itchy skin ◆ Poor skin turgor ◆ Dry mucous membranes ◆ Dehydration ◆ Decreased peripheral pulses ◆ Cool skin temperature ◆ Decreased reflexes ◆ Orthostatic hypotension ◆ Muscle wasting ◆ Loss of subcutaneous fat ◆ Fruity breath odor from ketoacidosis	◆ Fasting plasma glucose level is 126 mg/dl or greater, or a random blood glucose level is 200 mg/dl or greater on at least two occasions. ◆ Blood glucose level is 200 mg/dl or greater 2 hours after ingestion of 75 grams of oral dextrose. ◆ An ophthalmologic examination may show diabetic retinopathy.
Heart failure (complication)	◆ Cough that produces pink, frothy sputum ◆ Cyanosis of the lips and nail beds ◆ Pale, cool, clammy skin ◆ Diaphoresis ◆ Jugular vein distention ◆ Ascites ◆ Pulsus alternans ◆ Tachycardia ◆ Hepatomegaly ◆ Decreased pulse pressure ◆ Third and fourth heart sounds ◆ Moist, basilar crackles ◆ Rhonchi ◆ Expiratory wheezing ◆ Decreased pulse oximetry ◆ Peripheral edema ◆ Decreased urinary output	◆ B-type natriuretic peptide immunoassay is elevated. ◆ Chest X-ray shows increased pulmonary vascular markings, interstitial edema, or pleural effusions and cardiomegaly. ◆ Electrocardiography reveals heart enlargement or ischemia, tachycardia, extrasystole, or atrial fibrillation. ◆ Pulmonary artery pressure, pulmonary artery wedge pressure, and left ventricular end-diastolic pressure are elevated in the presence of left-sided heart failure; right atrial or central venous pressure is elevated in right-sided heart failure.

trol. In some cases, panhypopituitarism develops and the endocrinologist can prescribe treatment for deficiencies of other endocrine hormones. An orthopedic surgeon or rheumatologist may be consulted to manage the damaging effects on the joints, cartilage, and bones. A psychological consult may be necessary to help the patient deal with his altered appearance.

TREATMENT AND CARE

■ The goal of treatment is to curb overproduction of GH by removing the underlying tumor. Removal is done by cranial or transsphenoidal hypophysectomy or pituitary radiation therapy. In acromegaly, surgery is mandatory when a tumor is compressing surrounding healthy tissue.

■ Postoperative therapy commonly requires replacement of thyroid, cortisone, and gonadal hormones.

TREATMENT AND CARE

◆ Check blood glucose levels periodically because steroid replacement may require adjustment of the insulin dosage.
◆ Keep a late-morning snack available in case the patient becomes hypoglycemic.
◆ Keep accurate records of vital signs, weight, fluid intake, urine output, and calorie intake.
◆ Monitor serum glucose and urine acetone levels.
◆ Monitor the patient for acute complications of diabetic therapy, especially hypoglycemia (vagueness, slow cerebration, dizziness, weakness, pallor, tachycardia, diaphoresis, seizures, and coma); immediately give carbohydrates in the form of fruit juice, hard candy, or honey; if the patient is unconscious, give glucagon or I.V. dextrose.
◆ Be alert for signs of hyperosmolar coma (polyuria, thirst, neurologic abnormalities, and stupor). This hyperglycemic crisis requires I.V. fluids and insulin replacement.
◆ Monitor the effects of diabetes on the cardiovascular system – such as cerebrovascular, coronary artery, and peripheral vascular impairment – and on the peripheral and autonomic nervous systems.
◆ Provide meticulous skin care, and watch for manifestations of urinary tract and vaginal infections.

◆ Administer supplemental oxygen and mechanical ventilation, if needed.
◆ Place the patient in Fowler's position.
◆ Administer diuretics, inotropic drugs, vasodilators, angiotensin-converting enzyme inhibitors, angiotensin receptor blockers, cardiac glycosides, beta-adrenergic blockers, and electrolyte supplements.
◆ Initiate cardiac monitoring.
◆ Recurrent heart failure from valvular dysfunction may require surgery.
◆ A ventricular assist device may be needed.
◆ Maintain adequate cardiac output and monitor hemodynamic stability.
◆ Assess for deep vein thrombosis and apply antiembolism stockings.

■ Adjunctive treatment may include bromocriptine (Parlodel), a dopamine antagonist that inhibits GH synthesis; and octreotide acetate (Sandostatin), a long-acting somatostatin analog that suppresses GH secretion in at least two-thirds of patients with acromegaly.

DRUG ALERT *Dopamine antagonists may cause hypotension, stroke, acute myocardial infarction, and peptic ulcer. Somatostatin analogs may cause cardiac arrhythmias, hypoglycemia, hyperglycemia, cholelithiasis, and hypothyroidism. These analogs may also interact with beta-adrenergic blockers and calcium channel blockers, increasing the risk of bradyarrhythmias and heart conduction defects.*

Hypertension

Hypertension, an elevation in diastolic or systolic blood pressure, occurs as two major types: essential (idiopathic) hypertension (the most common) and secondary hypertension, which results from renal disease or another identifiable cause. Malignant hypertension is a severe, fulminant form of hypertension common to both types.

Hypertension affects 15% to 20% of adults in the United States and it's a major cause of stroke, cardiac disease, and renal failure. The risk of hypertension increases with age and is higher in blacks and in those with less education and lower income. Men have a higher incidence of hypertension in young and early middle adulthood; thereafter, women have a higher incidence.

Essential hypertension usually begins insidiously as a benign disease, slowly progressing to a malignant state. If left untreated, initially mild cases can lead to severely elevated blood pressure (hypertensive crisis), causing major complications and, possibly, proving fatal. However, with carefully managed treatment, which may include lifestyle modifications and drug therapy, the prognosis is significantly improved.

ETIOLOGY

Scientists haven't been able to identify any single cause for essential hypertension. The disorder probably reflects an interaction of multiple homeostatic forces, including changes in renal regulation of sodium and extracellular fluids, aldosterone secretion and metabolism, and norepinephrine secretion and metabolism.

Secondary hypertension may be caused by renal vascular disease; pheochromocytoma; primary hyperaldosteronism; Cushing's syndrome; or dysfunction of the thyroid, pituitary, or parathyroid glands. It may also result from coarctation of the aorta, pregnancy, and neurologic disorders.

Certain risk factors appear to increase the likelihood of hypertension. These include:
■ family history of hypertension
■ race
■ gender
■ diabetes mellitus

■ stress
■ obesity
■ high dietary intake of saturated fats or sodium
■ tobacco use
■ hormonal contraceptive use
■ sedentary lifestyle
■ aging.

PATHOPHYSIOLOGY

Arterial blood pressure is a product of total peripheral resistance and cardiac output. Cardiac output is increased by conditions that increase heart rate, stroke volume, or both. Peripheral resistance is increased by factors that increase blood viscosity or reduce the lumen size of vessels, especially the arterioles.

Several theories help to explain the development of hypertension, including:
■ changes in the arteriolar bed, causing increased peripheral vascular resistance
■ abnormally increased tone in the sympathetic nervous system that originates in the vasomotor system centers, causing increased peripheral vascular resistance
■ increased blood volume, resulting from renal or hormonal dysfunction
■ increased arteriolar thickening caused by genetic factors, leading to increased peripheral vascular resistance
■ abnormal renin release, resulting in the formation of angiotensin II, which constricts the arteriole and increases blood volume.
(See *Understanding blood pressure regulation.*)

In secondary hypertension, damage to the kidney from chronic glomerulonephritis or renal artery stenosis interferes with sodium excretion, the renin-angiotensin-aldosterone system, or renal perfusion, causing blood pressure to increase.

Cardiovascular system

■ Prolonged hypertension increases the heart's workload as resistance to left ventricular ejection increases.
■ To increase contractile force, the left ventricle hypertrophies, raising the heart's oxygen demands and workload.
■ Cardiac dilation and failure may occur when hypertrophy can no longer maintain sufficient cardiac output.
■ Because hypertension promotes coronary atherosclerosis, the heart may be further

UNDERSTANDING BLOOD PRESSURE REGULATION

Hypertension may result from a disturbance in one of these intrinsic mechanisms.

Renin-angiotensin system
The renin-angiotensin system acts to increase blood pressure through these mechanisms:
◆ sodium depletion, reduced blood pressure, and dehydration stimulate renin release
◆ renin reacts with angiotensin, a liver enzyme, and converts it to angiotensin I, which increases preload and afterload
◆ angiotensin I converts to angiotensin II in the lungs; angiotensin II is a potent vasoconstrictor that targets the arterioles
◆ angiotensin II works to increase preload and afterload by stimulating the adrenal cortex to secrete aldosterone; this increases blood volume by conserving sodium and water.

Autoregulation
Several intrinsic mechanisms work to change an artery's diameter to maintain tissue and organ perfusion despite fluctuations in systemic blood pressure. These mechanisms include stress relaxation and capillary fluid shifts:

◆ in stress relaxation, blood vessels gradually dilate when blood pressure increases to reduce peripheral resistance
◆ in capillary fluid shift, plasma moves between vessels and extravascular spaces to maintain intravascular volume.

Sympathetic nervous system
When blood pressure drops, baroreceptors in the aortic arch and carotid sinuses decrease their inhibition of the medulla's vasomotor center. The consequent increases in sympathetic stimulation of the heart by norepinephrine increase cardiac output by strengthening the contractile force, raising the heart rate, and augmenting peripheral resistance by vasoconstriction. Stress can also stimulate the sympathetic nervous system to increase cardiac output and peripheral vascular resistance.

Antidiuretic hormone
The release of antidiuretic hormone can regulate hypotension by increasing reabsorption of water by the kidney. With reabsorption, blood plasma volume increases, thus raising blood pressure.

compromised by reduced blood flow to the myocardium, resulting in angina or myocardial infarction (MI).
■ Hypertension causes vascular damage, leading to accelerated atherosclerosis and target organ damage, such as retinal injury, renal failure, stroke, and aortic aneurysm and dissection. (See *Disorders affecting management of hypertension*, pages 200 to 203.)

Neurologic system
■ As organ damage occurs, cerebral perfusion decreases and stress on vessel walls increases.
■ Arterial spasm and ischemia lead to transient ischemic attacks.
■ Weakening of the vessel intima leads to possible aneurysm formation and intracranial hemorrhage.

ASSESSMENT
Assessment of the patient with a hypertensive emergency almost always reveals a history of hypertension that's poorly controlled or that has gone untreated. If secondary hypertension exists, signs and symptoms may be related to the cause. For example, Cushing's syndrome may cause truncal obesity and purple striae, whereas patients with pheochromocytoma may develop headache, nausea, vomiting, palpitations, pallor, and profuse perspiration.

Clinical findings
■ Occipital headache (may worsen on rising in the morning as a result of increased intracranial pressure) resulting from vascular changes
■ Nausea and vomiting
(*Text continues on page 202.*)

WATCHFUL EYE

DISORDERS AFFECTING
MANAGEMENT OF HYPERTENSION

This chart highlights disorders that affect the management of hypertension.

DISORDER	SIGNS AND SYMPTOMS	DIAGNOSTIC TEST RESULTS
Aortic aneurysm (complication)	◆ Pallor ◆ Diaphoresis ◆ Dyspnea ◆ Cyanosis ◆ Leg weakness or transient paralysis ◆ Abrupt onset of intermittent neurologic deficits ◆ Hoarseness ◆ Dyspnea ◆ Throat pain ◆ Dysphagia ◆ Dry cough *Dissecting ascending aneurysm* ◆ Pain most intense at its onset that may extend to neck, shoulders, lower back, and abdomen ◆ Boring, tearing, or ripping sensation in the thorax or the right anterior chest *Dissecting descending aneurysm* ◆ Sharp, tearing pain located between the shoulder blades that commonly radiates to the chest *Dissecting transverse aneurysm* ◆ Sharp, boring, and tearing pain that radiates to the shoulders	◆ Abdominal ultrasonography or echocardiography determines the size, shape, and location of the aneurysm. ◆ Aortography shows condition of vessels proximal and distal to aneurysm.
Chronic renal failure (complication)	◆ Muscle twitching ◆ Paresthesia ◆ Bone pain ◆ Pruritus ◆ Decreased urine output ◆ Stomatitis ◆ Lethargy ◆ Seizures ◆ Brittle nails and hair ◆ Kussmaul's respirations ◆ Uremic frost ◆ Ecchymosis ◆ Weight gain	◆ Glomerular filtration rate (GFR) is decreased or urinalysis shows albuminuria, proteinuria, glycosuria, erythrocytes, and leukocytes. ◆ Serum creatinine may increase by 2 mg/dl or more over a 2-week period. ◆ Creatinine clearance is decreased. ◆ Blood urea nitrogen (BUN) suddenly increases. ◆ Uric acid is elevated. ◆ Potassium level is elevated. ◆ Arterial blood gas (ABG) analysis may show metabolic acidosis.
Diabetes mellitus (coexisting)	◆ Weight loss ◆ Anorexia ◆ Polyphagia ◆ Acetone breath	◆ Fasting blood glucose is 126 mg/dl or higher, or a random blood glucose level is 200 mg/dl or higher on at least two occasions.

TREATMENT AND CARE

◆ Manage blood pressure with beta-adrenergic blockers, angiotensin-converting enzyme (ACE) inhibitors, and diuretics. For severe hypertensive episode, give nitroprusside.
◆ Monitor aneurysm growth with serial ultrasounds.
◆ Encourage lifestyle modifications, such as smoking cessation, weight loss, and diet modification, as appropriate.
◆ Advise the patient to seek medical attention for abdominal or back pain.

◆ ACE inhibitors and angiotensin receptor blockers are used to achieve target blood pressure of less than 130/80 mm Hg.
◆ Therapeutic goals are to reduce the deterioration of renal function and prevent stroke.
◆ Loop diuretics may be used in patients with advanced renal disease.
◆ Monitor creatinine clearance, BUN, uric acid, and GFR.
◆ Monitor potassium levels to detect hyperkalemia.
◆ Monitor ABG studies for metabolic acidosis.
◆ Be alert for drug toxicity and adverse reactions.
◆ Advise the patient taking loop diuretics about maintaining a sodium-restricted diet.

◆ Thiazide diuretics, ACE inhibitors, beta-adrenergic blockers, angiotensin receptor blockers, and calcium channel blockers help reduce the risk of cardiovascular disease and stroke.
◆ Encourage lifestyle modifications, such as smoking cessation, weight loss, and dietary modifications, as appropriate.
◆ Monitor blood glucose levels.

(continued)

DISORDERS AFFECTING
MANAGEMENT OF HYPERTENSION *(continued)*

DISORDER	SIGNS AND SYMPTOMS	DIAGNOSTIC TEST RESULTS
Diabetes mellitus *(continued)*	◆ Weakness ◆ Fatigue ◆ Dehydration ◆ Pain ◆ Paresthesia ◆ Polyuria ◆ Polydipsia ◆ Kussmaul's respirations ◆ Mottled extremities ◆ Blurred vision	◆ Blood glucose level is 200 mg/dl or higher 2 hours after ingestion of 75 grams of dextrose.

■ Epistaxis possibly caused by vascular involvement
■ Dizziness, confusion, and fatigue resulting from decreased tissue perfusion caused by vasoconstriction of blood vessels
■ Blurry vision resulting from retinal damage
■ Nocturia caused by an increase in blood flow to the kidneys and an increase in glomerular filtration
■ Elevated blood pressure readings on at least two consecutive occasions after initial screening (see *Blood pressure classifications*)
■ Bruits (which may be heard over the abdominal aorta or carotid, renal, and femoral arteries) caused by stenosis or aneurysm
■ Edema caused by increased capillary pressure

Diagnostic test results
■ *Serial blood pressure measurements* detect changes in baseline readings.
■ *Urinalysis* may show protein, casts, red blood cells, or white blood cells, suggesting renal disease; presence of catecholamines, suggesting pheochromocytoma; or glucose, suggesting diabetes.
■ *Blood studies* may reveal elevated blood urea nitrogen and serum creatinine levels, suggesting renal disease; or hypokalemia, indicating adrenal dysfunction (primary hyperaldosteronism); *complete blood count* may reveal other causes of hypertension, such as polycythemia or anemia.
■ *Excretory urography* may reveal renal atrophy, indicating chronic renal disease. One

kidney smaller than the other suggests unilateral renal disease.
■ *Electrocardiogram* may show left ventricular hypertrophy or ischemia.
■ *Chest X-rays* may show cardiomegaly.
■ *Echocardiography* may reveal left ventricular hypertrophy.

COLLABORATIVE MANAGEMENT
Because hypertension affects multiple body systems, a multidisciplinary approach to care is necessary. Medical and nursing health care providers focus on administering medications to treat hypertension and prevent potential complications. Surgeons may be needed to correct the underlying problem associated with secondary hypertension, such as removal of tumor in pheochromocytoma. Nutritional consultation may be necessary to help with lifestyle changes involving diet. If the patient experiences end-organ damage, additional specialists may be needed to address these problems. Social services may need to be consulted for a referral for home-care evaluation and follow-up.

TREATMENT AND CARE
■ Treatment is aimed at reducing systolic and diastolic blood pressure to less than 140/90 mm Hg. In the patient with coexisting disorders, such as diabetes or renal disease, the goal is to reduce blood pressure to less than 130/80 mm Hg.
■ Teach the patient about ways he can modify his lifestyle, including losing weight, following the Dietary Approaches to Stop

TREATMENT AND CARE

TREATMENT AND CARE

◆ Advise the patient to watch for changes in vision and signs of infection, diabetic neuropathy, and cardiac distress.
◆ Advise the patient to perform good foot care and to watch for altered skin integrity or delayed wound healing.
◆ Monitor potassium levels and assess for signs of dehydration, if a diuretic is prescribed.

Hypertension (DASH) diet (involves consuming a diet rich in fruits, vegetables, and low-fat dairy products with a reduced content of saturated and total fat), reducing intake of sodium, increasing physical activity (regular aerobic activity such as brisk walking), and moderating intake of alcohol.

■ For patients with a systolic blood pressure ranging from 140 to 159 mm Hg and a diastolic blood pressure ranging from 90 to 99 mm Hg, drug therapy initially involves thiazide diuretics. Other agents, such as angiotensin-converting enzyme (ACE) inhibitors, angiotensin receptor blockers, beta-adrenergic blockers, and calcium channel blockers may be used instead of, or in combination with, thiazide diuretics.

■ For patients with blood pressure *greater* than 160/100 mm Hg, combination drug therapy is used.

■ Combination drug therapy is also used for patients with hypertension as well as other underlying disorders, such as heart failure, history of previous MI, diabetes, chronic renal disease, or history of stroke.

■ Treatment of secondary hypertension focuses on correcting the underlying cause and controlling hypertensive effects.

■ Hypertensive emergencies typically require parenteral administration of a vasodilator or an adrenergic inhibitor, or oral administration of a drug such as nifedipine (Procardia), captopril (Capoten), clonidine (Catapres), or labetalol (Normodyne)to rapidly reduce blood pressure. The goal is to reduce mean arterial blood pressure first by no more than 25% (within minutes to hours), then to 160/110 mm Hg within 2 hours while avoiding excessive decreases in blood pressure that can precipitate renal, cerebral, or myocardial ischemia.

BLOOD PRESSURE CLASSIFICATIONS

This table classifies blood pressure according to systolic blood pressure (SBP) and diastolic blood pressure (DBP).

BP CLASSIFICATION	NORMAL	PREHYPERTENSION	STAGE 1	STAGE 2
SBP (mm Hg)	< 120	120 to 139	140 to 159	≥ 160
	and	or	or	or
DBP (mm Hg)	< 80	80 to 89	90 to 99	≥ 100

Hyperthermia

Hyperthermia, also known as heat syndrome, refers to an elevation in body temperature over 99° F (37.2° C). Hyperthermia results when environmental and internal factors increase heat production or decrease heat loss beyond the body's ability to compensate.

Hyperthermia affects males and females equally; however, incidence increases among elderly patients and neonates during excessively hot days. If not treated aggressively, patients with temperatures over 106° F (41.1° C) (for a prolonged time) may die.

Risk factors for hyperthermia include obesity, salt and water depletion, alcohol use, poor physical condition, age (very young or very old), and socioeconomic status.

ETIOLOGY

Hyperthermia may result from conditions that increase heat production, such as excessive exercise, infection, and use of certain drugs (for example, amphetamines). It can also stem from factors that impair heat loss, such as high temperatures or humidity, lack of acclimatization, excess clothing, cardiovascular disease, obesity, dehydration, and sweat gland dysfunction.

Hyperthermia can manifest (and be categorized) in three ways: heat cramps, heat exhaustion, and heatstroke. Heat cramps are painful muscle contractions in the calves, usually caused by heat, dehydration, and poor conditioning. Heat exhaustion is acute heat injury with hyperthermia caused by dehydration. Heatstroke is extreme hyperthermia with thermoregulatory failure.

Malignant hyperthermia is a specific complication that may occur as a result of certain medications, primarily anesthetic agents. (See *Malignant hyperthermia*.)

PATHOPHYSIOLOGY

Normally, the human body adjusts to excessive temperatures through complex cardiovascular and neurologic changes, which are coordinated by the hypothalamus. Heat loss offsets heat production to regulate the body temperature. It does this by evaporation of sweat or vasodilation, which cools the body's surface by radiation, conduction, and convection. However, if the temperature remains elevated for a prolonged period of time, multiple body systems may be affected.

Cardiovascular system

■ If body temperature remains elevated, blood flow is redistributed to the periphery, fluid and electrolyte losses occur through sweat, and cardiac output is decreased
■ If left untreated, excessive body temperature can lead to hypovolemic shock, cardiogenic shock, and cardiac arrhythmias.

Gastrointestinal system

■ Fulminant hepatic failure may result from massive destruction of liver tissue following prolonged hyperthermia. (See *Disorders affecting management of hyperthermia*, pages 206 and 207.)

Hematologic system

■ Disseminated intravascular coagulation may result from the extensive destruction of endothelial surfaces caused by hyperthermia, causing the direct release of tissue plasminogen activator (tPA) and generation of plasmin.

Neurologic system

■ Prolonged hyperthermia results in cerebral edema and cerebrovascular congestion; cerebral perfusion pressure increases and cerebral perfusion decreases.
■ Level of consciousness is altered.

Renal system

■ Prolonged hyperthermia may result in rhabdomyolysis related to the hypermetabolic state of muscles, resulting in myoglobinuria and, possibly, renal failure.

Respiratory system

■ Prolonged hyperthermia results in acidosis, central nervous system (CNS) stimulation, and hypoxia, causing respiratory failure.

ASSESSMENT

Assessment findings vary depending on the type of hyperthermia present.

Clinical findings

Heat cramps
- Painful cramps in the gastrocnemius (back of the calves) or hamstring muscles
- Profuse sweating
- Nausea
- Pale, moist, cool skin
- Tachycardia

Heat exhaustion
- Muscle cramps
- Nausea and vomiting
- Thirst
- Weakness
- Headache
- Fatigue
- Rectal temperature higher than 100° F (37.8° C)
- Pale skin
- Thready, rapid pulse
- Cool, moist skin
- Decreased blood pressure
- Irritability
- Impaired judgment
- Hyperventilation

Heatstroke
- Signs and symptoms of heat exhaustion
- Blurred vision
- Confusion
- Hallucinations
- Decreased muscle coordination
- Syncope
- Rectal temperature of at least 104° F (40° C)
- Red, diaphoretic, hot skin in early stages
- Gray, dry, hot skin in later stages
- Tachycardia
- Slightly elevated blood pressure in early stages
- Decreased blood pressure in later stages
- Signs of CNS dysfunction
- Altered mental status
- Hyperpnea
- Cheyne-Stokes respirations
- Anhydrosis (late sign)

Diagnostic test results
- *Serum electrolyte levels* may reveal hyponatremia, hypokalemia, hypocalcemia, and hypophosphatemia.
- *Arterial blood gas studies* may reveal respiratory alkalosis.

MALIGNANT HYPERTHERMIA

Malignant hyperthermia is an inherited condition of hypermetabolism that occurs after exposure to certain drugs, including anesthetic agents such as succinylcholine or halothane. Drugs such as cocaine, diuretics, barbiturates, hallucinogens, and tricyclic antidepressants may depress hypothalamus activity, produce skin vasoconstriction (thus decreasing the ability to dissipate heat, causing a systemwide blockage of sweat production), and block the body's cardiovascular responses to heat, which increases cardiac output.

The number of malignant hyperthermia cases has increased in part because of "designer drug" use. For example, people attending raves (dance parties that last from one to several days) use various illicit drugs to avoid sleeping. Many patients suffer water intoxication and malignant hyperthermia. Frequent monitoring of electrolyte levels in addition to controlling core temperature is crucial. Also, obtaining a sample of the drug taken allows for chemical analysis of the substance, which may help guide treatment.

- *Blood studies* reveal leukocytosis, elevated blood urea nitrogen levels, hemoconcentration, thrombocytopenia, increased bleeding and clotting times, fibrinolysis, and consumption coagulopathy.
- *Urinalysis* results show concentrated urine with elevated protein levels, tubular casts, and myoglobinuria.

COLLABORATIVE MANAGEMENT
The emergency medical service team begins the process of decreasing the patient's temperature. Emergency department personnel evaluate the degree of hyperthermia and proceed with treatment accordingly. A cardiologist may be consulted to manage cardiac arrhythmias and shock if the patient is severely compromised. A pulmonary specialist may be needed to provide respiratory therapy if the patient requires mechanical ventilation. A neurosurgeon or neurologist may be consulted if an underlying neurologic condition is involved. If the cause of hyperthermia involves environmental or psychosocial con-

DISORDERS AFFECTING MANAGEMENT OF HYPERTHERMIA

This chart highlights disorders that affect the management of hyperthermia.

DISORDER	SIGNS AND SYMPTOMS	DIAGNOSTIC TEST RESULTS
Acute renal failure (complication)	◆ Urine output less than 400 ml/day for 1 to 2 weeks followed by diuresis (excretion of 3 to 5 L/day) for 2 to 3 weeks ◆ Lethargy ◆ Drowsiness ◆ Stupor ◆ Coma ◆ Irritability ◆ Headache ◆ Costovertebral pain ◆ Numbness around the mouth ◆ Tingling extremities ◆ Anorexia ◆ Restlessness ◆ Weight gain ◆ Nausea and vomiting ◆ Pallor ◆ Epistaxis ◆ Ecchymosis ◆ Diarrhea or constipation ◆ Stomatitis ◆ Thick, tenacious sputum	◆ Blood urea nitrogen (BUN) and serum creatinine levels are increased. With rhabdomyolysis, a creatinine increase greater than 5 mg/dl/day may occur because muscle is a major source of creatine, which is the precursor of creatinine. ◆ Potassium levels are increased. ◆ Hematocrit, blood pH, bicarbonate, and hemoglobin levels are decreased. ◆ Urine casts and cellular debris are present; specific gravity is decreased.
Disseminated intravascular coagulation (complication)	◆ Petechiae ◆ Ecchymosis ◆ Prolonged bleeding after venipuncture ◆ Hemorrhage ◆ Oliguria ◆ Anxiety ◆ Restlessness ◆ Purpura ◆ Acrocyanosis ◆ Joint pain ◆ Dyspnea ◆ Hemoptysis ◆ Crackles	◆ Decreased platelet count, usually less than 100,000/µl, because platelets are consumed during thrombosis. ◆ Fibrinogen levels are less than 150mg/dl. ◆ Prothrombin time (PT) is greater than 15 seconds. ◆ Partial thromboplastin time (PTT) is greater than 60 seconds. ◆ Fibrin degradation products are increased, commonly greater than 45 mcg/ml. ◆ D-dimer test is positive at less than 1:8 dilution. ◆ Fibrin monomers are positive. ◆ Levels of factors V and VIII are diminished. ◆ Red blood cell smear shows fragmentation. ◆ Hemoglobin is less than 10 g/dl.

ditions, a social worker or case manager is needed for discharge planning and follow up in the home for preventive measures.

TREATMENT AND CARE

■ Treat mild to moderate hyperthermia by providing a cool, restful environment.

■ Give oral or I.V. fluid and electrolyte replacements.

If the patient is experiencing heat stroke:
■ Remove the patient's clothing as much as possible, and apply cool water to the skin; fan the patient with cool air.

- Expect treatment to continue until the patient's body temperature drops to 102.2° F (39° C).
- Assess oxygen saturation and administer supplemental oxygen as indicated. Monitor the patient's pulmonary status closely, including respiratory rate and depth and lung sounds; anticipate the need for endotracheal intubation and mechanical ventilation if respiratory status deteriorates.
- Monitor vital signs continuously, especially core body temperature. Although the goal is to reduce the patient's temperature rapidly, too rapid a reduction can lead to vasoconstriction, which can cause shivering. Shivering increases metabolic demand and oxygen consumption and should be avoided.
- Institute continuous cardiac monitoring to evaluate for arrhythmias secondary to electrolyte imbalances.
- Employ additional external cooling measures, such as cool, wet sheets and tepid baths.
- Monitor hemodynamic parameters, such as central venous pressure and pulmonary artery wedge pressure, and assess peripheral circulation, including skin color, peripheral pulses, and capillary refill.
- Monitor fluid and electrolyte balance and laboratory test results. Assess renal function studies to evaluate for rhabdomyolysis.

TREATMENT AND CARE

- Monitor fluid balance status, including skin turgor; evidence of peripheral, sacral, or periorbital edema; and intake and output. Monitor urine output every hour and assess daily weights.
- Anticipate insertion of a central venous catheter or pulmonary artery catheter to assess hemodynamic status.
- Insertion of temporary dialysis catheter may be necessary for hemodialysis or continuous renal replacement therapy, depending on the patient's condition.
- Monitor results of laboratory and diagnostic tests, especially BUN and creatinine levels, arterial blood gas studies, and serum electrolyte levels.

- Assess the patient for bleeding and blood loss. Administer fluid replacement and blood products as indicated.
- Be alert for signs of pulmonary emboli. Watch hemodynamic parameters closely; decreased values suggest hemorrhage, whereas increased values suggest emboli.
- Fresh frozen plasma administration allows for replacement of clotting factors and inhibitors. Cryoprecipitate is the drug of choice if the patient's fibrinogen levels are significantly decreased.
- Obtain serial hemoglobin and hematocrit levels; monitor results of coagulation studies, including PTT, PT, fibrinogen levels, fibrin split products, and platelet counts.
- Monitor intake and output hourly. Monitor renal status for signs of acute renal failure.

- Assess the patient's airway, breathing, and circulation and initiate emergency resuscitative measures as indicated.
- Administer diazepam (Valium) or chlorpromazine (Thorazine) to control shivering.
- Apply a hyperthermia blanket and ice packs to the groin and axillae.

Hyperthyroidism

Hyperthyroidism (also known as *Graves' disease, Basedow's disease,* or *thyrotoxicosis*) is a metabolic imbalance that results from thyroid hormone overproduction. The most common form of hyperthyroidism is Graves' disease, which increases thyroxine (T_4) production, enlarges the thyroid gland (goiter), and causes multiple system changes.

With treatment, most patients can lead normal lives. However, thyroid storm—an acute exacerbation of hyperthyroidism—is a medical emergency that may lead to life-threatening cardiac, hepatic, or renal failure.

ETIOLOGY

Hyperthyroidism may result from genetic and immunologic factors. An increased incidence of this disorder in monozygotic twins, for example, points to an inherited factor, most likely an autosomal recessive gene. This disease occasionally coexists with abnormal iodine metabolism and other endocrine abnormalities, such as diabetes mellitus, thyroiditis, and hyperparathyroidism. Hyperthyroidism is also associated with the production of autoantibodies (thyroid-stimulating immunoglobulin and thyroid-stimulating hormone [TSH]-binding inhibitory immunoglobulin), possibly due to a defect in suppressor–T-lymphocyte function that allows the formation of autoantibodies.

In latent hyperthyroidism, excessive dietary intake of iodine and, possibly, stress can precipitate clinical hyperthyroidism. In a person with inadequately treated hyperthyroidism, stress — including surgery, infection, toxemia of pregnancy, and diabetic ketoacidosis — can precipitate thyroid storm. (See *Types of hyperthyroidism*.)

Incidence of Graves' disease is highest in those older than age 20, especially in patients with family histories of thyroid abnormalities; only 5% of hyperthyroid patients are younger than age 15.

PATHOPHYSIOLOGY

Hyperthyroidism affects virtually every body system.

Cardiovascular system
■ Hyperthyroidism causes tachycardia; full, bounding pulse; wide pulse pressure; cardiomegaly; increased cardiac output and blood volume; visible point of maximal impulse; paroxysmal supraventricular tachycardia and atrial fibrillation (especially in elderly people); and occasionally, systolic murmur at the left sternal border.

Eyes
■ The combined effects of accumulation of mucopolysaccharides and fluids in the retro-orbital tissues may force the eyeball outward (exophthalmos), and the lid to retract, producing the characteristic staring gaze of hyperthyroidism.
■ Inflammation of conjunctivae, corneas, or eye muscles may occur.
■ Diplopia and increased tearing may occur.

■ The eyes may not be able to close, causing the exposed corneal surfaces to become dry and irritated.

Gastrointestinal system
■ Increased GI mobility and peristalsis may cause anorexia, nausea and vomiting, increased defecation, soft stools or, with severe disease, diarrhea, and liver and spleen enlargement.

Integumentary system
■ Skin becomes smooth, warm, and flushed; the patient sleeps with minimal covering and little clothing.
■ Fine, soft hair; premature graying; and increased hair loss occurs in both sexes.
■ Nails become friable, and onycholysis (distal nail becomes separated from the bed) develops.
■ Pretibial myxedema (dermopathy) produces thickened skin, accentuated hair follicles, and raised red patches of skin that are itchy and sometimes painful with occasional nodule formation. Microscopic examination shows increased mucin deposits.

Neurologic system
■ Increased T_4 secretion accelerates cerebral function, causing difficulty in concentrating.
■ Excitability or nervousness occurs because of an increased basal metabolic rate.
■ Increased activity in the spinal cord area that controls muscle tone leads to fine tremor, shaky handwriting, and clumsiness.
■ Emotional instability and mood swings range from occasional outbursts to overt psychosis.

Musculoskeletal system
■ Weakness, fatigue, and muscle atrophy may develop.
■ Generalized or localized paralysis is associated with hypokalemia.
■ Occasionally, acropachy — soft-tissue swelling, accompanied by underlying bone changes where new bone formation occurs — develops. (See *Disorders affecting management of hyperthyroidism*, pages 210 and 211.)

Reproductive system
■ In females, oligomenorrhea or amenorrhea, decreased fertility, and higher incidence of spontaneous abortions may occur.
■ In males, gynecomastia (due to increased estrogen levels) may occur.
■ In both sexes, libido is diminished.

Respiratory system
■ Cardiac decompensation and increased cellular oxygen use cause an increased respiratory rate and dyspnea on exertion and at rest.

ASSESSMENT
Although the diagnosis of hyperthyroidism is usually straightforward, it depends on a careful clinical history and physical examination, a high index of suspicion, and routine hormone determinations.

Clinical findings
■ Nervousness
■ Heat intolerance
■ Weight loss despite increased appetite
■ Sweating
■ Diarrhea
■ Poor concentration
■ Palpitations
■ Shaky handwriting
■ Emotional instability and mood swings
■ Fertility problems
■ Oligomenorrhea or amenorrhea
■ Enlarged thyroid (goiter)
■ Exophthalmos (considered most characteristic but is absent in many patients with hyperthyroidism)
■ Tremor
■ Smooth, warm, flushed skin
■ Fine, soft hair
■ Premature graying and increased hair loss
■ Friable nails and onycholysis
■ Pretibial myxedema
■ Thickened skin
■ Accentuated hair follicles
■ Tachycardia at rest
■ Full, bounding pulse
■ Arrhythmias, especially atrial fibrillation
■ Wide pulse pressure
■ Possible systolic murmur
■ Dyspnea
■ Hepatomegaly and splenomegaly

(*Text continues on page 212.*)

TYPES OF HYPERTHYROIDISM

Other forms of hyperthyroidism include toxic adenoma, thyrotoxicosis factitia, functioning metastatic thyroid carcinoma, thyroid-stimulating hormone (TSH)–secreting pituitary tumor, and subacute thyroiditis.

Toxic adenoma
The second most common cause of hyperthyroidism, toxic adenoma is a small, benign nodule in the thyroid gland that secretes thyroid hormone. The cause of toxic adenoma is unknown; its incidence is highest in elderly people. Clinical effects are similar to those of Graves' disease except that toxic adenoma doesn't induce ophthalmopathy, pretibial myxedema, or acropachy (clubbing of fingers or toes). A radioactive iodine (^{131}I) uptake and a thyroid scan show a single hyperfunctioning nodule suppressing the rest of the gland. Treatment includes ^{131}I therapy or surgery to remove the adenoma after antithyroid drugs restore normal gland function.

Thyrotoxicosis factitia
Thyrotoxicosis factitia results from chronic ingestion of thyroid hormone for TSH suppression in patients with thyroid carcinoma. It may also result from thyroid hormone abuse by people trying to lose weight.

Functioning metastatic thyroid carcinoma
This rare disease causes excess production of thyroid hormone.

TSH-secreting pituitary tumor
This form of hyperthyroidism causes excess production of thyroid hormone.

Subacute thyroiditis
A virus-induced granulomatous inflammation of the thyroid, subacute thyroiditis produces transient hyperthyroidism associated with fever, pain, pharyngitis, and tenderness of the thyroid gland.

DISORDERS AFFECTING MANAGEMENT OF HYPERTHYROIDISM

This chart highlights disorders that affect the management of hyperthyroidism.

DISORDER	SIGNS AND SYMPTOMS
Cardiac arrhythmias (complication)	*Supraventricular tachycardia* ◆ Rapid apical pulse rate ◆ Rapid peripheral pulse rate ◆ Regular or irregular rhythm, depending on the type of atrial tachycardia ◆ Sudden feeling of palpitations, especially with paroxysmal atrial tachycardia ◆ Decreased cardiac output and possible hypotension and syncope from persistent tachycardia and rapid ventricular rate *Atrial fibrillation* ◆ Irregularly irregular pulse rhythm with normal or abnormal heart rate ◆ Radial pulse rate slower than apical pulse rate ◆ Palpable peripheral pulse with the stronger contractions of atrial fibrillation ◆ Hypotension ◆ Light-headedness
Osteoporosis (complication)	◆ Dowager's bump (kyphosis) ◆ Back pain (thoracic and lumbar) ◆ Loss of height ◆ Unsteady gait ◆ Joint pain ◆ Weakness
Thyroid storm (complication)	◆ Marked tachycardia ◆ Vomiting ◆ Stupor ◆ Vascular collapse ◆ Hypotension ◆ Irritability ◆ Restlessness ◆ Visual disturbances (diplopia) ◆ Tremor ◆ Weakness ◆ Angina ◆ Shortness of breath ◆ Cough ◆ Swollen extremities ◆ Warm, moist, flushed skin ◆ Hyperthermia ◆ Coma ◆ Death

DIAGNOSTIC TEST RESULTS

♦ Electrocardiography reveals cardiac arrhythmias – usually paroxysmal supraventricular tachycardia or atrial fibrillation.
♦ Chest X-ray may show heart failure.

TREATMENT AND CARE

♦ Monitor heart rhythm continuously.
♦ Monitor vital signs.
♦ Chemical conversion may include administration of adenosine (Adenocard), diltiazem (Cardizem), procainamide (Procanbid), or amiodarone (Cordarone) I.V.
♦ Synchronized electrical conversion may be needed; premedicate the patient with sedatives and heparin as appropriate.
♦ Continue treatment with beta-adrenergic blockers, calcium channel blockers, digoxin, or antiarrhythmics.
♦ Administer anticoagulant treatment as appropriate.
♦ Encourage follow-up care with a cardiologist.

♦ X-ray reveals characteristic degeneration in the lower vertebrae.
♦ Parathyroid levels may be elevated.
♦ Bone biopsy allows direct examination of changes in bone cells and the rate of bone turnover.
♦ Dual photon or dual energy X-ray absorptiometry can detect bone loss; bone mineral density is 2.5 or more below the young adult reference mean.

♦ Provide supportive devices such as a back brace.
♦ Encourage lifestyle modifications, such as weight loss, exercise program, and dietary modifications, as appropriate.
♦ Offer analgesics and heat for pain relief.
♦ Give calcium and vitamin D supplements to help support normal bone metabolism.
♦ Give sodium fluoride to stimulate bone formation.
♦ Calcitonin may reduce bone resorption and slow the decline in bone mass.

♦ Diagnosis is based on clinical findings for immediate treatment.
♦ Triiodothyronine (T_3) and thyroxine (T_4) are elevated; free T_4 is elevated; T_3 resin uptake is increased.
♦ Thyroid-stimulating hormone is suppressed.
♦ 24-hour iodine uptake is elevated.

♦ Monitor patients with a history of hyperthyroidism for thyroid storm.
♦ Monitor vital signs.
♦ Provide supplemental oxygen and ventilation support as needed.
♦ Administer antiadrenergic and antithyroid drugs.
♦ Provide supportive, symptomatic care.

- Hyperactive bowel sounds
- Possible generalized weakness or paralysis
- Gynecomastia in males
- Increased tearing

In cases of thyroid storm:

- Extreme irritability
- Hypertension
- Tachycardia
- Vomiting
- Temperature up to 106° F (41.1° C)
- Delirium
- Seizures
- Coma

Diagnostic test results

- *Radioimmunoassay* shows increased serum T_4 and triiodothyronine (T_3)concentrations.
- *Thyroid scan* reveals increased uptake of radioactive iodine (^{131}I). This test is contraindicated if the patient is pregnant.
- *TSH levels* are decreased.
- *Ultrasonography* confirms subclinical ophthalmopathy.
- *Antithyroglobulin antibody* is positive in Graves' disease.

COLLABORATIVE MANAGEMENT

Because hyperthyroidism increases metabolic rate, all body systems may be affected, necessitating a multidisciplinary approach to care. An endocrinologist can help manage the patient's hormonal status. A surgeon may be consulted if a thyroidectomy is indicated. An ophthalmologist may be needed to treat exophthalmos. During thyrotoxic crisis, the patient needs critical care monitoring. A pulmonologist and respiratory therapist participate in care if the patient requires mechanical ventilation. Additional specialists, such as a nephrologist, gastroenterologist, or cardiologist, may be consulted if these systems are affected. Nutritional therapy may be needed to assist with diet planning. Social services may be involved to assist with financial concerns and follow-up and long-term planning, such as the need for home care or referrals for community support.

TREATMENT AND CARE

- Monitor vital signs, electrocardiogram (ECG), and cardiopulmonary status continuously

- Administer medications, such as an antithyroid drug (propylthiouracil [PTU]) or beta-adrenergic blockers (propranolol), to block sympathetic effects; a corticosteroid may be administered to inhibit the conversion of T_3 and T_4 and to replace depleted cortisol; and an iodide may be used to block the release of the thyroid hormones.
- Institute cooling measures, closely monitoring the patient's temperature
- Administer acetaminophen, but not aspirin, which may further increase the patient's metabolic rate.
- Provide supportive care, such as vitamins, nutrients, fluids, and sedatives.
- Treatment for hyperthyroidism may also include ^{131}I consisting of a single oral dose; it's the treatment of choice for women past reproductive age or men and women who don't plan to have children. In most patients, hypermetabolic symptoms diminish within 6 to 8 weeks after such treatment. However, some patients may require a second dose.
- Prepare patient for possible subtotal (partial) thyroidectomy (indicated for the patient under age 40 who has a very large goiter and whose hyperthyroidism has repeatedly relapsed after drug therapy).
- Preoperatively, expect to administer iodides (Lugol's solution or potassium iodide oral solution), antithyroid drugs, or high doses of propranolol to help prevent thyroid storm. If euthyroidism isn't achieved, surgery should be delayed and propranolol should be administered to decrease cardiac arrhythmias caused by hyperthyroidism.

Hypocalcemia

Hypocalcemia is characterized by a total serum calcium level below 8.9 mg/dl and an ionized serum calcium level below 4.6 mg/dl. Hypoalbuminemia is the most common cause. However, this condition is sometimes referred to as *pseudohypocalcemia* because the ionized calcium remains normal despite a low serum calcium level.

ETIOLOGY

Hypocalcemia occurs when a person doesn't consume enough calcium, when the body doesn't absorb the mineral properly, or when the body loses excessive amounts of calcium. A decreased level of ionized calcium can also cause hypocalcemia.

Inadequate calcium intake can be caused by inadequate intake secondary to chronic alcoholism, insufficient exposure to sunlight, and possibly breast-feeding. A breast-fed infant can develop low calcium and vitamin D levels if the mother's intake of these nutrients is insufficient. Elderly people are also at risk for hypocalcemia because of inadequate dietary intake of calcium, poor calcium absorption, and reduced activity or inactivity.

Conditions related to calcium malabsorption include severe diarrhea, laxative abuse, malabsorption syndrome, insufficient vitamin D, a high phosphorus level in the intestine, and reduced gastric acidity. Pancreatic insufficiency, acute pancreatitis, thyroid or parathyroid surgery, hypoparathyroidism or other parathyroid disorders, and certain drugs can lead to excess calcium loss.

DRUG ALERT *Drugs that can cause hypocalcemia include certain anticonvulsants, calcitonin, drugs that lower magnesium levels, edetate disodium, loop diuretics, certain radiographic contrast media, mithramycin, and phosphates.*

Other causes of hypocalcemia include severe burns and infections, hypoalbuminemia, hyperphosphatemia, alkalosis, and massive blood transfusions.

PATHOPHYSIOLOGY

Pathophysiologic processes involved in hypocalcemia vary depending on the cause. For example, surgery on the neck may damage the parathyroid glands, possibly causing ischemia. The ischemia, in turn, interferes with the glands' ability to produce parathyroid hormone (PTH) and regulate serum calcium levels.

Hypocalcemia occurs in 40% to 75% of patients with acute pancreatitis. Inflammation of the pancreas causes the release of proteinolytic and lipolytic enzymes, which, in turn, cause lipolysis. It's believed that calcium ions combine with fatty acids released by lipolysis, forming soaps and resulting in a decrease in serum calcium concentrations.

In addition, the amount of other substances in the body affects calcium absorption. For example, a low magnesium level can affect how the parathyroid gland functions, causing a decrease in calcium reabsorption from the GI tract and the kidneys. Additionally, high amounts of phosphorous in the body or a low serum albumin level can cause calcium levels to fall. For example, when phosphates are administered I.V., orally, or rectally, the phosphorus binds with calcium to form salts, which are then deposited in soft tissues, resulting in decreased serum calcium levels.

In cases of alkalosis, calcium can bind with albumin, thus decreasing ionized calcium levels. Use of blood products affects calcium levels because the citrate added to the blood products (to prevent clotting during storage) binds with calcium and renders it unavailable for use by the body. Thus, patients receiving numerous blood transfusions are at risk for hypocalcemia.

Patients with intestinal malabsorptive disorders, such as Crohn's disease and hepatobiliary disease, are at risk for hypocalcemia because of decreased absorption of vitamin D, bile salts, and calcium.

In neonates, two types of hypocalcemia may occur. The first type generally develops during the first 3 days of life as a result of an immature parathyroid gland, maternal hyperparathyroidism, or both conditions. These conditions lead to neonatal parathyroid gland suppression but generally resolves within the first week of life.

The second type of neonatal hypocalcemia occurs about 1 week after birth and is associated with hyperphosphatemia and hypomagnesemia. This type is commonly caused by feeding neonates formula containing excessive phosphorus. (See *Disorders affecting management of hypocalcemia,* pages 214 and 215.)

Cardiovascular system

■ Arrhythmias, palpitations, decreased cardiac output, and an irregular heart rate may occur because of the lack of calcium and the direct effect on the contractility of the cardiac muscle.

■ The presence of hypomagnesemia and hypokalemia can potentiate the cardiac and neurologic effects of hypocalcemia.

DISORDERS AFFECTING MANAGEMENT OF HYPOCALCEMIA

This chart highlights disorders that affect the management of hypocalcemia.

DISORDER	SIGNS AND SYMPTOMS	DIAGNOSTIC TEST RESULTS
Heart failure (complication)	◆ Cough that produces pink, frothy sputum ◆ Cyanosis of the lips and nail beds ◆ Pale, cool, clammy skin ◆ Diaphoresis ◆ Jugular vein distention ◆ Ascites ◆ Pulsus alternans ◆ Tachycardia ◆ Hepatomegaly ◆ Decreased pulse pressure ◆ Third and fourth heart sounds ◆ Moist, basilar crackles ◆ Rhonchi ◆ Expiratory wheezing ◆ Decreased pulse oximetry ◆ Peripheral edema ◆ Decreased urinary output	◆ B-type natriuretic peptide immunoassay is elevated. ◆ Chest X-ray shows increased pulmonary vascular markings, interstitial edema, or pleural effusions and cardiomegaly. ◆ Electrocardiography (ECG) reveals heart enlargement or ischemia, tachycardia, extrasystole, or atrial fibrillation. ◆ Pulmonary artery pressure, pulmonary artery wedge pressure, and left ventricular end-diastolic pressure are elevated in the presence of left-sided heart failure; right atrial or central venous pressure is elevated in right-sided heart failure.
Torsades de pointes (complication)	◆ Tachycardia ◆ Hypotension ◆ Poor peripheral pulse ◆ Possibly unconscious with no pulse or respirations	◆ ECG reveals irregular or regular ventricular rhythm, a ventricular rate of 150 to 250 beats/minute, an unidentifiable P wave, and a wide QRS complex that's usually a phasic variation in electrical polarity (shown by complexes that point downward for several beats).

Gastrointestinal system

■ Increased nervous system excitability can lead to diarrhea.

Integumentary system

■ Calcium-phosphate calcification can lead to soft-tissue calcification, causing dry, itchy skin with papular eruptions.

■ Calcification of the ocular vessels can lead to conjunctivitis and corneal haziness, which may progress to impaired vision.

Neuromuscular system

■ Hypocalcemia can lead to symptoms of tetany, which includes tingling (parasthesia) in the fingertips and around the mouth. Parasthesia may increase in severity and spread up the arms and to the face, leading to numbness, muscle spasms, and pain.

■ Hypocalcemia may lead to hyperreflexia, mental status changes, irritability, confusion, muscle weakness, or seizures.

■ Carpopedal spasms, laryngeal spasms, and abdominal muscle cramps or spasms may occur.

■ Fractures may occur because of the loss of calcium from the bones.

Renal system

■ Precipitation of calcium phosphate can lead to progressive renal impairment.

■ Oliguria related to acute or chronic renal failure may occur.

◆ Administer supplemental oxygen and mechanical ventilation, if needed.
◆ Place the patient in Fowler's position.
◆ Administer diuretics, inotropic drugs, vasodilators, angiotensin-converting enzyme inhibitors, angiotensin receptor blockers, cardiac glycosides, beta-adrenergic blockers, and electrolyte supplements.
◆ Initiate cardiac monitoring.
◆ Recurrent heart failure from valvular dysfunction may require surgery.
◆ A ventricular assist device may be needed.
◆ Maintain adequate cardiac output and monitor hemodynamic stability.
◆ Assess for deep vein thrombosis and apply antiembolism stockings.

◆ Monitor cardiac status.
◆ The condition may progress quickly to ventricular fibrillation. Monitor the patient's hemodynamic status, although the patient may be hemodynamically stable with a normal pulse and blood pressure.
◆ Anticipate that the physician will initiate mechanical overdrive pacing.
◆ Be prepared to administer magnesium.
◆ Electrical cardioversion may be used if the patient doesn't respond to other treatments.

Respiratory system
■ Hypocalcemia may cause respiratory compromise related to lung tissue calcification.

ASSESSMENT
Clinical manifestations of hypocalcemia vary and depend on severity, duration, and rate of progression.

Clinical findings
■ Paresthesia, especially in the fingertips and around the mouth
■ Anxiety
■ Confusion
■ Diarrhea
■ Impaired mental status and seizures
■ Muscle weakness, cramps, and spasms
■ Hypotension
■ Chvostek's sign or Trousseau's sign
■ Fractures
■ Decreased cardiac output
■ Tetany
■ Tremors and twitching
■ Hyperactive deep tendon reflexes
■ Dry, itchy skin and hair; brittle nails

Diagnostic test results
■ *Total serum calcium level* is less than 8.9 mg/dl; ionized calcium level is below 4.6 mg/dl.
■ *Electrocardiography* shows a prolonged ST segment and lengthened QT interval.

COLLABORATIVE MANAGEMENT
Because hypocalcemia can affect multiple body systems, a multidisciplinary approach to care is needed. A renal specialist or nephrologist can help evaluate, treat, and manage the patient's kidney function. Respiratory and cardiology specialists may be consulted, depending on the patient's history and complications he may develop. Nutritional therapy may be necessary for dietary planning. If a prolonged hospital stay is expected and the patient requires long-term care or home care, social services may be consulted early on in the patient's care.

TREATMENT AND CARE
■ When possible, treatment is directed at the underlying disorder.
■ If the patient is at increased risk for hypocalcemia (if he has had parathyroid or thyroid surgery or has received massive blood transfusions), assess him carefully. If the patient is breast-feeding, assess for adequate vitamin D intake and exposure to sunlight.
■ Assess for fractures.
■ Be prepared to administer parenteral calcium to a patient who has symptomatic hypocalcemia.
■ Calcium replacement may come in the form of calcium gluconate or calcium chloride; doses vary according to the specific drug.
■ Always administer I.V. calcium using an infusion pump; avoid rapid administration because it may lead to syncope, hypertension, and arrhythmias. Never mix I.V. calcium with sodium bicarbonate because it will

form a precipitate. Monitor the I.V. site closely because infiltration can lead to tissue necrosis and sloughing.

■ I.V. calcium should be administered with magnesium because hypocalcemia won't respond to calcium alone.

■ Monitor vital signs, respiratory status, and cardiac rate and rhythm.

■ Monitor laboratory values, including calcium levels and magnesium and albumin levels. Ionized calcium levels should be drawn with every fourth unit of blood administered.

■ Assess for the presence of Chvostek's sign or Trousseau's sign.

■ Keep a tracheotomy tray at the bedside and have resuscitation equipment readily available in the event of laryngospasms.

■ Monitor patients receiving I.V. calcium for cardiac arrhythmias, especially if they're also taking digoxin. Digoxin and calcium have similar effects on the heart.

■ If the patient is receiving oral calcium replacement or supplementation, give the calcium 1 to 1½ hours after a meal and provide it with milk if GI upset occurs.

■ Monitor for changes in mental status and risk of injury; institute seizure precautions as needed.

Hypochloremia

Hypochloremia is a deficiency of chloride in extracellular fluid. The condition occurs when serum chloride levels fall below 96 mEq/L. When serum chloride levels fall, levels of sodium, calcium, and other electrolytes may be affected.

ETIOLOGY

Serum chloride levels drop when chloride intake or absorption decreases or when chloride loss increases. Reduced chloride intake can occur in infants being fed chloride-deficient formula and in people on salt-restricted diets. Patients dependent on I.V. fluids are also at risk if the fluids lack chloride, such as a dextrose solution without electrolytes. Losses may occur through the GI tract, the kidneys, or the skin (chloride is found in sweat). Changes in sodium levels

or acid-base balance also alter chloride levels.

Prolonged vomiting, diarrhea, severe diaphoresis, gastric surgery, nasogastric suctioning, and other GI tube drains can cause excessive chloride loss. Patients with cystic fibrosis can lose more chloride than normal through the GI tract because of prolonged vomiting from pyloric obstruction and the presence of draining fistulas and ileostomies.

DRUG ALERT *Such medications as loop diuretics, osmotic or thiazide diuretics, ethacrynic acid, and hydrochlorothiazide can cause an excessive loss of chloride from the kidneys.*

Other causes of hypochloremia include sodium and potassium deficiency and metabolic alkalosis. In addition, conditions that affect acid-base or electrolyte balance, such as diabetic ketoacidosis and Addison's disease, and the rapid removal of fluid from ascites during paracentesis can cause chloride loss. Patients with heart failure are at risk for developing hypochloremia related to serum chloride levels that are diluted by excess fluid in the body.

PATHOPHYSIOLOGY

Chloride accounts for two-thirds of all serum anions. It's secreted by the stomach's mucosa as hydrochloric acid and provides an acid medium that aids digestion and activation of enzymes. Chloride also helps maintain acid-base balance and body water balances. Additionally, chloride influences the osmolality or tonicity of extracellular fluid, plays a role in the exchange of oxygen and carbon dioxide in red blood cells, and helps activate salivary amylase, which leads to activation of the digestive tract.

Cardiovascular system
■ As the pH increases, myocardial function may be affected, leading to arrhythmias.

Endocrine and metabolic systems
■ Accumulation of bicarbonate ions in the extracellular fluid raises the pH level, leading to hypochloremic metabolic alkalosis.

Gastrointestinal system
■ Excessive loss of fluid through the GI tract can lead to hypochloremic metabolic alkalosis.

Integumentary system
■ Excessive diaphoresis can cause hypochloremia.

Neurologic system
■ Hypochloremia can affect the neurologic system by increasing excitability, irritability, or agitation, leading to hyperactive deep tendon reflexes; muscle hypertonicity; tetany; muscle cramps; twitching; and weakness.
■ Late-developing neurologic signs of hypochloremia include seizures and coma. (See *Disorder affecting management of hypochloremia*, pages 218 and 219.)

Respiratory system
■ Hyperchloremic metabolic alkalosis results in a high pH. To compensate, respirations become slow and shallow as the body attempts to retain carbon dioxide and restore the pH level to a normal range.
■ Untreated hypochloremia may lead to respiratory arrest.

ASSESSMENT
Hypochloremia rarely produces signs and symptoms on its own. The signs and symptoms associated with hypochloremia are generally related to acid-base and electrolyte abnormalities. Signs of hyponatremia, hypokalemia, or metabolic alkalosis may occur.

Clinical findings
■ Agitation and irritability
■ Muscle cramps and weakness
■ Cardiac arrhythmias
■ Laboratory results indicating metabolic alkalosis
■ Excessive GI losses of fluid
■ Excessive diaphoresis
■ Twitching and tremors
■ Shallow, depressed respirations or respiratory arrest
■ Hyperactive deep tendon reflexes
■ Seizures or coma

Diagnostic test results
■ *Serum chloride level* is below 96 mEq/L.
■ *Serum sodium level* is below 135 mEq/L, indicating hyponatremia.
■ *Serum pH* is greater than 7.45 and *serum bicarbonate* level is greater than 26 mEq/L, indicating metabolic alkalosis.

COLLABORATIVE MANAGEMENT
Because hypochloremia can affect multiple body systems, a multidisciplinary approach to care is needed. A renal specialist or nephrologist can help evaluate, treat, and manage the patient's kidney function and metabolic status. Respiratory and cardiology specialists may be consulted, depending on the patient's history and complications he may develop. Nutritional therapy may be necessary for dietary assistance. If a prolonged hospital stay is expected and the patient requires long-term care or home care, social services may be consulted early on in the patient's care.

TREATMENT AND CARE
■ Treatment for hypochloremia includes correcting the underlying cause and restoring fluid, electrolyte, and acid-base balance.
■ Chloride may be replaced through fluid administration or drug therapy, or orally through salty broth or oral supplements.
■ If the patient can't tolerate oral replacement, he may require I.V. normal saline solution.
■ The patient may require treatment for metabolic alkalosis or electrolyte imbalances such as hypokalemia.
■ Detection and correction of diaphoresis, vomiting, and other GI and renal losses typically corrects the associated metabolic alkalosis. Occasionally, however, metabolic alkalosis requires the administration of ammonium chloride.
■ Monitor cardiac rhythm, vital signs, level of consciousness, muscle strength, respiratory rate and function, serum electrolytes, and arterial blood gas results.
■ Provide foods rich in chloride.
■ Avoid allowing the patient to consume large quantities of water, which can lead to the excretion of large amounts of chloride.
■ Avoid administering ammonium chloride to patients with hepatic disease because this drug is metabolized by the liver.
■ Flush the patient's nasogastric tube with normal saline. Avoid using tap water — doing so leads to the excretion of large amounts of chloride.
■ Carefully monitor and record intake and output, including loss of fluid through vomiting or other GI losses.
■ Provide a safe environment, and monitor patients at risk for injury.

DISORDER AFFECTING
MANAGEMENT OF HYPOCHLOREMIA

This chart highlights how a seizure can affect the management of hypochloremia.

DISORDER	SIGNS AND SYMPTOMS	DIAGNOSTIC TEST RESULTS
Seizure (complication)	◆ Aura ◆ Loss of consciousness ◆ Dyspnea ◆ Fixed and dilated pupils ◆ Incontinence	◆ EEG shows abnormal wave patterns and the focus of the seizure activity. ◆ Magnetic resonance imaging may show pathologic changes. ◆ Brain mapping identifies seizure areas.

Hypokalemia

In hypokalemia, the serum potassium level drops below 3.5 mEq/L. Because the normal range for a serum potassium level is narrow (3.5 to 5 mEq/l), a slight decrease has significant consequences for the patient.

ETIOLOGY

Inadequate intake and excessive output of potassium can cause a moderate drop in its level, upsetting the balance and causing a potassium deficiency in the body. The body's inability to conserve potassium also contributes to potassium imbalance. Such conditions as prolonged intestinal suctioning, recent ileostomy, and villous adenoma can also cause a decrease in potassium levels.

Intestinal fluids contain large amounts of potassium. Therefore, any condition that causes GI loss of fluid, such as suction, lavage, or prolonged vomiting, can lead to hypokalemia. Diarrhea, fistulas, laxative abuse, and severe diaphoresis can also contribute to potassium loss.

Potassium can also be lost through diuresis. Diuresis following a kidney transplant or osmotic diuresis resulting from high urine glucose levels can lower potassium levels. Other renal-related potassium losses are seen in renal tubular acidosis, magnesium depletion, Cushing's syndrome, and periods of high stress.

Other disorders associated with hypokalemia include hepatic disease, hyperaldosteronism, acute alcoholism, heart failure, malabsorption syndrome, nephritis, and Bartter's syndrome. In addition, hypothermia can contribute to hypokalemia because of the stimulation of the cellular uptake of extracellular potassium in the presence of a low body temperature. Hypothermic-related hypokalemia can be reversed by warming the body.

DRUG ALERT *Such drugs as diuretics, corticosteroids, laxatives, insulin, cisplatin, and certain antibiotics can lead to potassium loss. Excessive secretion of insulin, whether endogenous or exogenous, may shift potassium into the cells. Insulin is then released from the body and leads to hypokalemia in patients receiving large amounts of dextrose solutions. Potassium levels also drop when adrenergics, such as albuterol (Albuterol), are used for asthma.*

PATHOPHYSIOLOGY

Potassium is a major cation in the intracellular fluid; therefore, a deficit in this electrolyte can have a significant impact on the body. (See *Disorders affecting management of hypokalemia,* pages 220 and 221.)

Cardiovascular system

■ Abnormalities of the electrophysiology and contractility of the heart muscle lead to orthostatic hypotension and a weak and irregular pulse, possibly resulting in cardiac arrest.

Endocrine and metabolic systems

■ Hypokalemia impairs insulin release and organ sensitivity to insulin, which contributes to worsening hyperglycemia in patients with diabetes.
■ Vomiting can lead to metabolic alkalosis related to gastric acid loss and the movement of potassium ions into the cell as hydrogen ions move out of the cell.

Gastrointestinal system

■ Anorexia, nausea, vomiting, prolonged gastric emptying, and paralytic ileus may result from a weakness of the GI tract's smooth muscle.

Neuromuscular system

■ Neurologic involvement includes muscle weakness, especially in the legs, which eventually leads to paresthesia and leg cramps.
■ Deep tendon reflexes may be decreased or absent.

Renal system

■ The patient may experience polyuria, nocturia, dilute urine, and polydipsia related to the inability to concentrate urine.
■ Cell function is affected, which can produce rhabdomyolysis — a breakdown of muscle fibers leading to myoglobin in the urine.

Respiratory system

■ The effects on the neurologic system can lead to paralysis of the respiratory muscles and to respiratory failure.

ASSESSMENT

Symptoms usually don't occur unless the potassium level drops below 3 mEq/L.

Clinical findings

■ Abdominal cramps, nausea, and vomiting
■ Muscle weakness
■ Irritability, malaise, and confusion
■ Paresthesia and progression to paralysis
■ Decreased cardiac output and possible cardiac arrest
■ Respiratory paralysis
■ Metabolic alkalosis
■ Orthostatic hypotension
■ Irregular heart rate
■ Decreased bowel sounds
■ Speech changes

Diagnostic test results

■ *Serum potassium level* is below 3.5 mEq/L.
■ *Bicarbonate levels* and *pH* are elevated.
■ *Serum glucose levels* are slightly elevated.
■ *Electrocardiography* (ECG) shows a flattened T wave, a depressed ST segment, and a characteristic U wave.

COLLABORATIVE MANAGEMENT

Because hypokalemia can affect multiple body systems, a multidisciplinary approach to care is needed. A renal specialist or nephrologist can help evaluate, treat, and manage the patient's kidney function and metabolic status. Cardiology and neurology specialists may be consulted, depending on the patient's history and complications he may develop. Nutritional therapy may be necessary for dietary assistance. Physical therapy and occupational therapy may be needed to assist with muscle strengthening and activities of daily living. If a prolonged

DISORDERS AFFECTING
MANAGEMENT OF HYPOKALEMIA

This chart highlights disorders that affect the management of hypokalemia.

DISORDER	SIGNS AND SYMPTOMS	DIAGNOSTIC TEST RESULTS
Respiratory arrest (complication)	◆ Absence of spontaneous breathing ◆ No rise or fall of the chest ◆ Inability to feel the movement of air from the mouth or nose ◆ Cyanosis	◆ Aterial blood gas analysis identifies hypoxemia or hypercapnia.
Rhabdomyolysis (complication)	◆ Abnormal urine color (dark, red, or cola colored) ◆ Muscle tenderness ◆ Weakness of the affected muscle ◆ Muscle stiffness or aching (myalgia) ◆ Unintentional weight gain ◆ Seizures ◆ Joint pain ◆ Fatigue	◆ Urine myoglobin level exceeds 0.5 mg/dl. ◆ Creatinine kinase level is elevated (0.5 to 0.95 mg/dl) from muscle damage. ◆ Blood urea nitrogen, creatinine, creatine, and phosphate levels are elevated. ◆ Intracompartmental venous pressure measurements are elevated. ◆ Computed tomography, magnetic resonance imaging, and bone scintigraphy are used to detect muscle necrosis. ◆ Urinalysis may reveal casts. ◆ Serum potassium is elevated.

hospital stay is expected and the patient requires long-term care or home care, social services may be consulted early on in the patient's care.

TREATMENT AND CARE

■ Treatment for hypokalemia focuses on restoring a normal potassium balance, preventing serious complications, and eliminating or treating the underlying cause.

■ After hypokalemia develops, dietary potassium intake alone may not be effective because most potassium consumed orally is metabolized into bicarbonate. Therefore, patients should also be treated with I.V. potassium chloride.

■ I.V. potassium chloride should be administered with an infusion pump—never as a bolus—to prevent cardiac arrhythmias and cardiac arrest. Infusion rates are generally 10 mEq/hour and shouldn't exceed 40 to 60 mEq/hour.

■ Provide continuous cardiac monitoring during I.V. potassium chloride infusions. Report irregularities and toxic reactions immediately.

■ Assess the I.V. site for signs and symptoms of infiltration, phlebitis, or tissue necrosis.

■ Advise the patient that I.V. potassium chloride administration can cause a burning sensation at the infusion site.

■ Monitor vital signs, ECG, heart rate and rhythm, respiratory status, serum potassium levels, and intake and output.

■ Monitor the patient for signs of metabolic alkalosis.

■ Provide a safe environment and assess the patient's risk of injury.

■ Assess for constipation and gastric distention, but avoid using laxatives because of potassium losses associated with these medications.

TREATMENT AND CARE

- Assess for respirations, circulation, and airway patency. Initiate basic life support in the absence of circulation and respirations and in the presence of a patent airway.
- Assess breath sounds; observe for "seesaw" respirations.
- Administer oxygen; monitor oxygen saturation using pulse oximetry.
- Continually assess for stridor, cyanosis, and changes in level of consciousness.
- Prepare for endotracheal intubation or a tracheostomy if the airway can't be established.
- Anticipate cardiac arrest; initiate or continue cardiac monitoring.
- Place an I.V. line for fluid and medication administration if one isn't already in place.
- Administer medications.

- Treat the underlying disorder.
- Assess for and prevent renal failure.
- Place the patient on bed rest to prevent further muscle breakdown.
- Administer I.V. fluids.
- Monitor intake and output.
- Monitor renal studies, urine myoglobin levels, electrolytes, and acid-base balance.
- If renal failure occurs, prepare the patient for dialysis or slow, continuous renal replacement therapy.
- Administer anti-inflammatory agents, diuretics, corticosteroids, and analgesics, as appropriate.
- Prepare the patient for an immediate fasciotomy and debridement if compartment venous pressures exceed 25 mm Hg.

- Avoid crushing slow-release potassium supplements.
- After the potassium has returned to a normal level, the patient may need further dietary counseling and a prescription for a sustained-release oral potassium supplement.
- The patient taking a diuretic should be switched to a potassium-sparing diuretic to prevent excessive loss of potassium in the urine.
- The patient with hypokalemia who's also taking digoxin should be monitored closely because the risk of drug toxicity increases.

Hypomagnesemia

In hypomagnesemia, the body's serum magnesium level falls below 1.5 mEq/L. This imbalance is fairly common and likely underdiagnosed. Hypomagnesemia affects approximately 10% of all hospitalized patients.

ETIOLOGY

Hypomagnesemia can be caused by any condition that impairs the GI system or the renal system (the body's magnesium regulators). These conditions fall into four main categories: poor dietary intake of magnesium, poor magnesium absorption by the GI tract, excessive magnesium loss from the GI tract, and excessive magnesium loss from renal excretion.

Inadequate magnesium intake may be related to chronic alcoholism, prolonged I.V. therapy, or use of total parenteral nutrition or enteral feeding formulas without sufficient magnesium. Inadequate GI absorption of magnesium can be caused by malabsorption syndrome, steatorrhea, ulcerative colitis, Crohn's disease, GI surgery or bowel re-

DISORDERS AFFECTING
MANAGEMENT OF HYPOMAGNESEMIA

This chart highlights disorders that affect the management of hypomagnesemia.

DISORDER	SIGNS AND SYMPTOMS	DIAGNOSTIC TEST RESULTS
Cardiac arrhythmias (complication)	◆ May be asymptomatic ◆ Dizziness ◆ Hypotension ◆ Syncope ◆ Weakness ◆ Cool, clammy skin ◆ Altered level of consciousness (LOC) ◆ Reduced urine output ◆ Shortness of breath ◆ Chest pain	◆ Electrocardiography detects arrhythmias as well as ischemia and infarction that may result in arrhythmias. ◆ Laboratory testing may reveal electrolyte abnormalities, acid-base abnormalities, or drug toxicities that may cause arrhythmias. ◆ Holter monitoring, event monitoring, and loop recording can detect arrhythmias and effectiveness of drug therapy during a patient's daily activities. ◆ Exercise testing may detect exercise-induced arrhythmias. ◆ Electrophysiologic testing identifies the mechanism of an arrhythmia and the location of accessory pathways; it also assesses the effectiveness of antiarrhythmic drugs, radiofrequency ablation, and implanted cardioverter-defibrillators.
Seizures (complication)	◆ Aura ◆ Loss of consciousness ◆ Dyspnea ◆ Fixed and dilated pupils ◆ Incontinence	◆ EEG shows abnormal wave patterns and the focus of the seizure activity. ◆ Magnetic resonance imaging may show pathologic changes. ◆ Brain mapping identifies seizure areas.

section, cancer, pancreatic insufficiency, or excessive calcium or phosphorus in the GI tract.

Prolonged diarrhea, fistula drainage, laxative abuse, nasogastric tube suctioning, or acute pancreatitis may lead to an excessive loss of magnesium. Excessive magnesium loss may also be caused by loss of fluid from sweating, diuretic abuse, breast-feeding, serious burns, or chronic diarrhea. Excessive renal excretion of magnesium may be a result of such conditions as primary aldosteronism, hyperparathyroidism or hypoparathyroidism, diabetic ketoacidosis, or renal disorders, including glomerulonephritis, pyelonephritis, and renal tubular acidosis. Other causes of hypomagnesemia may be related to hemodialysis, sepsis, hypothermia, hypercalcemia, inappropriate secretion of antidiuretic hormone, or wounds requiring debridement.

DRUG ALERT *Certain drugs can cause or contribute to hypomagnesemia, including aminoglycoside antibiotics,* *such as amikacin (Amikin), gentamicin (Garamycin), or tobramycin (Nebcin); amphotericin B (Amphocin); cisplatin (Platinol); cyclosporine (Neoral); insulin; laxatives; loop diuretics, such as bumetanide (Bumex) and furosemide (Lasix); thiazide diuretics, such as chlorothiazide (Diuril) and hydrochlorothiazide (HydroDIURIL); and pentamidine isethionate (Pentacarinate).*

PATHOPHYSIOLOGY

Magnesium is the second most abundant intracellular cation. It's active in cellular metabolism and is important for neuromuscular transmission. Magnesium is also closely related to calcium, phosphorus, and potassium; thus, changes in magnesium levels can affect multiple body systems.

Cardiovascular system

■ Myocardial irritability can lead to cardiac arrhythmias, which can cause a decrease in cardiac output. (See *Disorders affecting management of hypomagnesemia.*)

TREATMENT AND CARE

◆ When life-threatening arrhythmias develop, rapidly assess LOC, respirations, and pulse rate.
◆ Initiate cardiopulmonary resuscitation, if indicated.
◆ Evaluate cardiac output resulting from arrhythmias.
◆ If the patient develops heart block, prepare for cardiac pacing.
◆ Administer antiarrhythmics; prepare to assist with medical procedures, if indicated.
◆ Assess intake and output every hour; insert an indwelling urinary catheter as indicated to ensure accurate urine measurement.
◆ Document arrhythmias in a monitored patient and assess for possible causes and effects.
◆ If the patient's pulse is abnormally rapid, slow, or irregular, watch for signs of hypoperfusion, such as hypotension and diminished urine output.
◆ Monitor for predisposing factors, such as fluid and electrolyte imbalance, or possible drug toxicity.

◆ Observe and record the seizure activity (initial movement, respiratory pattern, duration of seizure, loss of consciousness, aura, incontinence, and pupillary changes).
◆ Assess postictal state.
◆ Protect the patient from falls.
◆ Assess neurologic and respiratory status.
◆ Administer anticonvulsants.
◆ Maintain seizure precautions.
◆ Monitor and record vital signs, intake and output, neurovital signs, and laboratory studies.

■ Arrhythmias triggered by a low serum magnesium level include atrial fibrillation, heart block, paroxysmal atrial tachycardia, premature ventricular contractions, supraventricular tachycardia, torsades de pointes, ventricular fibrillation, and ventricular tachycardia.

Gastrointestinal system
■ Insufficient magnesium can cause anorexia, dysphagia, and nausea and vomiting.

Neurologic system
■ Decreased serum magnesium increases the irritability of nerve tissue, possibly leading to altered level of consciousness (LOC), ataxia, confusion, delusions, depression, emotional lability, hallucinations, insomnia, psychosis, seizures, or vertigo.

Neuromuscular system
■ As the body compensates for low serum magnesium levels, magnesium moves out of the cells, affecting the neuromuscular sys-

tem. Skeletal muscles become weak and nerves become hyperirritable.
■ Increased nerve irritability can lead to leg and foot cramps, hyperactive deep tendon reflexes, twitching, tremors, tetany, Chvostek's sign, and Trousseau's sign.

Renal system
■ Hypokalemia is a common finding with hypomagnesemia because the kidneys can't conserve potassium in the presence of a magnesium deficiency.

Respiratory system
■ Respiratory muscles may be affected, possibly leading to respiratory difficulties, respiratory failure, or laryngeal stridor.

ASSESSMENT
Signs and symptoms of hypomagnesemia can range from mild to severe and life-threatening. Generally, signs and symptoms associated with hypomagnesemia resemble those seen with potassium or calcium imbal-

ances. Occasionally, a patient may have a serum magnesium level less than 1.5 mEq/L but remain asymptomatic.

Clinical findings
- Altered LOC, hallucinations, or seizures
- Anorexia or dysphagia
- Arrhythmias, such as atrial fibrillation, heart block, paroxysmal atrial tachycardia, premature ventricular contractions, supraventricular tachycardia, torsades de pointes, ventricular fibrillation, and ventricular tachycardia
- Hypertension
- Foot and leg cramps
- Muscle weakness, twitching, tremors, or tetany
- Nausea and vomiting
- Dysphagia
- Chvostek's sign and Trousseau's sign
- Hyperactive deep tendon reflexes
- Respiratory difficulties
- Twitching and tremors

Diagnostic test results
- *Serum magnesium level* is below 1.5 mEq/L (possibly with a below-normal serum albumin level).
- *Electrocardiography* reveals a prolonged PR interval; a widened QRS complex; a prolonged QT interval; a depressed ST segment; a broad, flattened T wave; and a prominent U wave.

COLLABORATIVE MANAGEMENT
Because hypomagnesemia can affect multiple body systems, a multidisciplinary approach to care is needed. A renal specialist or nephrologist can help evaluate, treat, and manage the patient's kidney function and metabolic status. Cardiology and neurology specialists may be consulted, depending on the patient's history and complications he may develop. Nutritional therapy may be needed for dietary assistance. If a prolonged hospital stay is expected and the patient requires long-term care or home care, social services may be consulted for assistance with discharge planning and follow-up.

TREATMENT AND CARE
- Treatment for hypomagnesemia depends on the underlying cause and the patient's clinical signs and symptoms.

- Dietary replacement and teaching may correct a mild magnesium deficiency.
- Oral supplementation with magnesium chloride may be prescribed. Magnesium oxide is rarely prescribed because it's poorly absorbed and can cause alkalosis.
- Because it takes several days to fully restore magnesium balance and stores, replacement may continue for several days (even after achieving a normal magnesium balance) to ensure long-term balance.
- Patients with severe hypomagnesemia may require I.V. or deep I.M. injections of magnesium sulfate. (*Note:* Before administering magnesium sulfate, assess renal function. Report urine output less than 100 ml over 4 hours.)
- Magnesium sulfate comes in three concentrations: 10%, 12.5%, and 50%. Always check the order and drug label to ensure that the correct dose and concentration are given.
- Monitor the patient's serum magnesium level after each bolus of magnesium sulfate or at least every 6 hours. When using an infusion pump, magnesium sulfate administration shouldn't exceed 150 mg/minute.
- Keep calcium gluconate readily available to counteract adverse reactions to magnesium sulfate, if needed.
- Monitor the patient's vital signs, cardiac rhythm, mental status, respiratory status, and neuromuscular status.
- Assess for dysphagia before providing food, oral fluids, or oral medications to prevent choking.
- Replace lost fluids and closely monitor intake and output, electrolyte levels, and renal function studies.
- Provide a safe environment and assess the patient's risk of injury.
- Monitor patients receiving digoxin for signs of toxicity. A low magnesium level may increase a patient's retention of the drug. Suspect toxicity if the patient has anorexia, arrhythmias, nausea, vomiting, and yellow-tinged vision.

Hyponatremia

Hyponatremia occurs when the serum sodium level is less than 135 mEq/L. It's the most common electrolyte imbalance. Body fluids are diluted and cells swell from decreased extracellular fluid osmolality. Hyponatremia occurs in approximately 1% of all hospitalized patients. It most commonly affects children and elderly people and occurs in males and females equally.

ETIOLOGY

Hyponatremia results from a loss of sodium, gain of water (dilutional hyponatremia), or inadequate sodium intake (depletion hyponatremia). It may be classified according to whether extracellular fluid volume is abnormally decreased (hypovolemic hyponatremia), abnormally increased (hypervolemic hyponatremia), or equal to intracellular fluid volume (isovolumic hyponatremia).

In hypovolemic hyponatremia, nonrenal causes include vomiting, diarrhea, fistulas, gastric suctioning, excessive sweating, cystic fibrosis, burns, and wound drainage. Renal causes include osmotic diuresis, salt-losing nephritis, adrenal insufficiency, and diuretic use. Drinking large volumes of water can worsen hyponatremia, and sodium deficiencies can be more extreme if the patient is on a sodium-restricted diet. Diuretics can cause potassium loss, which is linked to hyponatremia.

Causes of hypervolemic hyponatremia include heart failure, liver failure, nephrotic syndrome, excessive administration of hypotonic I.V. fluids, and hyperaldosteronism. Causes of isovolumic hyponatremia include glucocorticoid deficiency, hypothyroidism, and renal failure.

Syndrome of inappropriate antidiuretic hormone (SIADH) can cause isovolumic hyponatremia because the excessive release of antidiuretic hormone (ADH) disrupts fluid and electrolyte balance. ADH is released when the body doesn't need it, which results in water retention and sodium excretion. SIADH occurs with cancers of the duodenum, pancreas, and lung; acquired immunodeficiency syndrome (AIDS), central nervous system disorders, such as trauma and stroke; and pulmonary disorders, such as asthma and chronic obstructive pulmonary disease.

DRUG ALERT *Drugs can contribute to the development of hyponatremia by potentiating the action of ADH, thus causing SIADH, or by inhibiting sodium reabsorption in the kidney. Drugs associated with hyponatremia include anticonvulsants (such as carbamazepine [Tegretol]), antidiabetics (such as chlorpropamide [Diabenese] and tolbutamide [Orinase]), antineoplastics (such as cyclophosphamide [Cytoxan] and vincristine [Oncovin]), antipsychotics (such as fluphenazine [Prolixin], thioridazine [Mellaril], and thiothixene [Navane]), diuretics (such as bumetanide [Bumex], ethacrynic acid [Edecrin], furosemide [Lasix], and thiazides), and sedatives (such as barbiturates and morphine).*

PATHOPHYSIOLOGY

Sodium is the major cation in extracellular fluid. Potassium is the major cation in intracellular fluid. To maintain normal sodium and potassium levels, the sodium-potassium pump is constantly at work with every body cell to maintain balance across the cell's membrane. During repolarization, the sodium-potassium continually shifts sodium into the cells; during depolarization, the reverse occurs.

Sodium cations help maintain the tonicity and concentration of extracellular fluid, acid-base balance, nerve conduction and neuromuscular function, glandular secretion, and water balance. Thus, hyponatremia has extensive effects on the body's systems.

Cardiovascular system

- Associated hypovolemia results in hypotension, tachycardia, vasomotor collapse, and a thready pulse. Central venous pressure and pulmonary artery pressure may be decreased.
- Patients with associated hypervolemia may exhibit edema, jugular vein distention, hypertension, and a rapid, bounding pulse. Central venous pressure and pulmonary artery pressure may be elevated.

Integumentary system

- Hypovolemia with depletional hyponatremia can cause dry mucous membranes

DISORDERS AFFECTING MANAGEMENT OF HYPONATREMIA

This chart highlights disorders that affect the management of hyponatremia.

DISORDER	SIGNS AND SYMPTOMS	DIAGNOSTIC TEST RESULTS
Cerebral edema (complication)	◆ Headache (especially new onset) ◆ Irritability ◆ Altered behavior ◆ Drowsiness ◆ Decreasing level of consciousness ◆ Bradycardia ◆ Hypertension	◆ Computed tomography scan and magnetic resonance imaging (MRI) rule out herniation or neoplasms that would cause altered mental status and may show evidence of brain edema.
Seizures (complication)	◆ Aura ◆ Loss of consciousness ◆ Dyspnea ◆ Fixed and dilated pupils ◆ Incontinence	◆ EEG shows abnormal wave patterns and the focus of the seizure activity. ◆ MRI may show pathologic changes. ◆ Brain mapping identifies seizure areas.

and poor skin turgor related to fluid volume deficits.

Metabolic and endocrine systems
■ Loss or gain of body fluids may result in weight gain from fluid retention or loss of weight from a fluid volume deficit.
■ Excessive release of ADH from a disorder of the posterior pituitary leads to SIADH.

Neuromuscular system
■ Hyponatremia leads to nerve conduction problems, such as headache, twitching, tremors, and muscle weakness.
■ Changes in level of consciousness (LOC) may start as a shortened attention span and progress to lethargy and confusion; as the condition worsens, stupor, seizures, and coma may develop. (See *Disorders affecting management of hyponatremia*.)

Renal system
■ Oliguria or anuria may occur related to renal failure or decreased renal function.

Respiratory system
■ Severe hyponatremia may lead to cyanosis from inadequate oxygenation.

ASSESSMENT
Signs and symptoms of hyponatremia vary among patients, depending on how quickly the sodium level drops. If the sodium level drops rapidly, the patient will be more symptomatic (even in patients with initial sodium levels above 125 mEq/L) than if the level drops slowly.

Clinical findings
■ Headache
■ Nausea, vomiting, and abdominal pain
■ Change in LOC that may progress to stupor, seizures, and coma
■ Bounding pulse, dyspnea, pulmonary edema, and hypertension resulting from hypervolemia
■ Dry mucous membranes, poor skin turgor, tachycardia, and orthostatic hypotension related to hypovolemia
■ Twitching, tremors, seizures, or coma

■ Muscle weakness and muscle irritability related to neuromuscular effects of hyponatremia

■ Cold, clammy skin

Diagnostic test results

■ *Serum osmolality* is less than 280 mOsm/kg.

■ *Serum sodium level* is less than 135 mEq/L.

■ *Urine specific gravity* is less than 1.010 or increased in patients with SIADH.

■ *Urine sodium level* is above 20 mEq/L in patients with SIADH.

■ *Hematocrit and serum protein levels* are elevated.

COLLABORATIVE MANAGEMENT

Because hyponatremia can affect multiple body systems, a multidisciplinary approach to care is needed. Cardiology and neurology specialists may be consulted, depending on the patient's history and clinical findings. A renal specialist or nephrologist can help evaluate, treat, and manage the patient's kidney function and metabolic status. Nutritional therapy may be needed for dietary assistance. If a prolonged hospital stay is expected and the patient requires long-term care or home care, social services may be consulted for assistance with discharge planning and follow-up.

TREATMENT AND CARE

■ Treatment for mild hyponatremia associated with hypervolemia or isovolemia commonly consists of restricted fluid intake and, possibly, oral sodium supplements.

■ If hypovolemia is related to hyponatremia, isotonic I.V. fluids, such as normal saline solution, are administered to restore fluid volume. Foods high in sodium may also be provided to this patient.

■ Severe cases of hyponatremia (the serum sodium level falls below 110 mEq/L) require intensive treatment. Care may include I.V. administration of a hypertonic saline solution. Carefully monitor the patient for signs and symptoms of volume overload and diminished neurologic status.

■ Patients with hypervolemia shouldn't receive a hypertonic saline solution, except in rare circumstances of severely symptomatic hyponatremia. During administration of hypertonic sodium chloride administration, monitor serum sodium levels closely.

■ Monitor vital signs, intake and output, neurologic status, daily weight, skin turgor, electrolyte and renal function studies, and the patient's risk of injury.

■ Provide dietary counseling or consult the dietitian if the patient has been instructed to increase his dietary intake of sodium.

Hypophosphatemia

Hypophosphatemia occurs when the serum phosphorus level falls below 2.5 mg/dl (or 1.8 mEq/L). Although this condition generally indicates a deficiency of phosphorus, it can also occur when total body stores of phosphorus are normal. Severe hypophosphatemia occurs when the serum phosphorus level drops below 1 mg/dl and the body can't support its energy demands.

DISORDERS AFFECTING
MANAGEMENT OF HYPOPHOSPHATEMIA

This chart highlights disorders that affect the management of hypophosphatemia.

DISORDER	SIGNS AND SYMPTOMS	DIAGNOSTIC TEST RESULTS
Cardiac arrhythmias (complication)	◆ Possibly asymptomatic ◆ Dizziness ◆ Hypotension ◆ Syncope ◆ Weakness ◆ Cool, clammy skin ◆ Altered level of consciousness (LOC) ◆ Reduced urine output ◆ Shortness of breath ◆ Chest pain	◆ Electrocardiography (ECG) detects arrhythmias as well as ischemia and infarction that may result in arrhythmias. ◆ Laboratory testing may reveal electrolyte abnormalities, acid-base abnormalities, or drug toxicities that may cause arrhythmias. ◆ Holter monitoring, event monitoring, and loop recording can detect arrhythmias and effectiveness of drug therapy during a patient's daily activities. ◆ Exercise testing may detect exercise-induced arrhythmias. ◆ Electrophysiologic testing identifies the mechanism of the arrhythmia.
Metabolic acidosis (complication)	◆ Confusion ◆ Decreased deep tendon reflexes ◆ Dull headache ◆ Hyperkalemic signs and symptoms (including abdominal cramping, diarrhea, muscle weakness, and ECG changes) ◆ Hypotension ◆ Kussmaul's respirations ◆ Lethargy ◆ Warm, dry skin	◆ Arterial blood gas (ABG) analysis reveals a pH below 7.35. Partial pressure of arterial carbon dioxide may be less than 35 mm Hg. ◆ Serum potassium levels are usually elevated. ◆ Blood glucose and serum ketone levels rise in patients with diabetic ketoacidosis (DKA). ◆ Plasma lactate levels rise in patients with lactic acidosis. ◆ The anion gap is increased. (Normal anion gap is 8 to 14 mEq/L.) ◆ ECG reveals changes associated with hyperkalemia, such as tall T waves, prolonged PR intervals, and widened QRS complexes.
Rhabdomyolysis (complication)	◆ Abnormal urine color (dark, red, or cola colored) ◆ Muscle tenderness ◆ Weakness of the affected muscle ◆ Muscle stiffness or aching (myalgia) ◆ Unintentional weight gain ◆ Seizures ◆ Joint pain ◆ Fatigue	◆ Urine myoglobin level exceeds 0.5 mg/dl. ◆ Creatinine kinase level is elevated (0.5 to 0.95 mg/dl) from muscle damage. ◆ Blood urea nitrogen, creatinine, creatine, and phosphate levels are elevated. ◆ Intracompartmental venous pressure measurements are elevated. ◆ Computed tomography, magnetic resonance imaging, and bone scintigraphy detect muscle necrosis. ◆ Urinalysis may reveal casts. ◆ Serum potassium is elevated.

ETIOLOGY

Three underlying mechanisms can lead to hypophosphatemia: a shift of phosphorus from extracellular fluid to intracellular fluid, a decrease in intestinal absorption of phosphorus, and an increased loss of phosphorus through renal excretion. Some causes may involve more than one of these mechanisms.

Respiratory alkalosis stemming from hyperventilation, sepsis, alcohol withdrawal, heatstroke, or acute salicylate poisoning can lead to hypophosphatemia; however, the

TREATMENT AND CARE

- When life-threatening arrhythmias develop, rapidly assess LOC, respirations, and pulse rate.
- Initiate cardiopulmonary resuscitation, if indicated.
- Evaluate cardiac output resulting from arrhythmias.
- If the patient develops heart block, prepare for cardiac pacing.
- Administer antiarrhythmics; prepare to assist with medical procedures, if indicated.
- Assess intake and output every hour; insert an indwelling urinary catheter as indicated to ensure accurate urine measurement.
- Document arrhythmias in a monitored patient and assess for possible causes and effects.
- If the patient's pulse is abnormally rapid, slow, or irregular, watch for signs of hypoperfusion, such as hypotension and diminished urine output.
- Monitor for predisposing factors, such as fluid and electrolyte imbalance, or possible drug toxicity.

- Monitor vital signs and assess cardiac rhythm.
- Prepare for mechanical ventilation or dialysis as required.
- Monitor the patient's neurologic status closely because changes can occur rapidly. Notify the physician of changes in the patient's condition.
- Insert an I.V. line and maintain patent I.V. access. Have a large-bore catheter in place for emergency situations.
- Administer I.V. fluid, a vasopressor, an antibiotic, and other medications (such as sodium bicarbonate).
- Position the patient to promote chest expansion and facilitate breathing. If the patient is stuporous, turn him frequently.
- Take steps to help eliminate the underlying cause. For example, administer insulin and I.V. fluids to reverse DKA.
- Watch for secondary changes that hypovolemia may cause, such as declining blood pressure.
- Monitor the patient's renal function by recording intake and output.
- Watch for changes in the serum electrolyte levels, and monitor ABG results throughout treatment to check for over-correction.
- Orient the patient as needed. If he's confused, take steps to ensure his safety, such as keeping his bed in the lowest position.

- Treat the underlying disorder.
- Assess for and prevent renal failure.
- Place the patient on bed rest to prevent further muscle breakdown.
- Administer I.V. fluids.
- Monitor intake and output.
- Monitor renal studies, urine myoglobin levels, electrolytes, and acid-base balance.
- In the presence of renal failure, prepare the patient for dialysis or slow, continuous renal replacement therapy.
- Administer anti-inflammatory agents, diuretics, corticosteroids, and analgesics.
- Prepare patient for an immediate fasciotomy and debridement if compartment venous pressures exceed 25 mm Hg.

mechanism for respiratory alkalosis–induced hypophosphatemia is unknown.

Such conditions as hyperglycemia, malnutrition, refeeding syndrome, and hypothermia can cause the release of insulin, which transports glucose and phosphorus into the cell. This phosphorus shift can produce hypophosphatemia.

Malabsorption syndromes, starvation, and prolonged or excessive use of phosphorus-binding medications can lead to impaired absorption of phosphorus. Because vitamin D contributes to intestinal absorption of phosphorus, inadequate vitamin D intake or synthesis can also inhibit phosphorus absorption. GI losses of phosphorus through vomiting, diarrhea, or GI suctioning can lead to hypophosphatemia.

Increased renal excretion of phosphorus is generally related to diuretic use or diabetic ketoacidosis (DKA). In DKA, an osmotic diuresis is induced from high glucose levels.

A build-up of parathyroid hormone (PTH), which occurs with hyperparathyroidism and hypocalcemia, leads to hypophosphatemia. The extensive diuresis of salt and water after a burn incident can also lead to hypophosphatemia.

DRUG ALERT *Several drugs, such as acetazolamide, loop diuretics, phosphate-binding medications, thiazide diuretics, antacids, insulin, and laxatives, can cause hypophosphatemia.*

PATHOPHYSIOLOGY

Hypophosphatemia affects many body systems.

Cardiovascular system
■ The heart's contractility is decreased because of low energy stores of adenosine triphosphate (ATP) and hypotension, possibly resulting in low cardiac output.
■ Severe hypophosphatemia may lead to cardiomyopathy, which can be reversed with treatment.
■ The patient may experience chest pain due to mechanisms that lead to decreased oxygen delivery to the myocardium.

Immune and hematologic systems
■ Because of structural and functional changes to the red blood cells, hypophosphatemia may lead to hemolytic anemia.
■ Lack of ATP results in decreased leukocyte production, making the patient susceptible to infection.
■ Chronic hypophosphatemia affects platelet function, resulting in bruising and bleeding.

Musculoskeletal system
■ Osteomalacia, loss of bone density, and bone pain may occur with prolonged hypophosphatemia and can result in pathological fractures.

Neuromuscular system
■ Lack of ATP may lead to muscle weakness, malaise, slurred speech, dysphagia, and a weakened hand grasp. The patient may also experience myalgia.
■ Lack of ATP may affect the central nervous system, causing paresthesia, irritability, apprehension, and confusion that may progress to seizures and coma.
■ Severe cases of hypophosphatemia may alter muscle cell activity by inhibiting the release of muscle enzymes from the cells into the extracellular fluid, resulting in rhabdomyolysis. (See *Disorders affecting management of hypophosphatemia, pages 228 and 229.*)

Respiratory system
■ Respiratory failure may result from weakened respiratory muscles and poor contractility of the diaphragm.
■ Respirations may be shallow and ineffective, leading to poor oxygenation and cyanosis.

ASSESSMENT

Signs and symptoms of hypophosphatemia may develop acutely following a rapid decrease in phosphorus, or gradually, as a result of a slow, continuous decrease. Because phosphorus is required to make high-energy ATP, many of the signs and symptoms of hypophosphatemia are related to low energy stores.

Clinical findings
■ Respiratory failure
■ Decreased cardiac output
■ Cardiomyopathy
■ Rhabdomyolysis
■ Myalgia
■ Seizures and coma
■ Hemolytic anemia
■ GI bleeding
■ Hypotension
■ Cyanosis
■ Weakened hand grasp, muscle weakness, and malaise
■ Dysphagia
■ Slurred speech
■ Bruising and bleeding
■ Fractures

Diagnostic test results

- *Serum phosphorus level* is less than 2.5 mg/dl (or 1.8 mEq/L).
- *Creatine kinase level* is elevated if rhabdomyolysis is present.
- *X-ray studies* reveal skeletal muscle changes, types of osteomalacia, or bone fractures.
- *White blood cell count* is decreased.

COLLABORATIVE MANAGEMENT

Because hypophosphatemia can affect multiple body systems, a multidisciplinary approach to care is needed. Cardiology and neurology specialists may be consulted, depending on the patient's history and clinical findings. A hematologist may be required if the patient experiences hemolytic anemia or clotting problems. Infection control may be necessary to institute measures to prevent infection. A renal specialist or nephrologist can help evaluate, treat, and manage the patient's kidney function and metabolic status. Nutritional therapy may be needed for dietary assistance. If a prolonged hospital stay is expected and the patient requires long-term care or home care, social services may be consulted for assistance with discharge planning and follow-up.

TREATMENT AND CARE

- Treatment varies with the severity and underlying cause of the imbalance.
- Treatment for a mild to moderate phosphorus imbalance includes a diet high in phosphorus-rich foods, such as eggs, nuts, whole grains, meat, fish, poultry, and milk products. If the patient can't tolerate milk or if calcium is restricted, oral phosphorus supplements should be prescribed; adverse effects of oral phosphorus supplements include nausea and diarrhea.
- Patients with severe hypophosphatemia or a nonfunctioning GI tract should receive I.V. phosphorus replacement in the form of I.V. potassium phosphate or I.V. sodium phosphate. Adverse effects of I.V. phosphorus replacement may include hyperphosphatemia and hypocalcemia.
- Administer I.V. phosphorus supplements slowly at a rate not to exceed 10 mEq/hour.
- Monitor vital signs, intake and output, level of consciousness, neurologic status, respiratory status, white blood cell count, hemoglobin and hematocrit, electrolytes, and muscle strength.
- Monitor the patient for signs and symptoms of rhabdomyolysis or heart failure.
- Be aware that weaning a patient with hypophosphatemia from the ventilator is difficult because of ineffective respiration and muscle contractility.
- Provide a safe environment and monitor the patient for risk of injury.
- Consult a dietitian for dietary counseling and nutritional support.

Hypothermia

Hypothermia — core body temperature below 95° F (35° C) — effects chemical changes in the body. It may be classified as mild (89.6° to 95° F [32° to 35° C]), moderate (86° to 89.6° F [30° to 32° C]), or severe, which may be fatal (77° to 86° F [25° to 30° C]).

Risk factors that contribute to serious cold injury, especially hypothermia, include lack of insulating body fat, wet or inadequate clothing, drug abuse, cardiac disease, smoking, fatigue, malnutrition and depletion of caloric reserves, and excessive alcohol intake. The incidence of hypothermia is highest in children and elderly people.

ETIOLOGY

Hypothermia commonly results from cold-water near drowning and prolonged exposure to cold temperatures. It can also occur in normal temperatures if disease or debility alters the patient's homeostasis. The administration of large amounts of cold blood or blood products can also cause hypothermia.

PATHOPHYSIOLOGY

In hypothermia, metabolic changes slow the functions of most major organ systems. For example, renal blood flow and glomerular filtration are decreased. Hypothermia also has a physiologic effect on vital organs. Severe hypothermia results in depression of cerebral blood flow, diminished oxygen requirements, reduced cardiac output, and decreased arterial pressure.

(*Text continues on page 234.*)

DISORDERS AFFECTING
MANAGEMENT OF HYPOTHERMIA

This chart highlights disorders that affect the management of hypothermia.

DISORDER	SIGNS AND SYMPTOMS	DIAGNOSTIC TEST RESULTS
Aspiration pneumonia (complication)	◆ Fever ◆ Chills ◆ Sweats ◆ Pleuritic chest pain ◆ Cough ◆ Sputum production ◆ Hemoptysis ◆ Dyspnea ◆ Headache ◆ Fatigue ◆ Bronchial breath sounds over areas of consolidation ◆ Crackles ◆ Increased tactile fremitus ◆ Unequal chest wall expansion	◆ Chest X-rays show infiltrates, confirming the diagnosis. ◆ Sputum specimen for Gram stain and culture and sensitivity tests show acute inflammatory cells. ◆ White blood cell count indicates leukocytosis in bacterial pneumonia and a normal or low count in viral or mycoplasmal pneumonia. ◆ Blood cultures reflect bacteremia and help determine the causative organism. ◆ Arterial blood gas (ABG) levels vary depending on the severity of pneumonia and the underlying lung state. ◆ Bronchoscopy or transtracheal aspiration allows the collection of material for culture. Pleural fluid culture may also be obtained. ◆ Pulse oximetry may show a reduced level of arterial oxygen saturation.
Pancreatitis (complication)	◆ Steady epigastric pain centered close to the umbilicus, radiating between the 10th thoracic and 6th lumbar vertebrae ◆ Pain unrelieved by vomiting *In severe attack* ◆ Extreme pain ◆ Persistent vomiting ◆ Abdominal rigidity ◆ Diminished bowel activity ◆ Crackles at lung bases ◆ Left pleural effusion ◆ Extreme malaise ◆ Restlessness ◆ Mottled skin ◆ Tachycardia ◆ Low-grade fever (100° to 102° F [37.8° to 38.9° C]) ◆ Possible ileus ◆ Cold, sweaty extremities	◆ Serum amylase level is dramatically elevated (in many cases over 500 U/L), which confirms pancreatitis and rules out perforated peptic ulcer, acute cholecystitis, appendicitis, and bowel infarction or obstruction. ◆ Urine and pleural fluid analysis amylase is dramatically elevated in ascites. Characteristically, amylase levels return to normal 48 hours after onset of pancreatitis, despite continuing symptoms. ◆ Serum lipase levels are increased, which rise more slowly than serum amylase. ◆ Serum calcium levels are decreased (hypocalcemia) from fat necrosis and formation of calcium soaps. ◆ White blood cell counts range from 8,000 to 20,000/µl, with increased polymorphonuclear leukocytes. ◆ Glucose levels will be elevated — as high as 500 to 900 mg/dl, indicating hyperglycemia. ◆ Abdominal X-rays or CT scans show dilation of the small or large bowel or calcification of the pancreas. ◆ An ultrasound or CT scan reveals an increased pancreatic diameter and helps distinguish acute cholecystitis from acute pancreatitis.
Renal failure (complication)	◆ Oliguria (initially) ◆ Azotemia ◆ Anuria (rare) ◆ Electrolyte imbalance ◆ Metabolic acidosis ◆ Anorexia ◆ Nausea and vomiting ◆ Diarrhea or constipation ◆ Dry mucous membranes	◆ Blood urea nitrogen, serum creatinine, and potassium levels are elevated. ◆ Bicarbonate level, hematocrit, hemoglobin, and pH are decreased. ◆ Urine studies show casts, cellular debris, and decreased specific gravity; in glomerular diseases proteinuria, and urine osmolality that's close to serum osmolality; urine sodium level is less than 20 mEq/L if oliguria results from decreased perfusion, or more than 40 mEq/L if the cause is intrarenal.

TREATMENT AND CARE

◆ Maintain a patent airway and adequate oxygenation. Measure the patient's ABG levels, especially if he's hypoxic. Administer supplemental oxygen if his partial pressure of arterial oxygen falls below 55 to 60 mm Hg. If he has an underlying chronic lung disease, give oxygen cautiously.

◆ In severe pneumonia that requires endotracheal intubation or a tracheostomy with or without mechanical ventilation, provide thorough respiratory care and suction often, using sterile technique, to remove secretions.

◆ Obtain sputum specimens as needed. Use suction if the patient can't produce a specimen.

◆ Administer antibiotics and pain medication. Administer I.V. fluids and electrolyte replacement for fever and dehydration.

◆ Provide a high-calorie, high-protein diet of soft foods to offset the calories the patient uses to fight the infection. If necessary, supplement oral feedings with nasogastric (NG) tube feedings or parenteral nutrition.

◆ To prevent aspiration during NG tube feedings, elevate the patient's head, check the tube position, and administer the feeding slowly. Don't give large volumes at one time because this can cause vomiting.

◆ If the patient has an endotracheal tube, inflate the tube cuff before feeding. Keep his head elevated after feeding.

◆ Monitor the patient's fluid intake and output.

◆ Institute infection control precautions.

◆ Provide a quiet, calm environment, with frequent rest periods.

◆ After the emergency phase, continue I.V. therapy for 5 to 7 days to provide adequate electrolytes and protein solutions that don't stimulate the pancreas.

◆ If the patient can't tolerate oral feedings, total parenteral nutrition (TPN) or nonstimulating elemental gavage feedings may be needed.

◆ In extreme cases, laparotomy to drain the pancreatic bed, 95% pancreatectomy, or a combination of cholecystectomy-gastrostomy, feeding jejunostomy, and drainage may be needed.

◆ Give plasma or albumin, if ordered, to maintain blood pressure.

◆ Record intake and output, check urine output hourly, and monitor electrolyte levels.

◆ Watch for signs of calcium deficiency, such as tetany, cramps, carpopedal spasm, and seizures.

◆ If you suspect hypocalcemia, keep airway and suction apparatus readily available and pad the side rails.

◆ Administer analgesics as needed to relieve the patient's pain and anxiety.

◆ Watch for complications of TPN, such as sepsis, hypokalemia, overhydration, and metabolic acidosis.

◆ Measure intake and output, including body fluids, NG output, and diarrhea; weigh the patient daily.

◆ Measure hemoglobin level and hematocrit, and replace blood components.

◆ Monitor vital signs; check and report for signs of pericarditis (pleuritic chest pain, tachycardia, pericardial friction rub), inadequate renal perfusion (hypotension), and acidosis.

◆ Maintain proper electrolyte balance. Monitor potassium levels, and monitor for hyperkalemia (malaise, anorexia, paresthesia or muscle weakness) and ECG changes.

◆ If the patient receives hypertonic glucose and insulin infusions, monitor potassium and glucose levels. If giving sodium polystyrene sulfonate rectally, make sure the patient doesn't retain it and become constipated; doing so prevents bowel perforation.

(continued)

DISORDERS AFFECTING
MANAGEMENT OF HYPOTHERMIA *(continued)*

DISORDER	SIGNS AND SYMPTOMS	DIAGNOSTIC TEST RESULTS
Renal failure *(continued)*	◆ Headache ◆ Confusion ◆ Seizures ◆ Drowsiness ◆ Irritability ◆ Coma ◆ Dry skin ◆ Pruritus ◆ Pallor ◆ Purpura ◆ Uremic frost ◆ Hypotension (early) ◆ Hypertension with arrhythmias (later) ◆ Fluid overload ◆ Heart failure ◆ Systemic edema ◆ Anemia ◆ Altered clotting mechanisms ◆ Pulmonary edema ◆ Kussmaul's respirations	◆ Creatinine clearance tests measuring glomerular filtration rate reflect the number of remaining functioning nephrons. ◆ Electrocardiography (ECG) reveals tall, peaked T waves; widening QRS; and disappearing P waves if hyperkalemia is present. ◆ Ultrasonography, abdominal and kidney-ureter-bladder X-rays, excretory urography, renal scan, retrograde pyelography, CT scan, and nephrotomography reveal abnormalities of the urinary tract.

Cardiovascular system

■ Peripheral vasoconstriction, an increase in cardiac afterload, and elevated myocardial oxygen consumption result in initial tachycardia then bradycardia and myocardial depression, which lead to decreased cardiac output and hypotension.
■ Hypothermia causes metabolic changes that induce cardiac arrhythmias such as ventricular fibrillation.

Endocrine system

■ Cold stimulates the release of catecholamines, which produce thermogenesis.
■ Corticosteroid levels become elevated.
■ Hyperglycemia may result from an increase in catecholamines, a decrease in insulin activity, and a decrease in renal excretion of glucose.

Gastrointestinal system

■ GI smooth-muscle motility decreases, resulting in acute gastric dilation, paralytic ileus, and distention of the colon.
■ GI secretions and free acid production are decreased.

■ Cold-associated hemorrhages called *Wischnevsky's lesions* develop in the pancreatic and gastric mucosa.
■ Liver function decreases, eventually leading to an impaired ability to metabolize drugs, metabolites, or conjugate steroids.

Immune system

■ Cold temperatures inhibit immune function, resulting in cold-induced immunosuppression.

Renal system

■ Renal function is depressed because of a fall in systemic blood pressure. (See *Disorders affecting management of hypothermia*, pages 232 to 235.)
■ Renal vascular resistance rises, leading to a further decrease in renal flow and glomerular filtration.

Respiratory system

■ The brain stem is impaired by hypothermia, which results in respiratory compromise and diminished oxygen requirements and a decreased respiratory minute volume.

TREATMENT AND CARE

◆ Maintain nutritional status with a high-calorie, low-protein, low-sodium, and low-potassium diet and vitamin supplements.
◆ Monitor the patient carefully during peritoneal dialysis.
◆ If the patient requires hemodialysis, monitor the venous access site and assess the patient and laboratory work carefully.

■ Tissues retain carbon dioxide, resulting in respiratory acidosis.
■ Respiratory ciliary motility decreases.
■ Lung compliance decreases.
■ The potential for noncardiogenic pulmonary edema increases.
■ Elasticity of the thorax decreases.
■ Physiologic and anatomic dead spaces are increased.

ASSESSMENT

The history of a patient with a cold injury reveals the cause, the temperature to which the patient was exposed, and the length of exposure.

The patient with mild hypothermia will have amnesia; the patient with moderate hypothermia is unresponsive; the patient with severe hypothermia appears to be lifeless. A patient with a body temperature below 86° F (30° C) is at risk for cardiopulmonary arrest.

RED FLAG If a patient has hypothermia, use an esophageal or rectal probe that reads as low as 77° F (25° C) to determine an accurate core body temperature. Core body temperature can also be determined using a pulmonary artery catheter.

Clinical findings

Assessment findings in a patient with hypothermia vary with the patient's body temperature.

Mild hypothermia
■ Severe shivering
■ Slurred speech

Moderate hypothermia
■ Unresponsive
■ Peripheral cyanosis
■ Muscle rigidity
■ Signs of shock

Severe hypothermia
■ No palpable pulse
■ No audible heart sounds
■ Possible dilated pupils
■ State of rigor mortis
■ Ventricular fibrillation
■ Loss of deep tendon reflexes

Diagnostic test results

■ *Technetium pertechnetate scanning* shows perfusion defects and deep-tissue damage and can be used to identify nonviable bone.

■ *Doppler and plethysmographic studies* help determine pulses and the extent of frostbite after thawing.

■ *Laboratory testing* during treatment of moderate or severe hypothermia includes a complete blood count, coagulation profile, urinalysis, and serum amylase, electrolyte, hemoglobin, glucose, liver enzyme, blood urea nitrogen, creatinine, and arterial blood gas levels.

COLLABORATIVE MANAGEMENT

Depending on the severity of the patient's condition, he may require the services of a pulmonary specialist (for mechanical ventilation), neurosurgeon (if he remains obtunded when rewarmed), renal specialist (for renal involvement), or cardiologist (for cardiac involvement).

TREATMENT AND CARE

■ Specific rewarming techniques include passive rewarming (the patient rewarms on his own); active external rewarming (using heating blankets, warm-water immersion, heated objects such as water bottles, and radiant heat), and active core rewarming (using heated I.V. fluids, genitourinary tract irrigation, extracorporeal rewarming, hemodialysis, and peritoneal, gastric, and mediastinal lavage). Arrhythmias that develop usually convert to a normal sinus rhythm with rewarming.

■ If the patient has no pulse or respirations, cardiopulmonary resuscitation is needed until rewarming raises the core temperature to at least 89.6° F (32° C).

■ Administration of oxygen, endotracheal intubation, controlled ventilation, I.V. fluids, and treatment of metabolic acidosis depend on test results and careful patient monitoring.

Hypothyroidism

Hypothyroidism results from hypothalamic, pituitary, or thyroid insufficiency or resistance to thyroid hormone. The disorder can progress to life-threatening myxedema coma, if left untreated. In the United States, the incidence is increasing significantly in patients older than age 50 and is more prevalent in women than in men.

ETIOLOGY

Hypothyroidism in adults may be caused by inadequate production of thyroid hormone, which usually occurs after thyroidectomy or radiation therapy (particularly with iodine 131). Other causes include inflammation, chronic autoimmune thyroiditis (Hashimoto's disease), or such conditions as amyloidosis and sarcoidosis (rare). Hypothyroidism is also caused by pituitary failure to produce thyroid-stimulating hormone (TSH), hypothalamic failure to produce thyrotropin-releasing hormone (TRH), inborn errors of thyroid hormone synthesis, iodine deficiency (usually dietary), or use of such antithyroid medications.

PATHOPHYSIOLOGY

Hypothyroidism may reflect a malfunction of the hypothalamus, pituitary gland, or thyroid gland, all of which are part of the same negative-feedback mechanism. Primary hypothyroidism, a disorder of the thyroid gland itself, is most common. Disorders of the hypothalamus and pituitary gland rarely cause hypothyroidism.

The thyroid gland synthesizes and secretes the iodinated hormones, thyroxine (T_4) and triiodothyronine (T_3). Thyroid hormones are necessary for normal growth and development and act on many tissues to increase metabolic activity and protein synthesis.

Chronic autoimmune thyroiditis, also called chronic lymphocytic thyroiditis, occurs when autoantibodies destroy thyroid gland tissue. Chronic autoimmune thyroiditis associated with goiter is called Hashimoto's thyroiditis. Although the exact cause of this autoimmune process is unknown, heredity may play a role. Additionally, specific human leukocyte antigen subtypes are associated with greater risk.

Outside the thyroid, antibodies can reduce the effect of thyroid hormone in two ways. First, antibodies can block the TSH receptor, preventing TSH production. Second, cytotoxic antithyroid antibodies may attack thyroid cells.

Subacute thyroiditis, painless thyroiditis, and postpartum thyroiditis are self-limited conditions that usually follow an episode of hyperthyroidism. Untreated, subclinical hypothyroidism in adults is likely to increase at a rate of 5% to 20% per year.

Cardiovascular system
■ Cardiovascular involvement includes decreased cardiac output resulting in slow pulse rate, signs of poor peripheral circulation and, occasionally, an enlarged heart, eventually leading to heart failure.
■ Fluid retention may lead to periorbital edema.

Gastrointestinal system
■ Unexplained weight gain may be attributed to fluid retention in the myxedematous tissues.
■ Constipation, anorexia, and abdominal distention occur; these conditions may eventually lead to megacolon.

Genitourinary system
■ Menorrhagia and decreased libido occur because of altered prolactin levels; these conditions may lead to infertility.

Integumentary system
■ Decreased sweating occurs.
■ The epidermis thins and hyperkeratosis occurs.
■ Increased dermal glycoaminoglycan content traps water and gives rise to skin thickening without pitting (myxedema).
■ Dry, flaky, inelastic skin develops.
■ Hair patterns and eyebrows change.
■ Nails become dry and brittle.

Musculoskeletal system
■ Ataxia, nystagmus, and reflexes with delayed relaxation time (especially in the Achilles tendon) occur because of endocrine effects.

Neurologic system
■ Metabolic effects disrupt the central nervous system (CNS), leading to weakness, fatigue, forgetfulness, sensitivity to the cold, and decreased mental stability.
■ CNS effects can progress to myxedema coma. Progression is usually gradual but may develop abruptly. Such stresses as hypoventilation, hypoglycemia, hyponatremia, hypotension, and hypothermia in those with

severe or prolonged hypothyroidism increase the risk. (See *Disorders affecting management of hypothyroidism,* pages 238 and 239.)

ASSESSMENT
Assessment findings in a patient with hypothyroidism may vary. Accurate diagnosis requires a thorough history and physical examination in conjunction with hormone level determinations.

Clinical findings
■ Cold intolerance
■ Constipation
■ Somnolence
■ Menstrual disorders
■ Anemia
■ Bradycardia
■ Arthritis
■ Muscle cramps
■ Delayed relaxation of reflexes
■ Dementia and slow speech
■ Decreased sociability
■ Memory impairment
■ Psychosis
■ Drowsiness and fatigue
■ Brittle hair and nails and loss of lateral third of eyebrow
■ Cool, dry skin and hypothermia
■ Gravelly voice and large tongue
■ Puffy face and hands
■ Weight gain

Diagnostic test results
■ *Radioimmunoassay* shows low T_3 and T_4 levels.
■ *TSH level* is increased if the cause is a thyroid disorder; decreased if the cause is a hypothalamic or pituitary disorder.
■ *Thyroid panel* differentiates primary hypothyroidism (thyroid gland hypofunction), secondary hypothyroidism (pituitary hyposecretion of TSH), tertiary hypothyroidism (hypothalamic hyposecretion of TRH), and euthyroid sick syndrome (impaired peripheral conversion of thyroid hormone due to a suprathyroidal illness such as severe infection).
■ *Serum cholesterol, alkaline phosphatase, and triglyceride levels* are elevated.
■ *Serum sodium levels* are low, *pH* is decreased, and *partial pressure of arterial car-*

DISORDERS AFFECTING MANAGEMENT OF HYPOTHYROIDISM

This chart highlights disorders that affect the management of hypothyroidism.

DISORDER	SIGNS AND SYMPTOMS	DIAGNOSTIC TEST RESULTS
Heart failure (complication)	◆ Cough that produces pink, frothy sputum ◆ Cyanosis of the lips and nail beds ◆ Pale, cool, clammy skin ◆ Diaphoresis ◆ Jugular vein distention ◆ Ascites ◆ Pulsus alternans ◆ Tachycardia ◆ Hepatomegaly ◆ Decreased pulse pressure ◆ Third and fourth heart sounds ◆ Moist, basilar crackles ◆ Rhonchi ◆ Expiratory wheezing ◆ Decreased pulse oximetry ◆ Peripheral edema ◆ Decreased urinary output	◆ B-type natriuretic peptide immunoassay is elevated. ◆ Chest X-ray shows increased pulmonary vascular markings, interstitial edema, or pleural effusions and cardiomegaly. ◆ Electrocardiography reveals heart enlargement or ischemia, tachycardia, extrasystole, or atrial fibrillation. ◆ Pulmonary artery pressure, pulmonary artery wedge pressure, and left ventricular end-diastolic pressure are elevated in the presence of left-sided heart failure; right atrial or central venous pressure is elevated in right-sided heart failure.
Myxedema coma (complication)	◆ Progressive stupor ◆ Hypoventilation ◆ Hypoglycemia ◆ Hyponatremia ◆ Hypotension ◆ Hypothermia	◆ Serum sodium levels are low, pH is decreased, and partial pressure of arterial carbon dioxide is increased.

bon dioxide is increased, indicating respiratory acidosis (myxedema coma).

COLLABORATIVE MANAGEMENT

Because hypothyroidism can affect multiple body systems, a multidisciplinary approach to care is needed. An endocrinologist may be needed to help the patient obtain and maintain normal thyroid levels. A cardiologist may be necessary to improve cardiac output.

A GI specialist may be consulted if the patient experiences chronic bowel problems. Counselors may be needed to assist the patient and his family with psychosocial needs.

TREATMENT AND CARE

■ Expect therapy for hypothyroidism to consist of gradual thyroid replacement with levothyroxine.

TREATMENT AND CARE

◆ Administer supplemental oxygen and mechanical ventilation, if needed.
◆ Place the patient in Fowler's position.
◆ Administer diuretics, inotropic drugs, vasodilators, angiotensin-converting enzyme inhibitors, angiotensin receptor blockers, cardiac glycosides, beta blockers, and electrolyte supplements.
◆ Initiate cardiac monitoring.
◆ Recurrent heart failure from valvular dysfunction may require surgery.
◆ A ventricular assist device may be needed.
◆ Maintain adequate cardiac output and monitor hemodynamic stability.
◆ Assess for deep vein thrombosis and apply antiembolism stockings.

◆ Check frequently for signs of decreased cardiac output (such as decreased urine output).
◆ Monitor the patient's temperature until he's stable. Provide extra blankets and clothing and a warm room to compensate for hypothermia. Rapid rewarming may cause vasodilatation and vascular collapse.
◆ Record intake and output and daily weight. As treatment begins, urine output should increase and body weight decrease; if not, report this immediately.
◆ Turn the edematous, bedridden patient every 2 hours and provide skin care, particularly around bony prominences, at lease once per shift.
◆ Avoid sedation when possible or reduce dosage of sedatives because hypothyroidism delays metabolism of many drugs.
◆ Monitor serum electrolyte levels carefully when administering I.V. fluids.
◆ Monitor vital signs carefully when administering levothyroxine because rapid correction of hypothyroidism can cause adverse cardiac effects. Report chest pain or tachycardia immediately. Watch for hypertension and heart failure in the older patient.
◆ Check arterial blood gas values for hypercapnia, metabolic acidosis, and hypoxia to determine whether the patient requires ventilatory assistance.
◆ Administer corticosteroids.
◆ Because myxedema coma may have been precipitated by an infection, check possible sources of the infection, such as blood and urine, and obtain sputum cultures.

■ Provide a high-bulk, low-calorie diet and encourage activity.
■ Administer cathartics and stool softeners as needed.
■ After thyroid replacement therapy begins, watch for signs of hyperthyroidism, such as restlessness, sweating, and excessive weight loss.

Hypovolemic shock

In hypovolemic shock, reduced intravascular blood volume causes circulatory dysfunction and inadequate tissue perfusion. Without sufficient blood or fluid replacement, hypovolemic shock syndrome may lead to irreversible cerebral and renal damage, car-

DISORDERS AFFECTING
MANAGEMENT OF HYPOVOLEMIC SHOCK

This chart highlights disorders that affect the management of hypovolemic shock.

DISORDER	SIGNS AND SYMPTOMS	DIAGNOSTIC TEST RESULTS
Disseminated intravascular coagulation (complication)	◆ Bleeding from puncture sites ◆ Petechiae ◆ Ecchymoses ◆ Hematoma ◆ Nausea and vomiting ◆ Severe muscle, back, and abdominal pain ◆ Chest pain ◆ Hemoptysis	◆ Platelet count is less than 100,000/µl. ◆ Fibrinogen level is less than 150 mg/dl. ◆ Prothrombin time is greater than 15 seconds. ◆ Fibrin degradation products level is greater than 45 mcg/ml. ◆ D-dimer is elevated. ◆ Blood urea nitrogen and creatinine levels are elevated.
Myocardial infarction (MI) (complication)	◆ Persistent, crushing, substernal chest pain that may radiate ◆ Cool extremities, perspiration, anxiety, and restlessness ◆ Initially, elevated blood pressure and pulse; if cardiac output is reduced, decreased blood pressure ◆ Bradycardia ◆ Fatigue and weakness ◆ Nausea and vomiting ◆ Shortness of breath and crackles ◆ Low-grade temperature ◆ Jugular vein distention ◆ Third (S_3) and fourth (S_4) heart sounds ◆ Loud, holosystolic murmur ◆ Reduced urine output	◆ Serial 12-lead electrocardiography (ECG) may reveal characteristic changes such as serial ST-segment depression in non–Q-wave MI and ST-segment elevation in Q-wave MI. ECG can also identify the location of MI, arrhythmias, hypertrophy, and pericarditis. ◆ Serial cardiac enzymes and proteins (CK-MB, troponin T and I, and myoglobin) may show a characteristic rise and fall. ◆ Laboratory testing may reveal elevated white blood cell count, C-reactive protein level, and erythrocyte sedimentation rate. ◆ Echocardiography may show ventricular wall motion abnormalities and may detect septal or papillary muscle rupture. ◆ Chest X-rays may show left-sided heart failure or cardiomegaly caused by ventricular dilation. ◆ Nuclear imaging scanning can identify areas of infarction. ◆ Cardiac catheterization may be used to identify the involved coronary artery and provide information on ventricular function and pressures and volumes within the heart.

diac arrest and, ultimately, death. Hypovolemic shock requires early recognition of signs and symptoms and prompt, aggressive treatment to improve the prognosis.

ETIOLOGY

Hypovolemic shock usually results from acute blood loss (about one-fifth of the total volume). Such massive blood loss may result from GI bleeding, internal hemorrhage (hemothorax and hemoperitoneum), external hemorrhage (accidental or surgical trauma), or conditions that reduce circulating intravascular plasma volume or other body fluids, such as severe burns. Other underlying causes of hypovolemic shock include intestinal obstruction, peritonitis, acute pancreatitis, ascites, and dehydration from excessive perspiration, severe diarrhea or protracted vomiting, diabetes insipidus, diuresis, or inadequate fluid intake.

PATHOPHYSIOLOGY

When fluid is lost from the intravascular space through external losses or the shift of fluid from the vessels to the interstitial or intracellular spaces, venous return to the heart is reduced. This reduction in preload decreases ventricular filling, leading to a drop in stroke volume and cardiac output, caus-

- Treat the underlying cause.
- Administer fresh frozen plasma, platelets, cryoprecipitate, and packed red blood cells to combat bleeding and blood loss.
- Monitor vital signs at least every 30 minutes.
- Administer supplemental oxygen as indicated.
- Assess level of consciousness hourly and when the patient's condition changes.
- Monitor serial hemoglobin, hematocrit, partial thromboplastin time, prothrombin time, fibrinogen levels, fibrinogen degradation products, and platelet counts.
- Administer low-dose heparin infusions, vitamin K, and folate.
- Institute safety precautions to minimize bleeding.

- Monitor and record the patient's ECG, blood pressure, temperature, and heart and breath sounds.
- Assess and record the severity and duration of pain, and administer analgesics. Avoid I.M. injections.
- Check blood pressure after giving nitroglycerin, especially the first dose.
- Frequently monitor ECG to detect rate changes or arrhythmias. Place rhythm strips in the patient's chart periodically for evaluation.
- During episodes of chest pain, obtain 12-lead ECG, blood pressure, and pulmonary artery measurements. Monitor for changes.
- Watch for signs and symptoms of fluid retention. Carefully monitor daily weight, intake and output, respirations, serum enzyme levels, and blood pressure.
- Auscultate for adventitious breath sounds periodically, for S_3 or S_4 gallops, and for new-onset heart murmurs.
- Organize care and activities to maximize periods of uninterrupted rest.
- Ask the dietary department to provide a clear liquid diet until nausea subsides. A low-cholesterol, low-sodium, low-fat, high-fiber diet may be prescribed.
- Provide a stool softener to prevent straining during defecation, which causes vagal stimulation and may slow the heart rate. Allow the patient to use a bedside commode, and provide as much privacy as possible.
- Assist the patient with range-of-motion exercises. If completely immobilized by a severe MI, turn him often.
- Antiembolism stockings help prevent venostasis and thrombophlebitis.
- Provide emotional support and help reduce stress and anxiety; administer sedatives as needed.

ing reduced perfusion of the tissues and organs.

Cardiovascular system
- Tachycardia and bounding pulse occur related to sympathetic stimulation.
- Hypotension occurs as compensatory mechanisms begin to fail.
- Narrowed pulse pressure is associated with reduced stroke volume.
- Weak, thready pulse is caused by decreased cardiac output.
- Rapidly falling blood pressure occurs as a result of decompensation.

Hematologic system
- Disseminated intravascular coagulation (DIC) may develop due to an imbalance of homeostasis mechanisms as coagulation factors are activated. (See *Disorders affecting management of hypovolemic shock.*)

Integumentary system
- Cool, pale skin is associated with vasoconstriction; continued shock results in cold, clammy skin.
- Cyanosis occurs as a result of hypoxia.

Neurologic system
■ Restlessness and irritability occur related to cerebral hypoxia.
■ Unconsciousness and absent reflexes are caused by reduced cerebral perfusion, acid-base imbalance, or electrolyte abnormalities.

Renal system
■ Reduced urinary output occurs secondary to vasoconstriction. Reduced urinary output continues to occur as a result of poor renal perfusion.
■ Anuria is related to renal failure.

Respiratory system
■ Tachypnea occurs to compensate for hypoxia.
■ Shallow respirations occur as the patient weakens.
■ Slow, shallow, or Cheyne-Stokes respirations occur secondary to respiratory center depression.
■ Metabolic acidosis with an accumulation of lactic acid develops as a result of tissue anoxia as cellular metabolism shifts from aerobic to anaerobic pathways.

ASSESSMENT
The specific signs and symptoms depend on the amount of fluid loss. As fluid loss increases, level of consciousness decreases.

Clinical findings
■ Shivering and feeling of being cold
■ Pain related to trauma
■ Hypotension with narrowing pulse pressure
■ Decreased sensorium
■ Tachycardia
■ Rapid, shallow respirations
■ Reduced urine output
■ Cold, pale clammy skin

Diagnostic test results
No single symptom or diagnostic test establishes the diagnosis or severity of shock. Characteristic laboratory findings include:
■ elevated potassium, serum lactate, and blood urea nitrogen levels
■ increased urine specific gravity (greater than 1.020) and urine osmolality
■ decreased blood pH and partial pressure of arterial oxygen and increased partial pressure of arterial carbon dioxide.

In addition, gastroscopy, aspiration of gastric contents through a nasogastric tube, and X-rays identify internal bleeding sites; coagulation studies may detect coagulopathy from DIC.

COLLABORATIVE MANAGEMENT
The patient in hypovolemic shock requires emergency team management to promptly and adequately replace blood and fluids to restore intravascular volume and raise blood pressure. Respiratory therapists may be needed if the patient requires intubation and mechanical ventilation. Surgeons may be brought in if internal bleeding is suspected. Orthopedic specialists may be consulted if bone trauma has occurred resulting in blood loss. Pulmonary specialists are needed if pulmonary sequelae have occurred (hemothorax or pulmonary contusion). Renal specialists are needed and dialysis required if the patient experiences renal failure. Neurologists or neurosurgeons may be needed if the patient continues to have decreased mentation despite adequate resuscitation. Other disciplines may be needed, depending on the severity of the patient's condition and the extent of treatment and rehabilitation required.

TREATMENT AND CARE
■ Treatment typically involves addressing the underlying cause and administering fluid replacement and vasopressors.
■ Assess the patient for the extent of fluid loss and begin fluid replacement. Obtain a type and crossmatching for blood component therapy. Emergency treatment relies on prompt fluid and blood replacement to restore intravascular volume and to raise blood pressure and maintain it above 80 mm Hg.
■ Expect to infuse normal saline or lactated Ringer's solution rapidly along with albumin (possible) or other plasma expanders until whole blood can be matched.
■ Assess airway, breathing, and circulation. If the patient experiences cardiac or respiratory arrest, start cardiopulmonary resuscitation.
■ Administer supplemental oxygen. Monitor oxygen saturation and arterial blood gas studies for evidence of hypoxemia, and anticipate the need for endotracheal intuba-

tion and mechanical ventilation should the patient's respiratory status deteriorate.

■ Place the patient in semi-Fowler's position to maximize chest expansion. Keep the patient as quiet and comfortable as possible to minimize oxygen demands.

■ Monitor vital signs, neurologic status, and cardiac rhythm continuously for such changes as cardiac arrhythmias or myocardial ischemia. Observe skin color and check capillary refill. Notify the physician if capillary refill is greater than 2 seconds.

■ Monitor hemodynamic parameters, including central venous pressure, pulmonary artery wedge pressure (PAWP), and cardiac output frequently — as often as every 15 minutes — to evaluate the patient's status and response to treatment.

■ Monitor intake and output closely. Insert an indwelling urinary catheter, and assess urine output hourly.

■ If bleeding from the GI tract is suspected as the cause, check all stools, emesis, and gastric drainage for occult blood. If output falls below 30 ml/hour in an adult, expect to increase the I.V. fluid infusion rate, but watch for signs of fluid overload such as elevated PAWP. Notify the physician if urine output doesn't increase.

■ Administer blood component therapy; monitor serial hemoglobin values and hematocrit to evaluate effects of treatment.

■ Administer dopamine (Intropin) or norepinephrine (Levophed) I.V. to increase cardiac contractility and renal perfusion.

■ Watch for signs of impending coagulopathy, such as petechiae, bruising, and bleeding or oozing from gums or venipuncture sites.

■ Provide emotional support and reassurance appropriately in the wake of massive fluid losses.

■ Prepare the patient for surgery as appropriate.

L

Lupus erythematosus

Lupus erythematosus is a chronic inflammatory disorder of the connective tissues that appears in two forms: discoid lupus erythematosus (DLE), which affects only the skin, and systemic lupus erythematosus (SLE), which affects multiple organ systems and the skin. (See *Discoid lupus erythematosus.*)

SLE is a potentially fatal disorder that's characterized by recurring remissions and exacerbations, which are especially common during the spring and summer. It strikes women 9 times more often than men (30 times more often during childbearing years). The disorder occurs worldwide but is most prevalent among Asians, Native Americans, Hispanics, and Blacks. Although the condition can occur in childhood and later in adult life, it most commonly occurs in patients between ages 15 and 45. The prognosis improves with early detection and treatment but remains poor for patients who develop cardiovascular, renal, or neurologic complications or severe bacterial infections. In about one-half of SLE cases, a major organ is affected.

ETIOLOGY

The exact cause of SLE remains unknown, but available evidence points to interrelated immunologic, environmental, hormonal, and genetic factors. Most people with SLE have a genetic predisposition. Other factors may include:

- physical or mental stress
- streptococcal or viral infections
- exposure to sunlight or ultraviolet light
- immunization
- pregnancy
- abnormal estrogen metabolism.

DRUG ALERT *Some drugs can cause symptoms that resemble those of SLE. Other drugs, such as procainamide (Procanbid), hydralazine (Apresoline), isoniazid (Nydrazid), methyldopa (Aldomet), and anticonvulsants, may actually trigger or activate it. Penicillins, sulfa drugs, and hormonal contraceptives are less common SLE triggers. Symptoms generally disappear when the drug is discontinued.*

PATHOPHYSIOLOGY

Autoimmunity is believed to be the prime mechanism linked to SLE. In autoimmune reactions, the body's normal defenses become self-destructive, recognizing self-antigens as foreign. What causes this misdirected response isn't clearly understood. For example, drugs or viruses have been implicated as causing some autoimmune reactions, but in SLE, the mechanism for misdirection is unclear.

Autoimmune reactions are believed to result from a combination of factors, including viruses and genetic, hormonal, and environmental influences, such as sunlight or stress. Many are characterized by B-cell hyperactivity and by hypergammaglobulinemia. B-cell hyperactivity may be related to T-cell abnormalities. Hormonal and genetic factors strongly influence the onset of some autoimmune disorders.

The body produces antibodies against components of its own cells, such as the antinuclear antibody (ANA), and immune complex disease follows. Once deposited, a local inflammatory response occurs, ultimately leading to tissue injury. Patients with SLE may produce antibodies against many different tissue components, such as red blood cells (RBCs), neutrophils, platelets, lymphocytes, or almost any organ or tissue in the body. (See *Disorders affecting management of lupus erythematosus,* pages 246 to 249.)

Cardiopulmonary system
■ Immune complexes may be deposited in the vascular tissue (of the heart and lungs), leading to pericarditis, myocarditis, valvular disease, pleural effusions, pleuritis, pneumonitis, chronic interstitial lung disease, and pulmonary embolism.
■ Raynaud's phenomenon may occur because of vasculitis.

Genitourinary system
■ Immune complexes may be deposited in the renal tissue, leading to glomerulonephritis, interstitial nephritis, nephritic syndrome and, possibly, renal failure.

Hematologic system
■ The development of autoantibodies against blood cell components – such as the red blood cells, white blood cells, platelets, and lymphocytes – and subsequent deposition of immune complexes can affect overall blood cell function, causing anemia, leukopenia, thrombocytopenia, and lymphopenia.
■ Immune complexes may be deposited in the lymph nodes, causing lymphadenopathy.

Integumentary system
■ As autoantibodies are produced and immune complexes are formed, they're deposited in the layers of the skin, causing an inflammatory response and tissue injury, resulting in the classic butterfly rash and lesions, such as hives and cyanotic discolorations.
■ Deposition of the immune complexes may cause erythema of the nailbeds, splinter hemorrhages, and hair loss.

Musculoskeletal system
■ Deposition of immune complexes into joint tissue may cause arthritis and arthralgias. As the disease progresses, tendons, ligaments, and joint capsules may become affected, leading to deformity and loss of function.

Neurologic system
■ SLE may cause acute vasculitis in the cerebral blood vessels, leading to impaired cerebral blood flow and, ultimately, hemorrhage or stroke.
■ Antibodies may be developed to specifically attack neuronal cells and phospho-

(*Text continues on page 248.*)

DISCOID LUPUS ERYTHEMATOSUS

Discoid lupus erythematosus (DLE) is a form of lupus erythematosus that's marked by chronic skin eruptions. DLE can cause scarring and permanent disfigurement if left untreated. About 5% of patients with DLE later develop systemic lupus erythematosus (SLE). An estimated 60% of patients with DLE are women in their late 20s or older. The disease seldom occurs in children. Its exact cause isn't known, but evidence suggests an autoimmune process.

Clinical findings
The patient with DLE has lesions that appear as raised, red, scaling plaques with follicular plugging and central atrophy. The raised edges and sunken centers give the lesions a coinlike appearance. Although these lesions can appear anywhere on the body, they usually erupt on the face, scalp, ears, neck, and arms or on any part of the body that is exposed to sunlight. Such lesions can resolve completely or may cause hypopigmentation or hyperpigmentation, atrophy, and scarring. Facial plaques sometimes assume the butterfly pattern characteristic of SLE. Hair becomes brittle and may fall out in patches.

Diagnostic test results
As a rule, the patient's history and the rash are enough to form the diagnosis. Positive findings in the LE cell test (in which polymorphonuclear leukocytes engulf cell nuclei to form so-called LE cells) occur in less than 10% of patients. Positive skin biopsy results of lesions typically disclose immunoglobulins or complement components. SLE must be ruled out.

Treatment and care
As in SLE, drug treatment consists of topical, intralesional, and systemic medications. In addition, patients require education about the following: avoiding prolonged exposure to the sun, fluorescent lighting, and reflected sunlight; use of protective clothing and sunscreens; avoidance of outdoor activity during peak sunlight periods (between 10 a.m. and 2 p.m.); and the need to report changes in the lesions.

DISORDERS AFFECTING
MANAGEMENT OF LUPUS ERYTHEMATOSUS

This chart highlights disorders that affect the management of lupus erythematosus.

DISORDER	SIGNS AND SYMPTOMS	DIAGNOSTIC TEST RESULTS
Acute renal failure (complication)	◆ Oliguria, azotemia and, rarely, anuria ◆ Electrolyte imbalance and metabolic acidosis ◆ Anorexia, nausea, vomiting, diarrhea or constipation, stomatitis, bleeding, hematemesis, dry mucous membranes, and uremic breath ◆ Headache, drowsiness, irritability, confusion, peripheral neuropathy, seizures, and coma ◆ Dry skin, pruritus, pallor, purpura and, rarely, uremic frost ◆ Hypotension (early); hypertension, arrhythmias, fluid overload, heart failure, systemic edema, anemia, and altered clotting mechanisms (later) ◆ Pulmonary edema ◆ Kussmaul's respirations	◆ Blood studies show elevated blood urea nitrogen (BUN), serum creatinine, and potassium levels; decreased bicarbonate level, hematocrit, and hemoglobin levels; and low blood pH. ◆ Urine studies show casts, cellular debris, and decreased specific gravity; urine sodium level is more than 40 mEq/L. ◆ Creatinine clearance test measures glomerular filtration rate and reflects the number of remaining functioning nephrons. ◆ Electrocardiography (ECG) shows tall, peaked T waves; widening QRS complex; and disappearing P waves if hyperkalemia is present.
Pericarditis (complication)	◆ Pericardial friction rub (best heard when the patient leans forward and exhales) ◆ Sharp and typically sudden pain, usually starting over the sternum and radiating to the neck (especially the left trapezius ridge), shoulders, back, and arms ◆ Shallow, rapid respirations ◆ Mild fever ◆ Dyspnea, orthopnea, and tachycardia as fluid builds up in the pericardial space ◆ Muffled and distant heart sounds ◆ Pallor, clammy skin, hypotension, pulsus paradoxus, neck vein distention and, eventually, cardiovascular collapse ◆ Fluid retention, ascites, hepatomegaly, jugular vein distention, and other signs of chronic right-sided heart failure ◆ Pericardial knock in early diastole along the left sternal border	◆ ECG may reveal diffuse ST-segment elevation in the limb leads and most precordial leads, downsloping PR segments and upright T waves present in most leads, QRS segments possibly diminished when pericardial effusion exists, and arrhythmias, such as atrial fibrillation and sinus arrhythmias. ◆ Laboratory testing may reveal an elevated erythrocyte sedimentation rate or a normal or elevated white blood cell count. ◆ BUN may detect uremia as a cause. ◆ Echocardiography may show an echo-free space between the ventricular wall and the pericardium and reduced pumping action of the heart. ◆ Chest X-rays may be normal with acute pericarditis. The cardiac silhouette may be enlarged with a water bottle shape caused by fluid accumulation, if pleural effusion is present.
Pleural effusion (complication)	◆ Dyspnea ◆ Dry cough ◆ Pleural friction rub ◆ Possible pleuritic pain that worsens with coughing or deep breathing ◆ Dullness on percussion ◆ Tachycardia ◆ Tachypnea ◆ Decreased chest motion and breath sounds	◆ Thoracentesis reveals pleural fluid with specific gravity greater than 1.02 and ratio of protein in pleural fluid to serum equal to or greater than 0.5. Pleural fluid lactate dehydrogenase (LD) is equal to or greater than 200 IU; ratio of LD in pleural fluid to LD in serum is equal to or greater than 0.6. ◆ Fluid aspiration is positive for LE cells. ◆ Chest X-ray shows radiopaque fluid in dependent regions.

TREATMENT AND CARE

◆ Measure and record intake and output, including body fluids; weigh the patient daily.
◆ Anticipate fluid restriction to minimize edema.
◆ Assess hemoglobin levels and hematocrit, and replace blood components.
◆ Monitor vital signs. Watch for and report signs of pericarditis, inadequate renal perfusion (hypotension), and acidosis.
◆ Maintain proper electrolyte balance. Strictly monitor potassium levels.
◆ Administer medications, such as diuretic therapy to treat oliguric phase; sodium polystyrene sulfonate (Kayexalate) to reverse hyperkalemia; and hypertonic glucose, insulin, and I.V. sodium bicarbonate for severe hyperkalemic symptoms.
◆ Prepare for hemodialysis or peritoneal dialysis to correct electrolyte and fluid imbalances.
◆ Assess the patient frequently, especially during emergency treatment to lower potassium levels.
◆ If the patient receives hypertonic glucose and insulin infusions, monitor potassium and glucose levels.
◆ If sodium polystyrene sulfonate is used rectally, make sure the patient doesn't retain it and become constipated, to prevent bowel perforation.
◆ Maintain nutritional status. Provide a high-calorie, low-protein, low-sodium, and low-potassium diet and vitamin supplements. Give the anorexic patient small, frequent meals.
◆ Encourage frequent coughing and deep breathing, and perform passive range-of-motion exercises.
◆ Provide good mouth care frequently.

◆ Maintain bed rest as long as fever and pain persist to reduce metabolic needs.
◆ Administer medications, such as nonsteroidal anti-inflammatory drugs (NSAIDs), to relieve pain and reduce inflammation; give corticosteroids if NSAIDs are ineffective and no infection exists.
◆ Prepare for pericardiocentesis to remove excess fluid from the pericardial space, or for partial or total pericardectomy, if indicated.
◆ Place the patient in an upright position to relieve dyspnea and chest pain.
◆ Administer supplemental oxygen as indicated.
◆ Monitor for signs of cardiac compression or cardiac tamponade and possible complications of pericardial effusion, which include decreased blood pressure, increased central venous pressure, and pulsus paradoxus.

◆ Prepare for thoracentesis and chest tube insertion, if indicated.
◆ Monitor vital signs closely during thoracentesis. If fluid is removed too quickly, the patient may experience bradycardia, hypotension, pain, pulmonary edema, or even cardiac arrest.
◆ Watch for respiratory distress or pneumothorax after thoracentesis.
◆ Administer oxygen.
◆ Encourage deep-breathing exercises to promote lung expansion and the use of incentive spirometry to promote deep breathing.
◆ Provide meticulous chest tube care (if inserted), and use sterile technique for changing dressings around the tube insertion site. Monitor chest tube patency.
◆ Record the amount, color, and consistency of tube drainage.

(continued)

DISORDERS AFFECTING
MANAGEMENT OF LUPUS ERYTHEMATOSUS *(continued)*

DISORDER	SIGNS AND SYMPTOMS	DIAGNOSTIC TEST RESULTS
Stroke (complication)	◆ Headache with no known cause ◆ Numbness or weakness of the face, arm, or leg, especially on one side of the body ◆ Confusion, trouble speaking or understanding ◆ Trouble seeing or walking, dizziness, and loss of coordination	◆ Magnetic resonance imaging or computed tomography scan shows evidence of thrombosis or hemorrhage. ◆ Brain scan reveals ischemia (may not be positive for up to 2 weeks after the stroke). ◆ Lumbar puncture may reveal blood in the cerebrospinal fluid (if hemorrhagic). ◆ Carotid ultrasound may detect a blockage, stenosis, or reduced blood flow. ◆ Angiography can help pinpoint the site of occlusion or rupture. ◆ EEG may help localize the area of damage.

lipids, damaging blood vessels and causing cerebral blood clots.

■ Seizure disorders, mental dysfunction (confusion, decreased cognition, and altered levels of consciousness), and psychosis (emotional lability involving extremes of euphoria and depression) may occur.

ASSESSMENT

The onset of SLE, which can be acute or insidious, produces no characteristic clinical pattern. The condition is commonly called the "great imitator" because it mimics other diseases. Although SLE may involve any organ system, clinical manifestations all relate to tissue injury and subsequent inflammation and necrosis resulting from the invasion by immune complexes. (See *Signs of systemic lupus erythematosus*, page 250.)

Clinical findings

■ Unexplained fever
■ Weight loss
■ Malaise
■ Extreme fatigue
■ Erythematous rash in areas exposed to light or a scaly, papular rash (mimics psoriasis), especially in sun-exposed areas of the skin
■ Butterfly rash (malar rash) over the nose and cheeks (occurs in less than 50% of patients) (see *Recognizing butterfly rash*, page 250)
■ Polyarthralgia
■ Painless mouth ulcers
■ Edema in legs or around the eyes
■ Photosensitivity
■ Anorexia
■ Abdominal or chest pain
■ Nausea and vomiting
■ Diarrhea and constipation
■ In about 90% of patients, joint involvement resembling rheumatoid arthritis (complaints of pain, joint tenderness, and muscle weakness)
■ Irregular menstruation or amenorrhea, particularly during flare-ups
■ In about 20% of patients, Raynaud's phenomenon
■ Chest pain (indicating pleuritis)
■ Dyspnea (suggesting parenchymal infiltrates and pneumonitis)
■ In about 50% of patients, cardiopulmonary manifestations, such as shortness of breath, skin color changes, and lightheadedness
■ Pleural effusions, pulmonary hypertension, and pericardial friction rub (signaling pericarditis)
■ Possible oliguria, urinary frequency, dysuria, and bladder spasms
■ Possible vasculitis, especially in the digits
■ Infarctive lesions, necrotic leg ulcers, and digital gangrene
■ Lymph node enlargement (diffuse or local and nontender)
■ Tachycardia and other signs of myocarditis and endocarditis

◆ Administer medications, such as antiplatelet agents to prevent recurrent stroke (but not in hemorrhagic stroke) and benzodiazepines or anticonvulsants to treat or prevent seizures.
◆ Maintain a patent airway and provide oxygen.
◆ If unconscious, the patient may aspirate saliva; place the patient in a lateral position to promote drainage, or suction as needed.
◆ Insert an artificial airway and start mechanical ventilation or supplemental oxygen, if needed.
◆ Check the patient's vital signs and neurologic status. Monitor blood pressure, level of consciousness, motor function (voluntary and involuntary movements), senses, speech, skin color, and temperature.
◆ Assess gag reflex before offering oral fluids. Maintain fluid intake orally or with I.V. therapy as appropriate.

■ Patchy alopecia and painless ulcers of the mucous membranes
■ Microscopic hematuria, pyuria, and urine sediment with cellular casts caused by glomerulonephritis, possibly progressing to kidney failure (particularly when untreated)
■ Seizure disorders and mental dysfunction
■ Central nervous system (CNS) involvement, such as emotional instability, psychosis, and organic brain syndrome
■ Headaches, irritability, and depression (common)

RED FLAG *Repeated arterial clotting manifests as tachycardia, central cyanosis, and hypotension. These signs and symptoms may indicate pulmonary emboli. Also, be alert for altered level of consciousness, weakness of the extremities, and speech disturbances, which point to stroke.*

Diagnostic test results
■ *Complete blood count* with differential may show anemia and a decreased white blood cell (WBC) count; platelet count may be decreased.
■ *Erythrocyte sedimentation rate* is commonly elevated.
■ *Serum electrophoresis* may show hypergammaglobulinemia.
   Other diagnostic tests include:
■ *ANA and lupus erythematosus cell tests* showing positive results in active SLE.
■ *Anti–double-stranded deoxyribonucleic acid (anti-dsDNA) antibody*, the most specific test

for SLE, correlates with disease activity (especially renal involvement) and helps monitor response to therapy; may be low or absent in remission.
■ *Urine studies* may show RBCs and WBCs, urine casts and sediment, and significant protein loss (more than 0.5 g/24 hours).
■ *Serum complement blood studies* show decreased serum complement (C3 and C4) levels, indicating active disease.
■ *Chest X-ray* may show pleurisy or lupus pneumonitis.
■ *Electrocardiography* may show a conduction defect with cardiac involvement or pericarditis.
■ *Kidney biopsy* determines the disease stage and extent of renal involvement.
■ *Lupus anticoagulant and anticardiolipin tests* may be positive in some patients (usually in patients prone to antiphospholipid syndrome of thrombosis, abortion, and thrombocytopenia).

COLLABORATIVE MANAGEMENT
Because SLE affects multiple body systems, a multidisciplinary approach to care is essential. Immunologists typically are consulted to address the underlying problems and manage drug therapy. Cardiopulmonary and renal specialists may be involved to minimize the effects on these body systems. Orthopedic specialists may be involved to assist with joint function. Neurologists may be consulted to assist with neurologic changes.

SIGNS OF SYSTEMIC LUPUS ERYTHEMATOSUS

Diagnosing systemic lupus erythematosus (SLE) is difficult because it often mimics other diseases; symptoms may be vague and vary greatly among patients.

For these reasons, the American Rheumatism Association issued a list of criteria for classifying SLE, to be used primarily for consistency in epidemiologic surveys. Usually, four or more of these signs are present at some time during the course of the disease:

◆ malar (over the cheeks of the face) or discoid (patch red) rash
◆ photosensitivity
◆ oral or nasopharyngeal ulcerations
◆ nonerosive arthritis (of two or more peripheral joints)
◆ pleuritis or pericarditis
◆ profuse proteinuria (more than 0.5 g/day) or excessive cellular casts in the urine
◆ seizures or psychoses
◆ hemolytic anemia, leukopenia, lymphopenia, or thrombocytopenia
◆ abnormal antinuclear antibody titer
◆ elevated anti–double-stranded deoxyribonucleic acid antibodies and anti-Smith antibodies
◆ positive anticardiolipin (or antiphospholipid) antibody test
◆ positive LE prep test
◆ positive lupus anticoagulant test
◆ false positive serologic test for syphilis.

RECOGNIZING BUTTERFLY RASH

In the classic butterfly rash of systemic lupus erythematosus, lesions appear on the cheeks and the bridge of the nose, creating a characteristic butterfly pattern. The rash may vary in severity from malar erythema (redness of the cheeks) to discoid lesions (plaques).

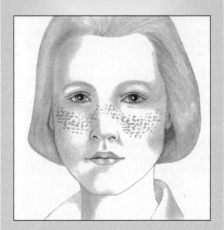

TREATMENT AND CARE

■ Treatment typically includes drug therapy, supportive measures, and patient education.
■ Drug therapy may include:
– nonsteroidal anti-inflammatory drugs, including aspirin, to control arthritis symptoms
– topical corticosteroid creams, such as hydrocortisone (Locoid)or triamcinolone (Kenalog), for acute skin lesions
– intralesional corticosteroids or antimalarials, such as hydroxychloroquine (Plaquentil), to treat refractory skin lesions
– systemic corticosteroids to reduce systemic symptoms of SLE; for acute generalized exacerbations; or for serious disease related to vital organ systems, such as pleuritis, pericarditis, lupus nephritis, vasculitis, and CNS involvement
– high-dose corticosteroids and cytotoxic therapy (such as cyclophosphamide [Cytoxan]) to treat diffuse proliferative glomerulonephritis

Respiratory therapy may be involved to assist with measures to improve respiratory muscle function and ventilation. Physical therapy may be consulted for assistance with exercises, muscle strengthening, and assistive devices for ambulation. Occupational therapy can help with adaptations needed for activities of daily living. Because SLE involves remissions and exacerbations, social services may be necessary to assist the patient with referrals to community support groups, financial concerns, and home care issues and equipment.

- If the patient develops renal involvement, administer antihypertensive drugs and make dietary changes to minimize effects.
- Dialysis or kidney transplant may be needed for renal failure.
- Warfarin (Coumadin) may be administered for antiphospholipid antibodies, which can cause clotting in vascular structures.
- Use heat application for pain relief.
- Perform exercises to maintain range of motion and prevent contractures.
- Physical and occupational therapy help to maintain joint function.
- Joint replacement may be necessary if chronic synovitis and pain are problematic.
- Patient teaching addresses dietary restrictions, medication therapy, skin care measures, activity and exercise, prevention of exposure to the sun, and adhering to routine follow-up.
- The patient may benefit from a referral to the Lupus Foundation of America, the Arthritis Foundation, or the National Institute of Arthritis and Musculoskeletal and Skin Diseases.

Lyme disease

Lyme disease is a multisystem disorder characterized by dermatologic, neurologic, cardiac, and rheumatic manifestations in various stages. Initially, Lyme disease was identified in a group of children in Lyme, Connecticut. Today, Lyme disease is known to occur primarily in three parts of the United States where certain ixodid ticks are located: the Northeast (from Massachusetts to Maryland), the Midwest (Wisconsin and Minnesota), and the West (California and Oregon). Although Lyme disease is endemic to these areas, cases have been reported in 43 states (with increased incidence over the past 8 years) and 20 other countries, including Germany, Switzerland, France, and Australia.

Individuals of all ages and both sexes are affected by Lyme disease. It usually manifests in summer or early fall as a skin lesion called erythema chronicum migrans. Weeks or months later, cardiac, neurologic, or joint abnormalities may develop, sometimes followed by arthritis.

ETIOLOGY

Lyme disease is caused by the spirochete *Borrelia burgdorferi,* which is carried by the minute tick *Ixodes dammini* or another type of tick in the Ixodidae family. The disease occurs when a tick injects spirochete-laden saliva into the bloodstream or deposits fecal matter on the skin; thus, it isn't contagious.

Animal studies show a tick must be attached for 24 hours to transmit the disease; this may also hold true in humans for contracting the disease. Incubation typically ranges from 7 to 14 days, but it may be as short as 3 days or as long as 30 days.

PATHOPHYSIOLOGY

Lyme disease occurs when a tick injects spirochete-laden saliva into the bloodstream or deposits fecal matter on the skin. After the incubation period, the spirochetes migrate out to the skin, causing a "bull's-eye" rash, called *erythema migrans.* The spirochetes then disseminate to other skin sites or organs by way of the bloodstream or lymph system. The spirochetes' life cycle isn't completely clear; they may survive for years in the joints, or they may trigger an inflammatory response in the host and then die.

Typically, Lyme disease has three stages. (See *Stages of Lyme disease,* page 254.)

Cardiovascular system
- Usually, weeks to months after the tick bite, the spirochete can disseminate through the blood stream and travel to the heart, causing myocarditis.
- The conduction system becomes damaged secondary to the myocarditis, resulting in atrioventricular block, possibly progressing to complete heart block.

Integumentary system
- Spirochetes migrate to the skin, where they set off an inflammatory response, producing the characteristic rash.

Musculoskeletal system
- Commonly, the spirochete invades the soft tissue and joint spaces of the musculoskeletal system, causing an inflammatory response that ultimately leads to the development of a chronic inflammatory infiltrate in the lining below the synovial fluid.

DISORDERS AFFECTING MANAGEMENT OF LYME DISEASE

This chart highlights disorders that affect the management of Lyme disease.

DISORDER	SIGNS AND SYMPTOMS	DIAGNOSTIC TEST RESULTS
Arthritis (complication)	◆ Fatigue ◆ Malaise ◆ Anorexia and weight loss ◆ Low-grade fever ◆ Lymphadenopathy ◆ Vague articular symptoms that become specific, localized, bilateral, and symmetric ◆ Stiffening of affected joints ◆ Joint pain and tenderness ◆ Feeling of warmth at joint ◆ Diminished joint function and deformities ◆ Stiff, weak, or painful muscles	◆ X-rays show bone changes, such as demineralization and soft-tissue swelling. ◆ Synovial fluid analysis shows increased volume and turbidity but decreased viscosity and elevated white blood cell counts. ◆ Serum protein electrophoresis possibly shows elevated serum globulin levels. ◆ Erythrocyte sedimentation rate (ESR) and C-reactive protein levels may be elevated. ◆ Complete blood count usually reveals moderate anemia, slight leukocytosis, and slight thrombocytosis.
Facial nerve palsy (complication)	◆ Unilateral facial weakness or paralysis, with aching at the jaw angle ◆ Drooping mouth, causing drooling on the affected side ◆ Distorted taste perception over the affected anterior portion of the tongue ◆ Markedly impaired ability to close the eye on the weak side ◆ Incomplete eye closure and Bell's phenomenon (eye rolling upward as eye is closed) ◆ Inability to raise the eyebrow, smile, show the teeth, or puff out the cheek on the affected side	◆ No specific diagnostic test findings are noted; diagnosis is based on clinical findings. ◆ After 10 days, electromyography helps predict the level of expected recovery by distinguishing temporary conduction defects from a pathologic interruption of nerve fibers.
Myocarditis (complication)	◆ Nonspecific symptoms, such as fatigue, dyspnea, palpitations, and fever ◆ Mild, continuous pressure or soreness in the chest (occasionally) ◆ Tachycardia ◆ Third and fourth heart sound gallops ◆ Possible murmur of mitral insufficiency ◆ Pericardial friction rub	◆ Laboratory testing may reveal elevated levels of creatine kinase (CK), CK-MB, troponin I, troponin T, aspartate aminotransferase, and lactate dehydrogenase. ◆ White blood cell count is increased. ◆ ESR is elevated. ◆ Electrocardiography may reveal diffuse ST-segment and T-wave abnormalities, conduction defects (prolonged PR interval, bundle-branch block, or complete heart block), supraventricular arrhythmias, and ventricular extrasystoles. ◆ Chest X-rays may show an enlarged heart and pulmonary vascular congestion. ◆ Echocardiography may demonstrate some degree of left ventricular dysfunction. ◆ Radionuclide scanning may identify inflammatory and necrotic changes characteristic of myocarditis.

TREATMENT AND CARE

◆ Administer salicylates or nonsteroidal anti-inflammatory drugs.
◆ Assess all joints carefully. Look for deformities, contractures, immobility, and an inability to perform everyday activities.
◆ Monitor vital signs. Note weight changes, sensory disturbances, and patient's level of pain.
◆ Administer analgesics and watch for adverse effects.
◆ Provide meticulous skin care. Check for pressure ulcers and skin breakdown.

◆ Administer prescribed prednisone therapy.
◆ Apply moist heat to the affected side of the face to reduce pain.
◆ Massage the patient's face with a gentle upward motion two to three times daily for 5 to 10 minutes, and teach him how to perform this massage.
◆ Apply a facial sling to improve lip alignment.
◆ Give the patient frequent and complete mouth care. Remove residual food that collects between the cheeks and gums.

◆ Administer antipyretics to reduce fever and decrease stress on the heart, diuretics to decrease fluid retention, antiarrhythmics, and anticoagulants to prevent thromboembolism.
◆ Institute bed rest to reduce oxygen demands and the heart's workload and restrict activity to minimize myocardial oxygen consumption.
◆ Administer supplemental oxygen therapy.
◆ Assess cardiovascular status frequently, watching for signs of heart failure, such as dyspnea, hypotension, and tachycardia. Check for changes in cardiac rhythm or conduction.
◆ Monitor sodium intake; anticipate sodium restriction to decrease fluid retention.
◆ Prepare for insertion of cardiac assist devices or transplantation as a last resort in severe cases that resist treatment.

■ Typically, only one joint or a few joints are affected, primarily the large weight-bearing joints such as the knees.
■ Recurrent attacks may lead to chronic arthritis with severe cartilage and bone erosion. (See *Disorders affecting management of Lyme disease.*)

Neurologic system

■ The spirochete can travel through the bloodstream to the nervous system, where an inflammatory response occurs in the meningeal lining of the peripheral and cranial nerves, resulting in lymphocytic meningitis; cranial neuropathy, including facial nerve palsy; and radiculoneuritis, which causes numbness, tingling, and aching pain.
■ The spirochete can invade the eye structures causing follicular conjunctivitis, keratitis, periorbital edema, photophobia, and subconjunctival hemorrhage.

ASSESSMENT

Signs and symptoms of Lyme disease vary in frequency and severity and may be deceptive. For example, the patient's complaints commonly mimic those of typical flulike symptoms. A complete patient history and thorough physical examination are necessary to aid in the diagnosis.

The patient's history may reveal recent exposure to ticks, especially if the patient lives, works, or plays in areas where Lyme disease is endemic. The patient may report the onset of signs and symptoms in warmer months.

Clinical findings

■ Erythema chronicum migrans, usually appearing on the axilla, thigh, or groin (lesion may be hot and pruritic)
■ Within a few days, a migratory, ringlike rash and conjunctivitis
■ In 3 to 4 weeks, small red blotches, which persist for several more weeks
■ Fatigue, malaise, and migratory myalgias and arthralgias
■ Bell's palsy in the second stage
■ Signs and symptoms of intermittent arthritis (joint swelling, redness, and limited movement) in the later stage
■ Tachycardia or irregular heartbeat
■ During the first or second stage, regional lymphadenopathy

STAGES OF LYME DISEASE

Lyme disease typically occurs in three stages. The signs and symptoms, however, may take years to develop. It may be impossible to delineate exactly when one stage ends and another stage starts. Additionally, not all patients pass through each stage.

Stage 1: Early, localized stage

Erythema migrans, or the "bull's-eye" rash, heralds stage 1 Lyme disease. It begins as a red macule or papule that typically develops at the site of a tick bite. This lesion tends to feel hot and itchy and may grow to more than 20" (51 cm) in diameter. Within a few days, more lesions may erupt along with a malar rash, conjunctivitis, or diffuse urticaria. In 3 to 4 weeks, lesions are replaced by small, red blotches, which persist for several more weeks.

Malaise and fatigue are constant, but other findings (headache, fever, chills, myalgias, and regional lymphadenopathy) are intermittent. Less common effects are meningeal irritation, mild encephalopathy, migrating musculoskeletal pain, and hepatitis. A persistent sore throat and dry cough may appear several days before erythema migrans.

Stage 2: Early, disseminated stage

Weeks to months later, the second stage begins with neurologic abnormalities—fluctuating meningoencephalitis with peripheral and cranial neuropathy—that usually resolve after days or months. Facial palsy is especially noticeable. Cardiac abnormalities, such as a brief, fluctuating atrioventricular heart block, may also develop.

Stage 3: Late stage

Characterized by arthritis, stage 3 begins weeks or years later. Migrating musculoskeletal pain leads to frank arthritis with marked swelling, especially in the large joints. Recurrent attacks may precede chronic arthritis with severe cartilage and bone erosion.

■ Tenderness in the skin lesion site or the posterior cervical area
■ Generalized lymphadenopathy (less common)

LYME DISEASE SEROLOGY

Serologic tests for Lyme disease, both indirect immunofluorescent and enzyme-linked immunosorbent assays, measure antibody response to the *Borrelia burgdorferi* spirochete and indicate current infection or past exposure. Serologic tests can identify 50% of patients with early-stage Lyme disease, all patients with later complications of carditis, neuritis, and arthritis, as well as patients in remission.

Positive serologic tests for Lyme disease can help confirm diagnosis, but their results aren't definitive because the tests can't detect infection until a sufficient amount of antibodies are produced, which may take as long as 2 to 4 months after the tick bite. In fact, more than 15% of patients with Lyme disease fail to develop any antibodies. Additionally, other treponemal diseases and high rheumatoid factor titers can cause false-positive results.

■ In nearly 10% of patients, cardiac symptoms, such as palpitations and mild dyspnea, especially in the early stage
If the patient has neurologic involvement:
■ Severe headache and stiff neck, suggestive of meningeal irritation
■ In the early stage, increased body temperature (104° F [40° C]) accompanied by chills (especially in children)
■ At a later stage, such symptoms as memory loss, absent Kernig's and Brudzinski's signs, and neck stiffness with extreme flexion

Diagnostic test results

■ *Enzyme-linked immunosorbent assay* may be positive for immunoglobulin G and M and *B. burgdorferi* antibodies; however, false-negatives can arise in first-stage infection or in late stages where patients received early antibiotic treatment. False-positives have been seen with Rocky Mountain spotted fever, syphilis, lupus, and rheumatoid arthritis. (See *Lyme disease serology*.)
■ *Cerebrospinal fluid and synovial fluid analyses* can be cultured for *B. burgdorferi*.

■ *Blood culture* or *skin biopsy* has less than a 40% detection rate for *B. burgdorferi* spirochetes and must be placed on Kelly's medium.

■ *Complete blood count* and *erythrocyte sedimentation rate* (ESR) may detect mild anemia, an elevated ESR and leukocyte count, and elevated aspartate aminotransferase levels.

■ *The PreVue* B. burgdorferi *antibody detection assay* can be performed and read in 1 hour. Positive results must be confirmed by the Western blot test.

COLLABORATIVE MANAGEMENT

Because Lyme disease can affect multiple body systems, a multidisciplinary approach to care is needed. Cardiologists may be consulted to treat myocarditis and damage to the conduction system. Neurologists may be involved to treat the problems associated with any peripheral and cranial nerve dysfunction. An ophthamalogist may be needed if the eye structures are affected. Orthopedists may be involved to maximize joint function and institute therapy to prevent cartilage and bone damage. Physical therapy may be consulted to promote joint function and mobility. Social services may be consulted for assistance with discharge planning, follow-up, and referrals for support.

TREATMENT AND CARE

■ Pharmacologic therapy includes a 14- to 21-day course of oral tetracycline (doxycycline) for adults. Beta-lactamase–inhibiting penicillins (amoxicillin [Amoxil]) and second-generation cephalosporins (cefuroxime [Ceftin]) are alternatives. Oral amoxicillin is usually prescribed for children. When given in the early stages, these drugs can minimize later complications. A short course of corticosteroids (prednisone [Deltasone]) may also be helpful.

■ Hospitalization may be necessary for stage 2 and stage 3 Lyme disease. Treatment involves either high-dose penicillin (penicillin G [Wycillin]) or third-generation cephalosporins (ceftriaxone [Rocephin], cefotaxime [Claforan]) for 2 to 4 weeks I.V.

■ Patient education includes how to prevent Lyme disease and information about the possible use of a vaccine.

■ Referrals to community support groups and organizations, such as the Lyme Disease Foundation (*www.lyme.org*) and the Arthritis Foundation (*www.arthritis.org*) are beneficial.

M

Marfan syndrome

Marfan syndrome is a rare multisystem disorder of the connective tissue. It results from microfibril defects and causes ocular, skeletal, and cardiovascular anomalies. Death can result at any point between early infancy and adulthood because of cardiovascular complications. The syndrome occurs in 1 out of every 5,000 to 10,000 people and affects males and females of all racial and ethnic groups equally.

ETIOLOGY

Marfan syndrome is inherited as an autosomal dominant trait of chromosome 15. It's caused by mutations in fibrillin-1 gene located on this chromosome. In 75% of patients, the syndrome is inherited from a biological parent. In the remaining 25%, mutation in the fibrillin-1 gene occurs spontaneously in the egg or sperm from which the patient was conceived.

PATHOPHYSIOLOGY

The gene on chromosome 15 is responsible for the genetic code for fibrillin — a glycoprotein component of connective tissue that comprises the extracellular matrix of many tissues. Many copies of fibrillin protein combine to make microfibrils, which are abundant in large blood vessels, the suspensory ligaments of the ocular lenses, and the bones. Fibrillin-1 mutations can lead to abnormal microfibrils and ultimately affect the elasticity or structure of connective tissues. Tissues subject to stress, such as in the aorta, eye, and skin, are especially vulnerable. Mutations of fibrillin-1 also cause overgrowth of long bones.

Cardiovascular system

■ The medial layer of the arteries, specifically the aorta, are weakened. The arterial wall shows a loss of elastic fibers and enlargement of smooth-muscle cells.
■ The aorta can't withstand the high-pressure blood flow. Subsequently, dilation of the aorta can occur, leading to an aneurysm that can rupture into the pericardial or retroperitoneal cavity.
■ The mitral valve leaflets may be affected, leading to mitral insufficiency and mitral valve prolapse. (See *Disorders affecting management of Marfan syndrome*, pages 258 and 259.)

Eyes

■ Suspensory fibers that hold the lens in place are weakened as a result of the disorder.
■ Other ocular structures may be affected because of the increased globe length, resulting from weakened connective tissue support. Subsequently, myopia and retinal detachment can occur.

Musculoskeletal system

■ Typically, the body is long and thin (especially the extremities) due to the overgrowth of bones.
■ The lower body from the pubis to the soles of the feet is usually longer than the upper body.
■ The skull bones are long, with a protruding frontal bone.
■ The ribs form pectus excavatum (funnel chest) or pectus carinatum (pigeon chest).
■ The laxity of the connective tissue leads to weakness in the tendons, ligaments, and joint capsules, resulting in hyperextensibility of the joints, dislocations, hernia, and kyphoscoliosis.

ASSESSMENT

Typically, diagnosis is based on a positive family history in one parent (75% of patients) and typical clinical features. In the absence of family history, diagnosis requires documentation of at least one major finding in two body systems and one minor finding in a third body system.

The patient may report a history of joint dislocations or "double-jointedness." Other complaints may involve visual problems, palpitations, or shortness of breath related to cardiac involvement.

Clinical findings

- Taller than average for his family (in the 95th percentile for his age), with the upper half of his body shorter than average and the lower half longer
- Long, slender fingers (arachnodactyly)
- Defects of sternum (funnel chest or pigeon breast), chest asymmetry, scoliosis, and kyphosis caused by effects on bone
- Loose, hyperextensible joints with possible dislocation
- Abnormal heart sounds suggesting valvular abnormalities (redundancy of leaflets, stretching of chordae tendineae, and dilation of valvulae annulus) from effects on cardiac connective tissue; mitral valve prolapse, caused by weakened connective tissue; or aortic insufficiency, caused by dilation of aortic root and ascending aorta
- Nearsightedness caused by an elongated ocular globe
- Possible lens displacement caused by altered connective tissue (the ocular hallmark of the syndrome)

Diagnostic test results

- *Skin culture* detects fibrillin.
- *X-rays* confirm skeletal abnormalities.
- *Echocardiogram* shows dilation of the aortic root.
- *Deoxyribonucleic acid linkage analysis* shows evidence of mutation. This test is performed if multiple family members are affected.

COLLABORATIVE MANAGEMENT

Because Marfan syndrome affects multiple body systems, a multidisciplinary approach to care is essential. Genetic specialists may be involved to assist with evaluating the genetic component of the disorder. Cardiopulmonary specialists may be involved to minimize the effects on the heart and blood vessels, such as mitral insufficiency and weakening of the vasculature. An ophthalmologist may be necessary if the eye structures are affected. Orthopedic specialists may be involved to assist with maximizing joint function and using braces. Respiratory therapy may be involved to assist with measures to improve respiratory muscle function and ventilation because of the development of funnel chest. Physical therapy may be consulted for assistance with exercises, muscle strengthening, and assistive devices such as braces. Occupational therapy can help with adaptations needed for activities of daily living. Social services may be necessary to assist the patient with referrals to community support groups, financial concerns, and home care issues and equipment.

TREATMENT AND CARE

- Treatment for Marfan syndrome is aimed at relieving symptoms.
- Anticipate surgical repair of aneurysms to prevent rupture and surgical correction of ocular deformities to improve vision

RED FLAG High school and college athletes (particularly basketball players) who fit the criteria for Marfan syndrome should undergo a careful clinical and cardiac examination before being allowed to play sports, to avoid sudden death from dissecting aortic aneurysm or other cardiac complications.

- Steroid and sex hormone therapy is used to induce early epiphyseal closure and limit adult height.
- Administer beta-adrenergic blockers to delay or prevent aortic dilation.
- Surgical replacement of the aortic valve and mitral valve allows for extreme dilation.
- For patients with scoliosis, mechanical bracing and physical therapy are needed if curvature is greater than 20 degrees; surgery is needed if curvature is greater than 45 degrees.
- Refer the woman with Marfan syndrome to genetic counseling because pregnancy and resultant increased cardiovascular workload can produce aortic rupture.
- Refer the patient to the National Marfan Foundation for additional information.

DISORDERS AFFECTING MANAGEMENT OF MARFAN SYNDROME

This chart highlights disorders that affect the management of Marfan syndrome.

DISORDER	SIGNS AND SYMPTOMS	DIAGNOSTIC TEST RESULTS
Dissecting aortic aneurysm (complication)	◆ Sudden, severe abdominal or lumbar pain that radiates to the flank and groin ◆ Severe and persistent abdominal pain mimicking renal or ureteral colic pain ◆ Massive hematemesis ◆ Melena ◆ Systolic bruit over the aorta ◆ Hypotension ◆ Tachycardia ◆ Cool, clammy skin	◆ Complete blood count (CBC) may reveal leukocytosis and decreased hemoglobin and hematocrit. ◆ Transesophageal echocardiogram provides visualization of the thoracic aorta and is usually combined with Doppler flow studies to provide information about blood flow. ◆ Abdominal ultrasonography or echocardiography can determine the aneurysm size, shape, length, and location. ◆ Anteroposterior and lateral X-rays of the chest or abdomen can detect aortic calcification and widened areas of the aorta. ◆ Computed tomography scan and magnetic resonance imaging can identify the aneurysm size and its effect on nearby organs. ◆ Aortography helps determine the aneurysm's approximate size and patency of the visceral vessels.
Mitral insufficiency (complication)	◆ Orthopnea and dyspnea ◆ Fatigue ◆ Angina, palpitations, and tachycardia ◆ Peripheral edema ◆ Jugular vein distention and hepatomegaly (right-sided heart failure) ◆ Crackles ◆ Pulmonary edema ◆ Holosystolic murmur at apex; a possible split second heart sound and third heart sound	◆ Cardiac catheterization reveals mitral insufficiency with increased left ventricular end-diastolic volume and pressure, increased atrial pressure and pulmonary artery wedge pressure, and decreased cardiac output. ◆ Chest X-rays show left atrial and ventricular enlargement and pulmonary venous congestion. ◆ Echocardiography reveals abnormal valve leaflet motion and left atrial enlargement. ◆ ECG may show left atrial and ventricular hypertrophy, sinus tachycardia, and atrial fibrillation.
Retinal detachment (complication)	◆ Floaters ◆ Light flashes ◆ Sudden, painless vision loss that may be described as a curtain that eliminates a portion of the visual field	◆ Ophthalmoscopic examination through a well-dilated pupil confirms the diagnosis. In severe detachment, examination reveals folds in the retina and a ballooning out of the area. ◆ Indirect ophthalmoscopy is used to search the retina for tears and holes. ◆ Ocular ultrasonography may be needed if the lens is opaque or if the vitreous humor is cloudy.

Metabolic acidosis

Metabolic acidosis is an acid-base disorder characterized by excess acid and deficient bicarbonate (HCO_3^-) caused by an underlying nonrespiratory disorder. Children are more vulnerable to metabolic acidosis because their metabolic rates are rapid and ratios of water to total-body weight are low.

Severe or untreated metabolic acidosis can be fatal. However, the prognosis improves with prompt treatment of the underlying cause and rapid reversal of the acidotic state.

TREATMENT AND CARE

◆ Insert or assist with insertion of an arterial line to allow for continuous blood pressure monitoring; assist with insertion of a pulmonary artery catheter to assess hemodynamic balance.
◆ Insert a large-bore I.V. catheter and begin fluid resuscitation.
◆ Administer nitroprusside (Nitropress) I.V., usually to maintain a mean arterial pressure of 70 to 80 mm Hg; also administer propranolol (Inderal) I.V. at a rate of 1 mg every 5 minutes (to a maximum initial dose not exceeding 0.15 mg/kg of body weight) to reduce left ventricular ejection velocity until the heart rate ranges from 60 to 80 beats/minute.
◆ If the patient is experiencing acute pain, administer morphine 2 to 10 mg I.V.
◆ Assess the patient's vital signs frequently, especially blood pressure; monitor blood pressure and pulse in extremities and compare findings bilaterally.
◆ Assess cardiovascular status frequently, including arterial blood gas (ABG) values, heart rate, rhythm, electrocardiogram (ECG), and cardiac enzyme levels. A myocardial infarction can occur if an aneurysm ruptures along the coronary arteries.
◆ Monitor urine output hourly.
◆ Evaluate CBC for evidence of blood loss, reflected in decreased hemoglobin level, hematocrit, and red blood cell count.
◆ Prepare the patient for emergency surgery.

◆ Assess the patient's vital signs, ABG values, pulse oximetry, intake and output, daily weights, blood chemistry studies, chest X-rays, and ECG.
◆ Promote measures to reduce activity level and decrease myocardial oxygen demands.
◆ Place the patient in an upright position to relieve dyspnea, if needed.
◆ Administer oxygen to prevent tissue hypoxia.
◆ Administer drug therapy, including digoxin, diuretics, and vasodilators to combat heart failure; anticoagulants to prevent thrombus formation; and nitroglycerin to relieve angina.
◆ Institute continuous cardiac monitoring to evaluate for arrhythmias if they occur; administer appropriate therapy per facility policy and physician's order.
◆ Observe for signs and symptoms of left-sided heart failure, pulmonary edema, and adverse reactions to drug therapy.
◆ Prepare for valvular surgery, if indicated.

◆ Restrict eye movements through bed rest and sedation.
◆ If the patient's macula is threatened, position his head so the tear or hole is below the rest of the eye before surgical intervention.
◆ Prepare patient for surgical repair (cryotherapy, laser therapy, scleral buckling, pneumatic retinopexy, or vitrectomy).
◆ Provide emotional support.
◆ Position the patient facedown if gas has been injected to maintain pressure on the retina.

ETIOLOGY

Metabolic acidosis usually results from excessive production of metabolic acids such as fat metabolism in the absence of usable carbohydrates. This can be caused by diabetic ketoacidosis, chronic alcoholism, malnutrition, or a low-carbohydrate, high-fat diet — all of which produce more ketoacids than the metabolic process can handle. Other causes include:

■ anaerobic carbohydrate metabolism (decreased tissue oxygenation or perfusion [as in cardiac pump failure after myocardial infarction, pulmonary or hepatic disease, shock, or anemia] forces a shift from aerobic to anaerobic metabolism, causing a corre-

UNDERSTANDING LACTIC ACIDOSIS

Lactate, produced as a result of carbohydrate metabolism, is metabolized by the liver. The normal lactate level is 0.93 to 1.65 mEq/L. With tissue hypoxia, however, cells are forced to switch to anaerobic metabolism and more lactate is produced. When lactate accumulates in the body faster than it can be metabolized, lactic acidosis occurs. It can happen at any time the demand for oxygen in the body is greater than its availability.

The causes of lactic acidosis include septic shock, cardiac arrest, pulmonary disease, seizures, and strenuous exercise.

The latter two cause transient lactic acidosis. Hepatic disorders can also cause lactic acidosis because the liver can't metabolize lactate.

Treatment

Treatment focuses on eliminating the underlying cause. If pH is below 7.1, sodium bicarbonate may be given. Use caution when administering sodium bicarbonate, however, because it may cause alkalosis.

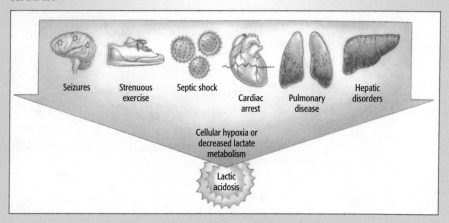

Seizures   Strenuous exercise   Septic shock   Cardiac arrest   Pulmonary disease   Hepatic disorders

Cellular hypoxia or decreased lactate metabolism

Lactic acidosis

---

sponding increase in lactic acid level) (see *Understanding lactic acidosis*)

■ underexcretion of metabolized acids or inability to conserve base caused by renal insufficiency and failure (renal acidosis)

■ diarrhea, intestinal malabsorption, or loss of sodium bicarbonate from the intestines, causing the bicarbonate buffer system to shift to the acidic side (for example, ureteroenterostomy and Crohn's disease can induce metabolic acidosis)

■ salicylate intoxication (overuse of aspirin); exogenous poisoning (inhalation of toluene or ingestion of methanol, ethylene glycol, paraldehyde, hydrochloric acid, or ammonium chloride); or, less frequently, addisonism (increased excretion of sodium and chloride and retention of potassium)

■ inhibited secretion of acid caused by hypoaldosteronism or the use of potassium-sparing diuretics.

PATHOPHYSIOLOGY

The underlying mechanisms in metabolic acidosis are a loss of HCO_3^- from extracellular fluid, an accumulation of metabolic acids, or a combination of the two. If the patient's anion gap (measurement of the difference between the amount of sodium and the amount of bicarbonate in the blood) is greater than 14 mEq/L, then the acidosis is due to an accumulation of metabolic acids (unmeasured anions). If the metabolic acidosis is associated with a normal anion gap (8 to 14 mEq/L), loss of HCO_3^- may be the cause. (See *What happens in metabolic acidosis*, pages 262 and 263.)

Metabolic acidosis is characterized by a gain in acids or a loss of bases from the plasma. The condition may be related to an overproduction of ketone bodies. Fatty acids are converted to ketone bodies when glucose supplies have been used and the body draws on fat stores for energy. Lactic acidosis can cause or worsen metabolic acidosis.

As acid (hydrogen) starts to accumulate in the body, chemical buffers (plasma HCO_3^- and proteins) in the cells and extracellular fluid bind the excess hydrogen ions. Excess hydrogen ions that the buffers can't bind lower the blood pH and stimulate chemoreceptors in the medulla to increase respiration. The consequent fall of partial pressure of arterial carbon dioxide ($Paco_2$) frees hydrogen ions to bind with HCO_3^-. Respiratory compensation occurs in minutes but isn't sufficient to correct the acidosis.

Healthy kidneys try to compensate by secreting excess hydrogen ions into the renal tubules, where these ions are buffered by either phosphate or ammonia and excreted into the urine in the form of weak acid. For each hydrogen ion secreted into the renal tubules, the tubules reabsorb and return to the blood one sodium ion and one HCO_3^- ion.

The excess hydrogen ions in extracellular fluid passively diffuse into cells. To maintain the balance of charge across the membranes, the cells release potassium ions. Excess hydrogen ions change the normal balance of potassium, sodium, and calcium ions and thereby impair neural excitability.

Cardiovascular system
■ As the pH drops and the balance of electrolytes is altered, membrane excitability in the cells of the heart muscle and blood vessels is altered, resulting in depressed myocardial function and decreased cardiac output and blood pressure.
■ Arrhythmias may occur because of the shifts in electrolytes (especially potassium and calcium).
■ Initially, vasodilation occurs as the blood vessels of the skin are less receptive to sympathetic stimuli. Skin is warm, flushed, and dry.
■ As metabolic acidosis progresses, shock ensues, leading to cold and clammy skin.

Gastrointestinal system
■ Excessive hydrogen ions diffuse into the cells of the GI system and potassium is released into the blood.
■ The elevated potassium levels disrupt the normal balance of electrolytes and ultimately affect nerve impulse transmission to the muscles of the GI tract, resulting in colic and diarrhea.

Neurologic system
■ As the pH drops, central nervous system (CNS) depression occurs.
■ Excessive hydrogen ions diffuse into the cells of the CNS and potassium is released into the blood.
■ Elevated potassium levels disrupt neuromuscular transmission. Subsequently, weakness or flaccid paralysis, numbness, and tingling in the extremities can occur.
■ The continued decrease in pH depresses the excitability of the cell membranes and disrupts the balance of other electrolytes, including sodium and calcium, leading to reduced excitability of the nerve cells. The patient's level of consciousness may deteriorate from confusion to stupor and coma.
■ A neuromuscular examination may show diminished muscle tone and deep tendon reflexes.

Respiratory system
■ As acid builds up in the bloodstream, the lungs compensate by blowing off carbon dioxide.
■ Hyperventilation, especially increased depth of respirations (Kussmaul's respirations), is the first clue to metabolic acidosis.
■ A patient with diabetes who experiences Kussmaul's respirations may have a fruity odor to his breath. The odor stems from catabolism of fats and excretion of acetone through the lungs.
■ If the pH remains low, stimulation of the chemoreceptors continues to maintain hyperventilation as a means to blow off carbon dioxide. If hyperventilation continues, respiratory failure may occur. (See *Disorders affecting management of metabolic acidosis*, pages 264 and 265.)

ASSESSMENT
Metabolic acidosis typically produces respiratory, neurologic, and cardiac signs and symptoms. The patient's history may point

WHAT HAPPENS IN METABOLIC ACIDOSIS

This series of illustrations shows how metabolic acidosis develops at the cellular level.

As hydrogen ions (H^+) start to accumulate in the body, chemical buffers (plasma bicarbonate [HCO_3^-] and proteins) in the cells and extracellular fluid bind with them. *No signs are detectable at this stage.*

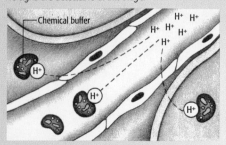

Excess H^+ that the buffers can't bind with decrease pH and stimulate chemoreceptors in the medulla to increase respiratory rate. Increased respiratory rate lowers partial pressure of arterial carbon dioxide ($Paco_2$), which allows more H^+ to bind with HCO_3^-. Respiratory compensation occurs within minutes but isn't sufficient to correct the imbalance. *Look for a pH level below 7.35, a bicarbonate level below 22 mEq/L, a decreasing $Paco_2$ level, and rapid, deeper respirations.*

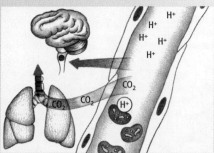

Healthy kidneys try to compensate for acidosis by secreting excess H^+ into the renal tubules. Those ions are buffered by phosphate or ammonia and then are excreted into the urine in the form of a weak acid. *Look for acidic urine.*

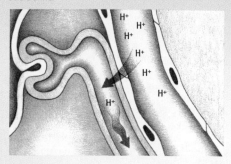

Each time a H^+ is secreted into the renal tubules, a sodium (Na) ion and an HCO_3^- are absorbed from the tubules and returned to the blood. *Look for pH and HCO_3^- levels that slowly return to normal.*

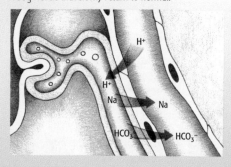

to the presence of risk factors, including associated disorders and the use of medications that contain alcohol or aspirin. Information about the patient's urine output, fluid intake, and dietary habits (including recent fasting) may help to establish the underlying cause and severity of metabolic acidosis.

The patient's history (obtained from a family member, if necessary) may also reveal CNS symptoms, such as changes in level of consciousness (LOC), ranging from lethargy,

Excess H+ in the extracellular fluid diffuse into cells. To maintain the balance of the charge across the membrane, the cells release potassium ions into the blood. *Look for signs and symptoms of hyperkalemia, including colic and diarrhea, weakness or flaccid paralysis, tingling and numbness in the extremities, bradycardia, a tall T wave, a prolonged PR interval, and a widened QRS complex.*

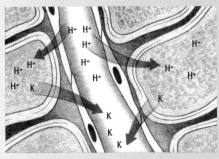

Excess H+ alter the normal balance of potassium (K), sodium (Na), and calcium ions (Ca), leading to reduced excitability of nerve cells. *Look for signs and symptoms of progressive central nervous system depression (lethargy, dull headache, confusion, stupor, and coma).*

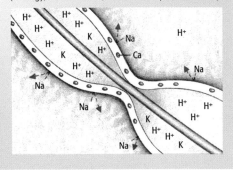

drowsiness, and confusion to stupor and coma.

Clinical findings
- Decreased deep tendon reflexes and muscle tone
- Dull headache

- Hyperkalemic signs and symptoms, including abdominal cramping, diarrhea, muscle weakness, and electrocardiogram changes
- Hypotension
- Arrhythmias
- Kussmaul's respirations
- Lethargy
- Warm, dry skin
- Fruity breath odor in patients with underlying diabetes mellitus
- Signs of dehydration, such as poor skin turgor and dry mucous membranes

Diagnostic test results
- *Arterial blood gas studies* reveal an arterial pH less than 7.35 (as low as 7.10 in severe acidosis), $Paco_2$ that's normal or less than 34 mm Hg as respiratory compensatory mechanisms take hold, and a HCO_3^- level of 22 mEq/L.
- *Urine pH* is less than 4.5 in the absence of renal disease (as the kidneys excrete acid to raise blood pH).
- *Potassium level* is greater than 5.5 mEq/L from chemical buffering.
- *Glucose level* is greater than 150 mg/dl.
- *Serum ketone bodies* are present in patients with diabetes.
- *Lactic acid level* is elevated in lactic acidosis.
- *Anion gap* is greater than 14 mEq/L in high anion gap metabolic acidosis, lactic acidosis, ketoacidosis, aspirin overdose, alcohol poisoning, renal failure, or other conditions characterized by accumulation of organic acids, sulfates, or phosphates; 12 mEq/L or less in normal anion gap metabolic acidosis from HCO_3^- loss, GI or renal loss, increased acid load (hyperalimentation fluids), rapid I.V. saline solution administration, or other conditions characterized by loss of bicarbonate.

COLLABORATIVE MANAGEMENT
Because metabolic acidosis can affect multiple body systems, a multidisciplinary approach to care is needed. A renal specialist or nephrologist can help evaluate, treat, and manage the patient's kidney function. Respiratory and cardiology specialists may be consulted to institute measures to promote optimal respiratory and cardiac function. A diabetic specialist may be involved if the underlying problem is related to diabetes. Nu-
(*Text continues on page 266.*)

DISORDERS AFFECTING
MANAGEMENT OF METABOLIC ACIDOSIS

This chart highlights disorders that affect the management of metabolic acidosis.

DISORDER	SIGNS AND SYMPTOMS	DIAGNOSTIC TEST RESULTS
Cardiac arrhythmias (complication)	◆ Palpitations ◆ Chest pain ◆ Dizziness ◆ Weakness and fatigue ◆ Irregular heart rhythm ◆ Hypotension ◆ Syncope ◆ Altered level of consciousness (LOC) ◆ Diaphoresis ◆ Pallor ◆ Cold, clammy skin	◆ 12-lead electrocardiogram (ECG) identifies specific waveform changes associated with the arrhythmia.
Hyperkalemia (complication)	◆ Abdominal cramping ◆ Diarrhea ◆ Hypotension ◆ Irregular pulse rate; tachycardia changing to bradycardia ◆ Irritability ◆ Muscle weakness, especially of the lower extremities ◆ Nausea ◆ Paresthesia	◆ Laboratory testing reveals hyperkalemia electrolyte abnormalities, hypoxemia, or acid-base abnormalities. ◆ Serum potassium level is greater than 5 mEq/L. ◆ ECG changes include a tall, tented T wave; widened QRS complex; prolonged PR interval; flattened or absent P wave; and depressed ST segment. ◆ Arterial blood gas (ABG) analysis reveals decreased pH and metabolic acidosis.
Respiratory failure (complication)	◆ Diminished chest movement ◆ Restlessness, irritability, and confusion ◆ Decreased LOC ◆ Pallor; possible cyanosis of lips, nail beds, or mucous membranes ◆ Tachypnea, tachycardia (strong and rapid initially, but thready and irregular in later stages) ◆ Cold, clammy skin and frank diaphoresis, especially around the forehead and face ◆ Diminished breath sounds; possible adventitious breath sounds ◆ Possible cardiac arrhythmias	◆ ABG analysis indicates early respiratory failure when partial pressure of arterial oxygen is low (usually less than 70 mm Hg) and partial pressure of arterial carbon dioxide is high (greater than 45 mm Hg). ◆ Serial vital capacity reveals readings less than 800 ml. ◆ ECG may demonstrate arrhythmias. ◆ Pulse oximetry reveals a decreased oxygen saturation level. Mixed venous oxygen saturation levels less than 50% indicate impaired tissue oxygenation.

TREATMENT AND CARE

◆ Evaluate the monitored patient's ECG regularly for arrhythmias, and assess hemodynamic parameters as indicated. Document arrhythmias and notify the physician immediately.

◆ Assess an unmonitored patient for rhythm disturbances. If the patient's pulse rate is abnormally rapid, slow, or irregular, watch for signs of hypoperfusion, such as hypotension and diminished urine output.

◆ As ordered, obtain an EGG tracing in an unmonitored patient to confirm and identify the type of arrhythmia present.

◆ Administer medications and monitor the patient for adverse effects.

◆ If a life-threatening arrhythmia develops, rapidly assess the patient's LOC, pulse and respiratory rates, and hemodynamic parameters. Monitor EGG continuously. Be prepared to initiate cardiopulmonary resuscitation or cardioversion if indicated.

◆ Assess vital signs. Anticipate continuous cardiac monitoring if the patient's serum potassium level exceeds 6 mEq/L.

◆ Monitor the patient's intake and output; report an output of less than 30 ml/hour.

◆ Administer a slow calcium gluconate I.V. infusion to counteract the myocardial depressant effects of hyperkalemia.

◆ For a patient receiving repeated insulin and glucose treatment, check for signs and symptoms of hypoglycemia, including muscle weakness, syncope, hunger, and diaphoresis.

◆ Administer sodium polystyrene sulfonate and monitor serum sodium levels, which may rise; assess for signs of heart failure. Encourage the patient to retain sodium polystyrene sulfonate enemas for 30 to 60 minutes. Monitor the patient for hypokalemia when administering the drug on 2 or more consecutive days.

◆ Monitor bowel sounds and the number and character of bowel movements.

◆ Monitor serum potassium level and related laboratory test results.

◆ If the patient has acute hyperkalemia that doesn't respond to other treatments, prepare for dialysis.

◆ If the patient has muscle weakness, implement safety measures.

◆ Assess for signs of hypokalemia after treatment.

◆ Institute oxygen therapy immediately.

◆ Prepare for endotracheal (ET) intubation and mechanical ventilation, if needed; anticipate the need for high-frequency or pressure ventilation to force airways open.

◆ Administer drug therapy, such as bronchodilators to open airways, corticosteroids to reduce inflammation, continuous I.V. solutions of positive inotropic agents (which increase cardiac output) and vasopressors (which induce vasoconstriction) to maintain blood pressure, and diuretics to reduce fluid overload and edema.

◆ Assess the patient's respiratory status at least every 2 hours, or more often, as indicated.

◆ Monitor the patient for a positive response to oxygen therapy, such as improved breathing, color, and ABG values. Monitor oximetry and capnography values to detect important changes in the patient's condition.

◆ Position the patient for optimal breathing.

◆ Maintain a normothermic environment to reduce the patient's oxygen demand.

◆ Monitor vital signs, heart rhythm, and fluid intake and output.

◆ If intubated, auscultate the lungs to check for accidental intubation of the esophagus or the mainstem bronchus.

◆ Perform suctioning using strict aseptic technique when the patient is intubated. Note the amount and quality of lung secretions, and look for changes in the patient's status.

◆ Check cuff pressure on the ET tube to prevent erosion from an overinflated cuff. Normal cuff pressure is about 20 mm Hg.

◆ Implement measures to prevent nasal tissue necrosis. Position and maintain the nasotracheal tube midline in the nostrils and reposition daily. Tape the tube securely, but use skin protection measures and nonirritating tape to prevent skin breakdown.

◆ Provide a means of communication for patients who are intubated and alert.

tritional therapy may be involved to help institute necessary restrictions or supplementations. A gastroenterologist may be consulted to address problems involving the GI tract.

TREATMENT AND CARE

■ Treatment aims to correct the acidosis as quickly as possible by addressing the symptoms and the underlying cause (for example, in diabetic ketoacidosis, administer continuous low-dose I.V. insulin infusion).
■ For severe high anion gap, administer I.V. sodium bicarbonate to neutralize blood acidity in patients with a pH less than 7.20 and HCO_3^- loss; monitor electrolyte levels, especially potassium, during sodium bicarbonate therapy. (Potassium level may fall as pH rises.)
■ I.V. lactated Ringer's solution is used to correct normal anion gap metabolic acidosis and extracellular fluid volume deficit.
■ Evaluate and correct electrolyte imbalances.
■ Institute mechanical ventilation to maintain respiratory compensation, if needed.
■ Administer antibiotic therapy to treat infection.
■ Prepare patients with renal failure or certain drug toxicities for dialysis.
■ Administer antidiarrheal agents for diarrhea-induced HCO_3^- loss.
■ Monitor for secondary changes caused by hypovolemia, such as falling blood pressure (in diabetic acidosis).
■ Frequently monitor the patient's vital signs, laboratory results, and LOC because changes can occur rapidly.
■ Assess respiratory function with proper positioning to facilitate chest expansion; turn the stuporous patient frequently.
■ Monitor intake and output to assess renal function. Watch for signs of excessive serum potassium, including weakness, flaccid paralysis, and arrhythmias, possibly leading to cardiac arrest. After treatment, check for overcorrection to hypokalemia.
■ Orient the patient frequently and reduce unnecessary environmental stimuli.
■ Implement such safety measures as raising side rails and placing the bed in the lowest position, especially if the patient is confused or comatose.
■ Provide patient teaching related to diabetes as appropriate.

Metabolic alkalosis

Metabolic alkalosis occurs when low levels of acid or high bicarbonate (HCO_3^-) levels cause metabolic, respiratory, and renal responses, producing characteristic symptoms (most notably, hypoventilation). This condition is always secondary to an underlying cause. With early diagnosis and prompt treatment, prognosis is good; however, untreated metabolic alkalosis may lead to coma and death.

ETIOLOGY

Metabolic alkalosis results from loss of acid, retention of base, or renal mechanisms linked to low potassium and chloride levels.
    Causes of critical acid loss include:
■ chronic vomiting
■ nasogastric tube drainage or lavage without adequate electrolyte replacement
■ fistulas
■ use of steroids or certain diuretics (furosemide [Lasix], thiazides, and ethacrynic acid [Edecrin])
■ massive blood transfusions
■ Cushing's syndrome, primary hyperaldosteronism, and Bartter's syndrome, which lead to sodium and chloride retention and urinary loss of potassium and hydrogen.
    Excessive HCO_3^- retention causing chronic hypercapnia can result from:
■ excessive intake of bicarbonate of soda or other antacids (usually for treatment of gastritis or peptic ulcer)
■ excessive intake of absorbable alkali (as in milk alkali syndrome, commonly seen in patients with peptic ulcers)
■ excessive amounts of I.V. fluids with high bicarbonate or lactate levels
■ respiratory insufficiency.
    Alterations in extracellular electrolyte levels that can cause metabolic alkalosis include:
■ low chloride level (as chloride diffuses out of the cell, hydrogen diffuses into the cell)
■ low potassium level, causing increased hydrogen ion excretion by the kidneys.

PATHOPHYSIOLOGY

In metabolic alkalosis, the underlying mechanisms include a loss of hydrogen ions (acid), a gain in HCO_3^-, or both. A partial pressure of arterial carbon dioxide (Pa_{CO_2})

level greater than 45 mm Hg (possibly as high as 60 mm Hg) indicates that the lungs are compensating for the alkalosis. The kidneys are more effective at compensating; however, they're far slower than the lungs. As a result, numerous body systems may be affected.

Metabolic alkalosis is commonly associated with hypokalemia, particularly from the use of thiazides, furosemide, ethacrynic acid, and other diuretics that deplete potassium stores. In hypokalemia, the kidneys conserve potassium. At the same time, the kidneys also increase the excretion of hydrogen ions, which prompts alkalosis from the loss of acid. Metabolic alkalosis may also occur with hypochloremia and hypocalcemia. (See *What happens in metabolic alkalosis,* pages 268 and 269.)

Cardiovascular system
■ As a result of electrolyte imbalances (such as hypokalemia) cardiac muscle contraction and electrical conductivity are altered, which may lead to the development of arrhythmias.
■ The risk of arrhythmias is further complicated by the decreased calcium influx in the cardiac muscle secondary to the accompanying hypocalcemia.

Genitourinary system
■ When the blood HCO_3^- rises to 28 mEq/L or more, the amount filtered by the renal glomeruli exceeds the reabsorptive capacity of the renal tubules.
■ Excess HCO_3^- is excreted in the urine, and hydrogen ions are retained.
■ To maintain electrochemical balance, sodium ions and water are excreted with the bicarbonate ions.

Neurologic system
■ When hydrogen ion levels in extracellular fluid are low, hydrogen ions diffuse passively out of the cells and, to maintain the balance of charge across the cell membrane, extracellular potassium ions move into the cells.
■ As intracellular hydrogen ion levels fall, calcium ionization decreases and nerve cells become more permeable to sodium ions.
■ As sodium ions move into the cells, they trigger neural impulses, first in the peripheral nervous system and then in the central nervous system. Subsequently, hypocalcemia

and seizures occur. (See *Disorders affecting management of metabolic alkalosis,* pages 270 and 271.)

Respiratory system
■ Chemical buffers in the extracellular fluid and intracellular fluid bind HCO_3^- that accumulates in the body.
■ Excess unbound HCO_3^- raises blood pH, which depresses chemoreceptors in the medulla, inhibiting respiration and raising $Paco_2$.
■ Carbon dioxide combines with water to form carbonic acid. Low oxygen levels limit respiratory compensation.

ASSESSMENT
The signs and symptoms of metabolic alkalosis are commonly associated with an underlying condition. The patient may be asymptomatic or demonstrate signs and symptoms associated with volume depletion or hypokalemia.

The patient's history (obtained from a family member, if necessary) may reveal risk factors such as excessive ingestion of alkali antacids. The history may also reveal conditions leading to extracellular fluid (ECF) volume depletion, such as vomiting or nasogastric tube suctioning. The patient or a family member may report irritability, belligerence, and paresthesia.

Clinical findings
■ Anorexia
■ Apathy
■ Confusion
■ Cyanosis
■ Hypotension
■ Loss of reflexes
■ Muscle twitching
■ Nausea and vomiting
■ Paresthesia
■ Polyuria
■ Weakness
■ Cardiac arrhythmias (occurring with hypokalemia)
■ Positive Trousseau's and Chvostek's signs
■ Tetany, if serum calcium levels are borderline or low
■ Decreased rate and depth of respirations (This mechanism is limited because of the development of hypoxemia, which stimulates ventilation.)

WHAT HAPPENS IN METABOLIC ALKALOSIS

This series of illustrations shows how metabolic alkalosis develops at the cellular level.

As bicarbonate ions (HCO_3^-) start to accumulate in the body, chemical buffers (in extracellular fluid and cells) bind with them. *No signs are detectable at this stage.*

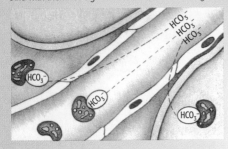

Excess HCO_3^- that doesn't bind with chemical buffers elevates serum pH levels, which in turn depresses chemoreceptors in the medulla. Depression of those chemoreceptors causes a decrease in respiratory rate, which increases partial pressure of arterial carbon dioxide ($Paco_2$). The additional carbon dioxide (CO_2) combines with water (H_2O) to form carbonic acid (H_2CO_3). *Note:* Lowered oxygen levels limit respiratory compensation. *Look for a serum pH level above 7.45, a HCO_3^- level above 26 mEq/L, a rising $Paco_2$, and slow, shallow respirations.*

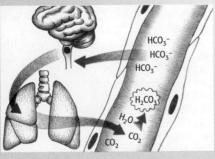

When the HCO_3^- level exceeds 28 mEq/L, the renal glomeruli can no longer reabsorb excess amounts. The excess HCO_3^- is excreted in urine; hydrogen ions ($H+$) are retained. *Look for alkaline urine and pH and bicarbonate levels that slowly return to normal.*

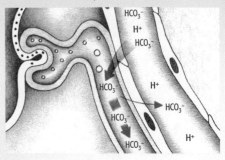

To maintain electrochemical balance, the kidneys excrete excess sodium ions (Na), water, and HCO_3^-. *Look for polyuria initially, then signs and symptoms of hypovolemia, including thirst and dry mucous membranes.*

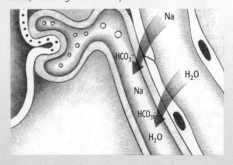

Diagnostic test results

■ *ABG studies* reveal a blood pH greater than 7.45, HCO_3^- greater than 26 mEq/L, and $Paco_2$ greater than 45 mm Hg (indicates attempts at respiratory compensation).
■ *Potassium level* is less than 3.5 mEq/L, *calcium level* is less than 8.9 mg/dl, and *chloride level* is less than 98 mEq/L.

■ *Urine pH* is about 7, and urine is alkaline after the renal compensatory mechanism begins to excrete bicarbonate.
■ *Electrocardiography* (ECG) may show a low T wave merging with a P wave and atrial or sinus tachycardia.

Lowered H+ levels in the extracellular fluid cause the ions to diffuse out of the cells. To maintain the balance of charge across the cell membrane, extracellular potassium ions (K) move into the cells. *Look for signs and symptoms of hypokalemia, including anorexia, muscle weakness, loss of reflexes, and others.*

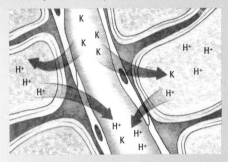

As H+ levels decline, calcium (Ca) ionization decreases. That decrease in ionization makes nerve cells more permeable to sodium ions. Sodium ions moving into nerve cells stimulate neural impulses and produce overexcitability of the peripheral and central nervous systems. *Look for tetany, belligerence, irritability, disorientation, and seizures.*

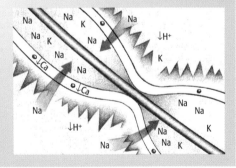

COLLABORATIVE MANAGEMENT

Because metabolic alkalosis can affect multiple body systems, a multidisciplinary approach to care is needed. A renal specialist or nephrologist can help evaluate, treat, and manage the patient's kidney function. Respiratory and cardiology specialists may be consulted to institute measures to promote optimal respiratory and cardiac function. Nutritional therapy may be involved to help institute necessary restrictions or supplementations. A gastroenterologist may be consulted to address problems involving the GI tract.

TREATMENT AND CARE

■ The goal of treatment is to correct the underlying cause.

■ Use ammonium chloride I.V. (rarely) or hydrochloric acid cautiously to restore ECF hydrogen and chloride levels

RED FLAG When administering ammonium chloride 0.9% I.V., limit the infusion rate to 1 L/4 hours. Faster administration may cause hemolysis of red blood cells. Avoid overdosage, which may cause overcorrection and result in metabolic acidosis. Don't give ammonium chloride to a patient with signs and symptoms of hepatic or renal disease.

■ Administer potassium chloride and normal saline solution (except in heart failure) to replace losses from gastric drainage.

RED FLAG Dilute potassium when giving the patient I.V. solutions containing potassium salts. Monitor the infusion rate to prevent damage to blood vessels, and use an I.V. infusion pump. Watch for signs of phlebitis.

■ Discontinue diuretics, and administer supplementary potassium chloride (metabolic alkalosis from potent diuretic therapy).

■ Administer oral or I.V. acetazolamide (Diamox; assists renal bicarbonate excretion) to correct metabolic alkalosis without rapid volume expansion (acetazolamide also enhances potassium excretion; therefore, potassium may be administered before the drug).

■ Frequently monitor vital signs, intake and output, and laboratory values, including pH, serum bicarbonate, serum potassium, and serum calcium.

■ Monitor ECG for arrhythmias; administer supplemental oxygen, if indicated.

■ Complete a neurologic assessment with reorientation as necessary.

■ Provide seizure precautions and safety measures for the patient with altered thought processes.

DISORDERS AFFECTING MANAGEMENT OF METABOLIC ALKALOSIS

This chart highlights disorders that affect the management of metabolic alkalosis.

DISORDER	SIGNS AND SYMPTOMS	DIAGNOSTIC TEST RESULTS
Hypocalcemia (complication)	◆ Anxiety ◆ Irritability ◆ Twitching around the mouth ◆ Laryngospasm ◆ Seizures ◆ Muscle cramps ◆ Paresthesias of the face, fingers, or toes ◆ Tetany ◆ Positive Chvostek's and Trousseau's signs ◆ Hypotension ◆ Arrhythmias ◆ Hyperactive deep tendon reflexes	◆ Serum calcium level is less than 8.5 mg/dl. ◆ Ionized calcium level is usually below 4.5 mg/dl. ◆ Platelet count is decreased. ◆ Electrocardiography shows lengthened QT interval, prolonged ST segment, and arrhythmias. ◆ Serum protein levels may reveal possible changes because half of the serum calcium is bound to albumin.
Seizures (generalized tonic-clonic) (complication)	◆ Loud cry upon start of seizure ◆ Changes in level of consciousness ◆ Body stiffening, alternating between muscle spasm and relaxation ◆ Tongue biting ◆ Incontinence ◆ Labored breathing, apnea, and cyanosis ◆ Upon wakening, possible confusion and difficulty talking ◆ Drowsiness, fatigue, and headache ◆ Muscle soreness and weakness	◆ EEG reveals paroxysmal abnormalities; high, fast voltage spikes are present in all leads. ◆ Serum chemistry blood studies may reveal hypoglycemia, electrolyte imbalances, elevated liver enzymes, or elevated alcohol levels. ◆ Arterial blood gas (ABG) analysis provides baseline levels for oxygenation and acid-base status.

Myocardial infarction

In myocardial infarction (MI), also known as a *heart attack*, reduced blood flow through one or more coronary arteries leads to myocardial ischemia and necrosis. Complications of MI include arrhythmias, cardiogenic shock, ventricular aneurysms, pericarditis, and myocardial rupture. Additional complications include pulmonary edema due to heart failure, cerebral or pulmonary emboli due to mural thrombi, and rupture of the atrial or ventricular septum, ventricular wall, or valves. Extensions of the original infarction may also occur.

Each year, about 900,000 people in the United States experience MI. Risk of death increases if treatment is delayed. Indeed, almost one-half of sudden deaths due to MI occur within 1 hour of the onset of symptoms and before hospitalization. Prognosis improves if vigorous treatment begins immediately.

ETIOLOGY

Predisposing risk factors for MI include:
■ positive family history
■ gender (men and postmenopausal women are more susceptible to MI than premenopausal women, although the incidence is increasing among women, especially those

TREATMENT AND CARE

◆ Assess cardiovascular status and neurologic status for changes; monitor vital signs frequently.
◆ Monitor respiratory status, including rate, depth, and rhythm. Watch for stridor, dyspnea, and crowing.
◆ Keep a tracheotomy tray and a handheld resuscitation bag at the bedside in case laryngospasm occurs.
◆ Institute cardiac monitoring and evaluate for changes in heart rate and rhythm.
◆ Assess for Chvostek's sign or Trousseau's sign.
◆ Administer I.V. calcium replacement therapy carefully. Check magnesium and phosphate levels because a low magnesium level must be corrected before I.V. calcium can be effective; if the phosphate level is too high, calcium won't be absorbed.
◆ Ensure the patency of the I.V. line because infiltration can cause tissue necrosis and sloughing.
◆ Give oral replacements.
◆ Give calcium supplements 1 to 1½ hours after meals. If GI upset occurs, give the supplement with milk.
◆ Monitor laboratory test results, including calcium levels, albumin, and magnesium levels. Remember to check the ionized calcium level after every 4 units of blood transfused.
◆ Institute seizure precautions and safety measures to prevent injury.

◆ Establish and maintain the patient's airway; assess respiratory status, including rate, depth, and rhythm of respirations. Observe for accessory muscle use or labored respirations.
◆ Assess neurologic status to establish a baseline and then frequently reassess the patient, at least every 5 to 10 minutes initially, until stabilized.
◆ Assess oxygen saturation with pulse oximetry and ABG sanalysis; administer supplemental oxygen as indicated; have endotracheal intubation equipment and ventilatory assistance readily available at the bedside.
◆ Monitor vital signs every 2 to 5 minutes; anticipate continuous direct intra-arterial blood pressure monitoring if appropriate.
◆ Institute continuous cardiac monitoring to evaluate for arrhythmias.
◆ Monitor blood glucose levels for hypoglycemia (a possible cause or effect of the patient's continued seizures) and administer glucose; prepare to treat the underlying cause (metabolic acidosis).
◆ Administer anticonvulsants I.V. Expect to administer fast-acting agents first, followed by long-acting agents. Monitor the patient's response.
◆ If seizures continue, prepare for general anesthesia with pentobarbital (Nembutal), propofol (Diprivan), or midazolam (Versed).
◆ Institute seizure precautions and safety measures.

who smoke and use hormonal contraceptives)
■ hypertension
■ smoking
■ elevated serum triglyceride, total cholesterol, and low-density lipoprotein levels
■ obesity
■ excessive intake of saturated fats
■ sedentary lifestyle
■ aging
■ stress or type A personality
■ drug use, especially cocaine and amphetamines.

PATHOPHYSIOLOGY

MI results from occlusion of one or more coronary arteries. Occlusion may be caused by atherosclerosis, thrombosis, platelet aggregation, or coronary artery stenosis or spasm. (See *Understanding MI*, pages 272 and 273.)

Coronary artery occlusion typically progresses through three stages:
■ ischemia — the first indication of an imbalance between blood flow and oxygen demand
■ injury — prolonged ischemia damages the heart
■ infarction — indicates death of myocardial cells.

UNDERSTANDING MI

In myocardial infarction (MI), blood supply to the myocardium is interrupted. Here's what happens:
Injury to the endothelial lining of the coronary arteries causes platelets, white blood cells, fibrin, and lipids to gather at the injured site, as shown below. Foam cells, or resident macrophages, gather beneath the damaged lining and absorb oxidized cholesterol, forming a fatty streak that narrows the arterial lumen.

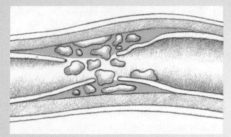

As the arterial lumen narrows, collateral circulation develops, which helps to maintain myocardial perfusion distal to the obstructed vessel lumen. The illustration below shows collateral circulation.

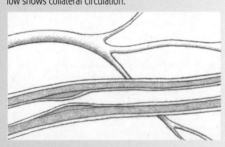

When myocardial demand for oxygen is more than the collateral circulation can supply, myocardial metabolism shifts from aerobic to anaerobic, producing lactic acid (A), which stimulates nerve endings, as shown below.

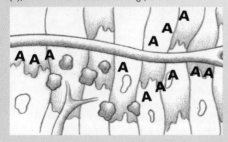

Lacking oxygen, the myocardial cells die, decreasing contractility, stroke volume, and blood pressure.

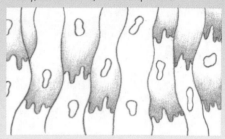

Hypotension stimulates baroreceptors, which in turn stimulate the adrenal glands to release epinephrine and norepinephrine as shown below. These catecholamines (C) increase heart rate and cause peripheral vasoconstriction, further increasing myocardial oxygen demand.

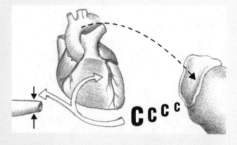

Damaged cell membranes in the infarcted area allow intracellular contents into the vascular circulation, as shown below. Ventricular arrhythmias then develop with elevated serum levels of potassium, creatine kinase (CK), CK-MB, aspartate, aminotransferase, and lactate dehydrogenase.

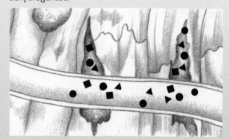

All myocardial cells are capable of spontaneous depolarization and repolarization, so the electrical conduction system may be affected by infarct, injury, or ischemia. The illustration below shows an injury site.

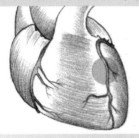

Extensive damage to the left ventricle may impair its ability to pump, allowing blood to back up into the left atrium and, eventually, into the pulmonary veins and capillaries, as shown in the illustration below. Crackles may be heard in the lungs on auscultation. Pulmonary artery wedge pressure is increased.

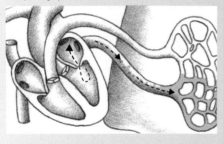

As back pressure rises, fluid crosses the alveolar-capillary membrane, impeding diffusion of oxygen (O_2) and carbon dioxide (CO_2). Arterial blood gas measurements may show decreased partial pressure of arterial oxygen and arterial pH and increased partial pressure of arterial carbon dioxide.

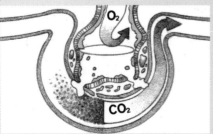

The site of an MI depends on the vessels involved. Occlusion of the circumflex branch of the left coronary artery can cause anterior, lateral, or posterior wall infarction; occlusion of the anterior descending branch of the left coronary artery can cause an anterior wall infarction. True posterior or inferior wall infarctions typically result from occlusion of the right coronary artery or one of its branches.

Right ventricular infarctions can also result from right coronary artery occlusion or accompany inferior infarctions. Right ventricular MI may lead to right-sided heart failure. In Q-wave or transmural MI, tissue damage extends through all myocardial layers; in non–Q-wave (subendocardial) MI, damage is less extensive, with decreased mortality. However, non–Q-wave MI affects a greater percentage of the myocardium, which places the patient at higher risk for reinfarction and recurrent angina.

All infarcts—areas of damage due to MI—consist of three zones: a central area of necrosis, a zone of injury surrounding the necrosis and consisting of potentially viable hypoxic injury, and an area of viable ischemic tissue surrounding the zone of injury. The outermost area—the viable ischemic tissue—may be salvaged if circulation is restored. If circulation isn't restored and myocardial oxygen demand remains higher than the supply, necrosis will occur in the zone of injury. Although ischemia begins immediately, the size of the infarct may be limited if circulation is restored within 6 hours.(See *Zones of myocardial infarction,* page 274.)

Although MI principally involves the heart, all body systems can be affected as a result of changes in heart contractility and blood flow. Many patients have coexisting disorders that place them at high risk for additional problems. (See *Disorders affecting management of MI,* pages 276 to 281.)

Cardiovascular system
■ After MI, the infarcted myocardial cells release cardiac enzymes and proteins.
■ Within 24 hours, the infarcted muscle becomes edematous and cyanotic.
■ During the next several days, leukocytes infiltrate the necrotic area and begin to remove necrotic cells, thinning the ventricular wall.

ZONES OF MYOCARDIAL INFARCTION

Characteristic electrocardiographic changes are associated with each of the three zones in myocardial infarction.

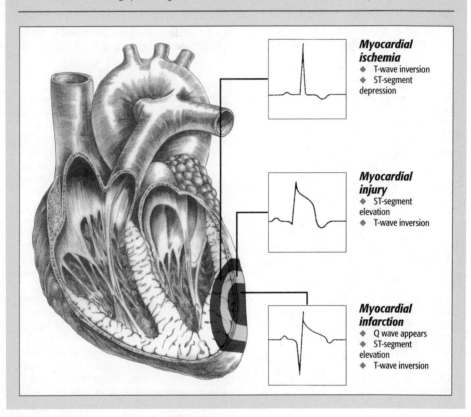

Myocardial ischemia
◆ T-wave inversion
◆ ST-segment depression

Myocardial injury
◆ ST-segment elevation
◆ T-wave inversion

Myocardial infarction
◆ Q wave appears
◆ ST-segment elevation
◆ T-wave inversion

■ Scar formation begins by the third week after MI. By the sixth week, scar tissue is well established.

■ The scar tissue that forms on the necrotic area inhibits contractility. When contractility is inhibited, the compensatory mechanisms (vascular constriction, increased heart rate, and renal retention of sodium and water) try to maintain cardiac output.

■ Ventricular dilation may occur in a process called *remodeling.*

■ Functionally, an MI may cause reduced contractility with abnormal wall motion, altered left ventricular compliance, reduced stroke volume, reduced ejection fraction, and elevated left ventricular end-diastolic pressure.

■ The backup of fluid results in heart failure.

Musculoskeletal system

■ Decreased perfusion to skeletal muscles results in fatigue and weakness of muscles.

■ Hypoxemia of the skeletal muscle tissue secondary to decreased perfusion leads to lactic acidosis.

Neurologic system

■ Anxiety and restlessness as well as cool extremities and perspiration may occur due to the release of catecholamines and stimulation of the sympathetic nervous system.

■ Stimulation of vasovagal reflexes or vomiting centers may cause nausea and vomiting.

Renal system
- Reduced urine output occurs secondary to reduced renal perfusion.
- Secretion of aldosterone and antidiuretic hormones increases, leading to fluid conservation.

Respiratory system
- Shortness of breath and crackles may occur due to heart failure and decreased oxygenation.
- The backup of fluid results in pulmonary edema and, possibly, acute respiratory distress syndrome.

ASSESSMENT
A swift and thorough assessment is essential for a patient with MI, especially if his condition seems unstable. After the patient is stabilized, additional information can be obtained about his lifestyle and possible risk factors.

Clinical findings
- Complaints of persistent, crushing substernal chest pain that may radiate to the arm, jaw, neck, or shoulder blades
- Complaints of atypical symptoms (in older patients or patients with diabetes), such as fatigue, dyspnea, falls, tingling of the extremities, nausea, vomiting, weakness, syncope, and confusion
- Light-headedness
- Fainting
- Sweating
- Nausea
- Shortness of breath
- Feeling of impending doom
- Cool extremities
- Anxiety and restlessness
- Initially elevated blood pressure as a result of sympathetic nervous system activation; may fall if cardiac output is reduced
- Bradycardia associated with conduction disturbances, particularly with damage to the inferior wall of the left ventricle
- Crackles
- Low-grade fever due to inflammatory response
- Jugular vein distention, reflecting right ventricular dysfunction and pulmonary congestion
- Audible third and fourth heart sounds, reflecting ventricular dysfunction

- Loud holosystolic murmur in apex, possibly caused by papillary muscle rupture
- Decreased urine output

Diagnostic test results
- *Serial 12-lead electrocardiography* may reveal characteristic ST-segment elevation. It can also identify the location of MI, arrhythmias, hypertrophy, and pericarditis.
- *Serial cardiac enzymes* and *proteins* (CK-MB, troponin T and I, and myoglobin) may show a characteristic rise and fall.
- *Laboratory testing* may reveal elevated white blood cell count, C-reactive protein level, and erythrocyte sedimentation rate.
- *Echocardiography* may show ventricular wall motion abnormalities and may detect septal or papillary muscle rupture.
- *Chest X-rays* may show left-sided heart failure or cardiomegaly due to ventricular dilation.
- *Nuclear imaging scanning* can identify areas of infarction.
- *Cardiac catheterization* and *coronary angiography* may be used to identify the involved coronary artery and provide information on ventricular function and pressures and volumes within the heart.

COLLABORATIVE MANAGEMENT
MI is an acute emergency that requires a multidisciplinary approach. Emergency teams, such as an advanced cardiac life support team, may stabilize the patient before his arrival at the facility or in the emergency department. A cardiologist will manage the patient's care directly related to the heart condition; a cardiothoracic surgeon may also be consulted. Nutritional specialists may provide education and meal-planning assistance after the patient's condition is stabilized. A pulmonary specialist or respiratory therapist may be involved if the patient requires endotracheal intubation or pulmonary care. A renal care specialist may be consulted if the patient requires dialysis.

TREATMENT AND CARE
Treatment of the patient with MI typically involves following the guidelines recommended by the American College of Cardiology/American Heart Association

(*Text continues on page 280.*)

DISORDERS AFFECTING MANAGEMENT OF MI

This chart highlights disorders that affect the management of myocardial infarction (MI).

DISORDER	SIGNS AND SYMPTOMS	DIAGNOSTIC TEST RESULTS
Cardiac arrhythmias (complication)	◆ May be asymptomatic ◆ Dizziness ◆ Hypotension ◆ Syncope ◆ Weakness ◆ Cool, clammy skin ◆ Altered level of consciousness ◆ Reduced urine output ◆ Shortness of breath ◆ Chest pain	◆ Electrocardiography (ECG) detects arrhythmias and ischemia and infarction that may result in arrhythmias. ◆ Laboratory testing may reveal electrolyte abnormalities, acid-base abnormalities, or drug toxicities that may cause arrhythmias. ◆ Holter monitoring, event monitoring, and loop recording can detect arrhythmias and effectiveness of drug therapy during a patient's daily activities. ◆ Exercise testing may detect exercise-induced arrhythmias. ◆ Electrophysiologic testing identifies the mechanism of an arrhythmia and the location of accessory pathways and assesses the effectiveness of antiarrhythmic drugs, radiofrequency ablation, and implanted cardioverter-defibrillators.
Cardiogenic shock (complication)	◆ Tachycardia and bounding pulse ◆ Restlessness, irritability, and hypoxia ◆ Tachypnea ◆ Reduced urinary output ◆ Cool, pale skin that progresses to cyanosis ◆ Hypotension ◆ Narrowed pulse pressure ◆ Weak, rapid, thready pulse ◆ Shallow respirations ◆ Reduced urinary output ◆ Unconsciousness and absent reflexes (in irreversible stages) ◆ Rapidly falling blood pressure with decompensation ◆ Anuria	◆ Coagulation studies may detect coagulopathy from disseminated intravascular coagulation (DIC). ◆ White blood cell count and erythrocyte sedimentation rate may be increased. ◆ Blood urea nitrogen and creatinine are elevated due to reduced renal perfusion. ◆ Serum lactate may be increased secondary to anaerobic metabolism. ◆ Serum glucose may be elevated in early stages. ◆ Cardiac enzymes and proteins may be elevated, indicating MI as the cause. ◆ Arterial blood gas (ABG) analysis may reveal respiratory alkalosis in early shock or respiratory acidosis in later stages. ◆ Urine specific gravity may be high. ◆ Chest X-rays may be normal in early stages; pulmonary congestion may be seen in later stages. ◆ Hemodynamic monitoring may reveal characteristic patterns of intracardiac pressures and cardiac output. ◆ ECG determines heart rate and detects arrhythmias, ischemic changes, and MI. ◆ Echocardiography determines left ventricular function and reveals valvular abnormalities.
Coagulation defects (complication)	◆ Signs and symptoms of shock if bleeding is severe (tachycardia, hypotension, and tachypnea) ◆ Bleeding (such as from endotracheal tube, wound, or I.V. sites)	◆ Coagulation studies may detect coagulopathy from DIC. ◆ Urinalysis may show red blood cells. ◆ Hemoglobin, hematocrit, and platelet count may be decreased.

TREATMENT AND CARE

◆ When life-threatening arrhythmias develop, rapidly assess level of consciousness, respirations, and pulse rate.
◆ Initiate cardiopulmonary resuscitation if indicated.
◆ Evaluate cardiac output.
◆ If the patient develops heart block, prepare for cardiac pacing.
◆ Administer antiarrhythmic agents as ordered.
◆ Prepare to assist with medical procedures if indicated.
◆ Assess intake and output every hour.
◆ Document arrhythmias in the monitored patient and assess for possible causes and effects.
◆ If the patients pulse is abnormally rapid, slow, or irregular, watch for signs of hypoperfusion, such as hypotension and diminished urine output.
◆ Monitor for predisposing factors, such as fluid and electrolyte imbalance, or possible drug toxicity.

◆ Assist in identifying and treating the underlying cause.
◆ Maintain a patent airway; prepare for intubation and mechanical ventilation if respiratory distress develops.
◆ Provide supplemental oxygen to increase oxygenation.
◆ Use continuous cardiac monitoring to detect changes in heart rate and rhythm; administer antiarrhythmics as necessary.
◆ Monitor vital signs every 15 minutes and assess hemodynamic parameters as indicated.
◆ Initiate and maintain at least two I.V. lines with large-gauge needles for fluid and drug administration.
◆ Administer I.V. fluids, crystalloids, colloids, blood products, inotropic drugs or vasodilators as ordered.
◆ Monitor intake, output, and daily weight. Administer diuretics to reduce preload if the patient has fluid volume overload.
◆ Initiate intra-aortic balloon pump (IABP) therapy to reduce the work of left ventricle by decreasing systemic vascular resistance. Monitor the patient carefully.
◆ Monitor the patient receiving thrombolytic therapy or coronary artery revascularization per facility protocol.
◆ Prepare for emergency surgery if the papillary muscle ruptures or if a ventricular septal defect is present.
◆ Monitor the patient with a ventricular assist device.

◆ Avoid I.M. injections and unnecessary I.V. sticks.
◆ Monitor the patient for signs of bleeding.
◆ Handle the patient gently to avoid bruising.
◆ Test all urine and stool for occult blood.
◆ Monitor vital signs and level of consciousness; report changes.
◆ Administer blood products, as ordered, and monitor for their effects.
◆ If patient is having a reaction to heparin, make sure heparin isn't given, especially in an arterial or pulmonary artery line.

(continued)

DISORDERS AFFECTING MANAGEMENT OF MI *(continued)*

DISORDER	SIGNS AND SYMPTOMS	DIAGNOSTIC TEST RESULTS
Coronary aneurysm (complication)	◆ Tachycardia and bounding pulse ◆ Restlessness and irritability ◆ Tachypnea ◆ Reduced urinary output ◆ Cool, pale skin ◆ Hypotension as compensatory mechanisms fail ◆ Narrowed pulse pressure ◆ Weak, rapid, thready pulse ◆ Shallow respirations ◆ Reduced urinary output as poor renal perfusion continues ◆ Anuria	◆ Cardiac enzymes and proteins may be elevated, indicating MI as the cause. ◆ ABG analysis may reveal respiratory alkalosis in early shock or respiratory acidosis in later stages. ◆ Urine specific gravity may be high. ◆ Chest X-rays may be normal in early stages; pulmonary congestion may be seen in later stages. ◆ Hemodynamic monitoring may reveal characteristic patterns of intracardiac pressures and cardiac output. ◆ ECG determines heart rate and detects arrhythmias, ischemic changes, and MI. ◆ Echocardiography determines left ventricular function and reveals valvular abnormalities.
Diabetes (coexisting)	◆ Polyuria and polydypsia ◆ Anorexia or polyphagia ◆ Weight loss ◆ Headaches, fatigue, lethargy, reduced energy levels, and impaired performance ◆ Muscle cramps ◆ Irritability; emotional imbalance ◆ Vision changes such as blurring ◆ Numbness and tingling ◆ Abdominal discomfort and pain ◆ Nausea, diarrhea, or constipation ◆ Slowly healing skin infections or wounds; itching of skin ◆ Recurrent monilial infections of the vagina or anus	◆ Two-hour postprandial blood glucose shows a level of 200 mg/dl or above. ◆ Fasting blood glucose level is 126 mg/dl or higher after at least an 8-hour fast.
Thyroid disease (coexisting)	◆ Tachycardia ◆ Hypertension ◆ Diaphoresis ◆ Irritability ◆ Nervousness	◆ Thyroid hormone levels are altered. ◆ ECG may show arrhythmias.
Valvular heart disease (complication)	*In mitral stenosis or insufficiency* ◆ Dyspnea on exertion ◆ Paroxysmal nocturnal dyspnea ◆ Orthopnea ◆ Weakness and fatigue ◆ Palpitations ◆ Peripheral edema ◆ Jugular vein distention ◆ Acites ◆ Hepatomegaly ◆ Crackles	◆ Cardiac catheterization can differentiate mitral stenosis or mitral insufficiency from aortic stenosis or aortic insufficiency. ◆ Chest X-rays show left atrial and ventricular enlargement, enlarged pulmonary arteries, and mitral valve calcification in mitral valve problems; left ventricular enlargement, pulmonary congestion, and valvular calcification in aortic valve problems. ◆ Echocardiography shows thickened valve leaflets. ◆ ECG reveals arrhythmias.

TREATMENT AND CARE

◆ Administer supplemental oxygen to increase oxygenation.
◆ Institute continuous cardiac monitoring to detect changes in heart rate and rhythm; administer antiarrhythmics as necessary.
◆ Monitor blood pressure, pulse rate, peripheral pulses, and other vital signs every 15 minutes; notify physician of changes.
◆ Monitor central venous pressure, pulmonary artery wedge pressure, and cardiac output as ordered; report changes.
◆ Initiate and maintain at least two I.V. lines with large-gauge needles for fluid and drug administration.
◆ Administer I.V. fluids, crystalloids, colloids, or blood products, as necessary, to maintain intravascular volume.
◆ Administer inotropic drugs, such as dopamine, dobutamine, and epinephrine, to increase heart contractility and cardiac output; monitor peripheral pulses and circulation and report changes.
◆ Administer vasodilators, such as nitroglycerin or nitroprusside, with a vasopressor to reduce the left ventricle's workload.
◆ Monitor intake, output, and daily weight. Administer diuretics to reduce preload if the patient has fluid volume overload.
◆ Initiate IABP therapy to reduce the work of left ventricle by decreasing systemic vascular resistance. Monitor the patient carefully.
◆ Monitor the patient receiving thrombolytic therapy or coronary artery revascularization per facility protocol.
◆ Prepare for emergency surgery if repair is required.

◆ Expect to administer two or more drugs, which are usually necessary to achieve target blood pressure of less than 130 mm Hg.
◆ Administer thiazide diuretics, angiotensin-converting enzyme inhibitors, beta-adrenergic blockers, angiotensin-receptor blockers, or calcium channel blockers as ordered.
◆ Monitor the patient's blood glucose level because beta-adrenergic blockers can cause hyperglycemia.
◆ Watch for signs of diabetic neuropathy (numbness or pain in the hands and feet, footdrop, impotence, neurogenic bladder), infection (increased temperature), cardiac distress (chest pain, palpitations, dyspnea, confusion), changes in vision, peripheral numbness or tingling, constipation, anorexia, and blisters or skin openings, particularly on the feet.
◆ Because thiazide and loop diuretic promote potassium excretion, monitor serum potassium levels for patients receiving diuretics.
◆ Monitor intake and output and watch for signs of dehydration.
◆ Review foods that are high and low in sodium and potassium with the patient.

◆ Monitor vital signs and administer antihypertensives and beta-adrenergic blockers; monitor the patient for drug effects.
◆ Monitor thyroid levels and the patient's response to thyroid medication.
◆ If the patient is on a low-iodine diet, teach him about avoiding products containing iodine (such as salt).

◆ Administer oxygen in acute situations to increase oxygenation.
◆ Monitor vital signs and effects of digoxin on heart rate.
◆ Instruct the patient on how to maintain a low-sodium diet.
◆ Monitor the effects of diuretics; record input and output and daily weights.
◆ Monitor the effects of antiarrhythmics and vasodilators.
◆ Monitor the patient taking anticoagulants for bleeding.
◆ Monitor the patient for signs of heart failure or pulmonary edema and for adverse effects of drug therapy.
◆ Administer nitroglycerine to relieve angina as ordered.

(continued)

DISORDERS AFFECTING MANAGEMENT OF MI *(continued)*

DISORDER	SIGNS AND SYMPTOMS	DIAGNOSTIC TEST RESULTS
Valvular heart disease *(continued)*	◆ Atrial fibrillation ◆ Signs of systemic emboli ◆ Loud first heart sound or opening snap and diastolic murmur at apex *In aortic stenosis or insufficiency* ◆ Dyspnea ◆ Cough ◆ Fatigue ◆ Palpitations ◆ Angina ◆ Syncope ◆ Pulmonary congestion ◆ Left-sided heart failure ◆ Pulsating nail beds ◆ Rapidly rising and collapsing pulses ◆ Cardiac arrhythmias ◆ Widened pulse pressure ◆ Third heart sound and diastolic blowing murmur at left sternal border ◆ Palpation and visualization of apical impulse (in chronic disease)	

(ACC/AHA) Task Force on Practice Guidelines. These include:

■ assessing the patient with chest pain in the emergency department within 10 minutes of symptom onset (At least 50% of deaths take place within 1 hour of the onset of symptoms; moreover, thrombolytic therapy is most effective when started within the first 3 hours after the onset of symptoms.)

■ oxygen by nasal cannula at 2 L/minute for at least 6 hours to increase blood oxygenation (see *Treating myocardial infarction,* pages 282 and 283)

■ nitroglycerin sublingually or I.V. for 24 to 48 hours to reduce afterload and preload and relieve chest pain (contraindicated if systolic blood pressure less than 90 mm Hg or heart rate less than 50 or greater than 100 beats/minute)

■ morphine I.V. at 5 to 10 minute intervals for analgesia because pain stimulates the sympathetic nervous system, leading to an increase in heart rate and vasoconstriction

■ aspirin every day indefinitely (to inhibit platelet aggregation)

■ continuous cardiac monitoring to detect arrhythmias and ischemia

■ I.V. fibrinolytic therapy for the patient with chest pain of at least 30 minutes' duration who reaches the hospital within 12 hours of the onset of symptoms (unless contraindications exist) and whose ECG shows new left bundle-branch block (LBBB) or ST-segment elevation of at least 1 to 2 mm in two or more ECG leads (The greatest benefit of reperfusion therapy, however, occurs when reperfusion takes place within 3 hours of the onset of chest pain.)

■ I.V. heparin for the patient who has received fibrinolytic therapy to increase the chances of patency in the affected coronary artery

■ percutaneous transluminal coronary angioplasty (PTCA), which is superior to fibrinolytic therapy if it can be performed in a timely manner in a facility with personnel skilled in the procedure

■ glycoprotein IIb/IIIa-receptor blocking agents, which strongly inhibit platelet aggregation (They're indicated as adjunct therapy

TREATMENT AND CARE

◆ Prepare for cardioversion if patient has atrial fibrillation.
◆ If the patient requires surgery, monitor for hypotension, arrhythmias, and thrombus formation. Monitor vital signs, ABG values, intake and output, daily weight, blood chemistries, chest X-rays, and pulmonary artery catheter readings.

with PTCA in acute ST-segment elevation MI and as a primary therapy in non-ST-segment elevation MI; their use in combination with fibrinolytic agents is controversial.)

■ limitation of physical activity for the first 12 hours to reduce cardiac workload, thereby limiting the area of necrosis

■ keeping atropine, amiodarone, transcutaneous pacing patches or a transvenous pacemaker, a defibrillator, and epinephrine readily available to treat arrhythmias (The ACC/AHA doesn't recommend the prophylactic use of antiarrhythmic drugs during the first 24 hours.)

■ I.V. nitroglycerin for 24 to 48 hours in the patient without hypotension, bradycardia, or excessive tachycardia to reduce afterload and preload and relieve chest pain

■ early I.V. beta-adrenergic blockers to the patient with an evolving acute MI followed by oral therapy, provided there are no contraindications, to reduce heart rate and myocardial contractile force, thereby reducing myocardial oxygen requirements

■ angiotensin-converting enzyme inhibitors for the patient with an evolving MI with ST-segment elevation or LBBB, but without hypotension or other contraindications, to reduce afterload and preload and prevent remodeling

■ magnesium sulfate for 24 hours to correct hypomagnesemia, if needed

■ angiography and possible percutaneous or surgical revascularization for the patient with spontaneous or provoked myocardial ischemia following an acute MI

■ exercise testing before discharge to determine the adequacy of medical therapy and to obtain baseline information for an appropriate exercise prescription (It can also determine functional capacity and assess the patient's risk of a subsequent cardiac event.)

■ cardiac risk modification program of weight control; a low-fat, low-cholesterol diet; smoking cessation; and regular exercise to reduce cardiac risk

■ lipid-lowering agents, as indicated by the fasting lipid profile.

TREATING MYOCARDIAL INFARCTION

This chart shows how treatments can be applied to myocardial infarction at various stages.

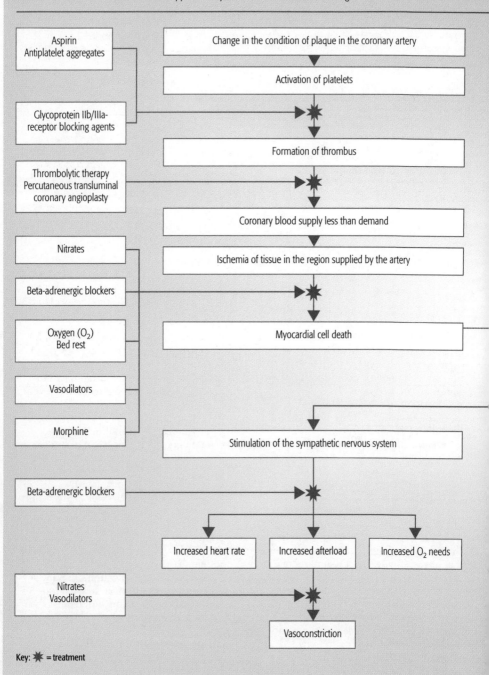

Aspirin
Antiplatelet aggregates

Glycoprotein IIb/IIIa-
receptor blocking agents

Thrombolytic therapy
Percutaneous transluminal
coronary angioplasty

Nitrates

Beta-adrenergic blockers

Oxygen (O₂)
Bed rest

Vasodilators

Morphine

Beta-adrenergic blockers

Nitrates
Vasodilators

Change in the condition of plaque in the coronary artery

Activation of platelets

Formation of thrombus

Coronary blood supply less than demand

Ischemia of tissue in the region supplied by the artery

Myocardial cell death

Stimulation of the sympathetic nervous system

Increased heart rate

Increased afterload

Increased O₂ needs

Vasoconstriction

Key: ✹ = treatment

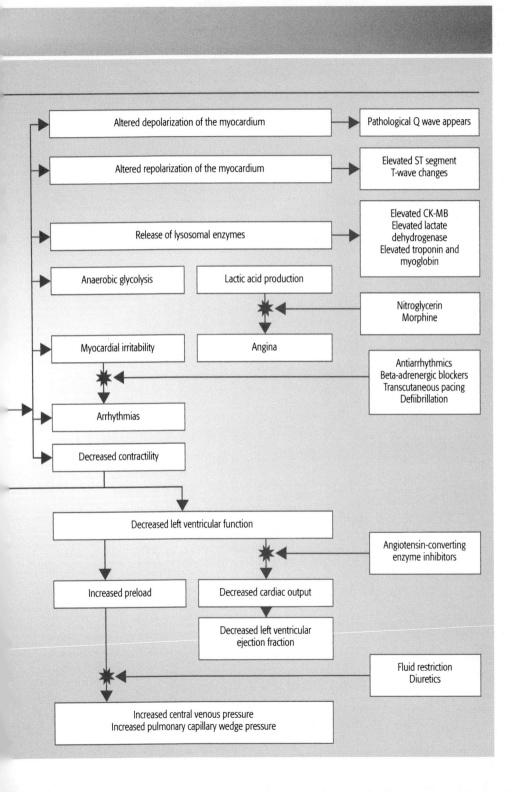

N-O

Near drowning

In near drowning, the victim survives (at least temporarily) the physiologic effects of submersion in fluid. Hypoxemia and acidosis are the primary effects of near drowning.

ETIOLOGY

Although inability to swim is the most obvious—and indeed, the most common—cause of near drowning, it isn't the only cause. Near drowning may be associated with panic, a boating accident, sudden acute illness (seizure or myocardial infarction), trauma to the head while in the water, venomous stings from aquatic animals, excessive alcohol consumption before swimming, a suicide attempt, or decompression sickness from deep-water diving.

PATHOPHYSIOLOGY

Near drowning occurs in three forms. In *dry near drowning,* which occurs in 10% to 20% of patients, the victim doesn't aspirate fluid; rather, he suffers respiratory obstruction or asphyxia. In *wet near drowning,* which occurs in about 80% to 90% of patients, the victim aspirates fluid and suffers from asphyxia or secondary changes from fluid aspiration. In *secondary near drowning,* the victim suffers recurrence of respiratory distress (usually aspiration pneumonia or pulmonary edema) within minutes or 1 to 2 days after a near-drowning incident. (See *Pathophysiologic changes in near drowning.*)

Regardless of the tonicity of the fluid aspirated, hypoxemia is the most serious consequence of near drowning, followed by metabolic acidosis. Other consequences depend on the type of water aspirated; for example, saltwater aspiration is considered more serious than freshwater aspiration because saltwater contains more disease-causing bacteria.

Cardiovascular system

■ Cold water submersion (exposure to temperatures below 69.8° F [21° C]) may lead to a protective effect (most pronounced in children and may be due to the large ratio of body surface area to mass). Rapid body cooling results in cardiac arrest and decreased tissue oxygen demand.

■ Hypothermia may occur because water rapidly conducts heat away from the body. (See *Disorders affecting management of near drowning,* pages 286 and 287.)

Neurologic system

■ The patient's level of consciousness (LOC) may be altered due to hypoxemia.

■ The release of catecholamines leads to vasoconstriction, decreasing cerebral oxygen consumption.

■ Submersion in cold water leads to decreased central blood flow and cooling of the blood that flows to the brain, resulting in mental confusion.

Respiratory system

■ In freshwater aspiration, water is absorbed across the alveolar-capillary membrane, resulting in destruction of surfactant and subsequent alveolar instability, atelectasis, and decreased compliance.

■ In saltwater aspiration, surfactant washout occurs and protein-rich exudates rapidly move into the alveoli and pulmonary interstitium. The hypertonicity of seawater pulls fluid from pulmonary capillaries into the alveoli. The resulting intrapulmonary shunt causes hypoxemia. The pulmonary capillary membrane may be injured, leading to pulmonary edema.

■ In wet and secondary near drowning, pulmonary edema and hypoxemia occur secondary to aspiration.

UP CLOSE

PATHOPHYSIOLOGIC CHANGES IN NEAR DROWNING

The chart below shows the primary cellular alterations that occur during near drowning. Separate pathways are shown for saltwater and freshwater incidents. Hypothermia presents a separate pathway that may preserve neurologic function by decreasing the metabolic rate. All pathways lead to diffuse pulmonary edema.

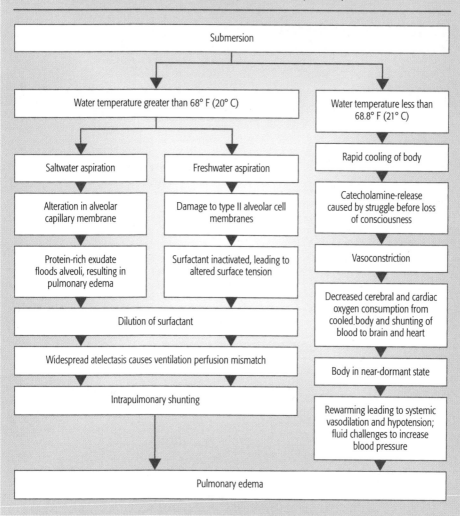

■ Aspiration of such contaminants as chlorine, mud algae, and weeds can occur, leading to obstruction, aspiration pneumonia, and pulmonary fibrosis.

ASSESSMENT

The patient's history and the cause of the near drowning are typically obtained from a family member, friend, or emergency personnel.

DISORDERS AFFECTING MANAGEMENT OF NEAR DROWNING

This chart highlights disorders that affect the management of near drowning.

DISORDER	SIGNS AND SYMPTOMS	DIAGNOSTIC TEST RESULTS
Acute respiratory distress syndrome (ARDS) (complication)	◆ Dyspnea on exertion ◆ Diminished breath sounds ◆ Tachypnea, tachycardia ◆ Increasing respiratory distress with use of accessory muscles ◆ Restlessness, apprehension ◆ Dry cough or frothy sputum ◆ Cool, clammy skin that progresses to pallor and cyanosis ◆ Basilar crackles, rhonchi ◆ Decreased mental status ◆ Arrhythmias such as premature ventricular contractions ◆ Labile blood pressure	◆ Arterial blood gas (ABG) analysis initially shows decreased partial pressure of arterial oxygen despite oxygen supplementation and decreased partial pressure of arterial carbon dioxide ($Paco_2$), causing an increase in blood pH. As ARDS worsens, $Paco_2$ increases and pH decreases as the patient becomes acidotic. ◆ Initially, chest X-rays may be normal. Basilar infiltrates begin to appear in about 24 hours. In later stages, lung fields have a ground glass appearance and, eventually, white patches appear. ◆ Pulmonary artery wedge pressure is 18 mm Hg or lower.
Hypothermia (complication)	*Mild hypothermia* ◆ Severe shivering, slurred speech, and amnesia *Moderate hypothermia* ◆ Unresponsiveness ◆ Peripheral cyanosis ◆ Muscle rigidity *Severe hypothermia* ◆ No palpable pulse or heart sounds ◆ Dilated pupils ◆ State of rigor mortis ◆ Ventricular fibrillation	◆ Technetium-99m pertechnetate scanning shows perfusion defects and deep tissue damage. ◆ Doppler and plethysmographic studies help determine pulses and the extent of frostbite after thawing. ◆ Laboratory studies determine the extent of tissue and organ damage.

Clinical findings

■ Variable LOC; patient initially unconscious, semiconscious, or awake (If he's awake, he usually appears apprehensive, irritable, restless, or lethargic, and complains of a headache or substernal chest pain.)
■ Fever
■ Confusion
■ Seizures

TREATMENT AND CARE

◆ Assess the patient's cardiopulmonary status, including lung sounds, heart rate, and blood pressure at least every 2 hours, or more often if indicated. Note respiratory rate, rhythm, and depth, reporting dyspnea and accessory muscle use. Be alert for inspiratory retractions. If the patient has injuries that affect his lungs, watch for adverse respiratory changes, especially in the first few days after the injury, when his condition may appear to be improving.

◆ Administer oxygen, assess oxygen saturation continuously, and monitor serial ABG levels.

◆ Check ventilator settings frequently if indicated; assess hemodynamic parameters if a pulmonary catheter is inserted.

◆ Institute continuous cardiac monitoring and watch for arrhythmias.

◆ Monitor the patient's level of consciousness, noting confusion or mental sluggishness.

◆ Be alert for signs of treatment-induced complications, including arrhythmias, disseminated intravascular coagulation, GI bleeding, infection, malnutrition, paralytic ileus, pneumothorax, pulmonary fibrosis, renal failure, thrombocytopenia, and tracheal stenosis.

◆ Give sedatives to reduce restlessness. Administer sedatives and analgesics at regular intervals if the patient is receiving neuromuscular blocking agents.

◆ Administer anti-infective agents if the underlying cause is sepsis or an infection.

◆ Place the patient in a comfortable position that maximizes air exchange, such as semi-Fowler's or high Fowler's position.

◆ Evaluate the patient's serum electrolyte levels frequently.

◆ Monitor urine output hourly to ensure adequate renal function. Measure intake and output. Weigh the patient daily.

◆ Record caloric intake. Administer tube feedings and parenteral nutrition.

◆ Assess airway, breathing, and circulation.

◆ Institute cardiopulmonary resuscitation until the patient's core body temperature increases to at least 86° F (30° C.)

◆ Assist in rewarming techniques; provide supportive measures such as mechanical ventilation and heated, humidified therapy to maintain tissue oxygenation and I.V. fluids that have been warmed with a warming coil to correct hypotension and maintain urine output.

◆ Insert an indwelling urinary catheter and assess urine output hourly.

◆ Continuously monitor core body temperature and other vital signs during and after initial rewarming. Monitor cardiac status with continuous cardiac monitoring for evidence of arrhythmias.

◆ If the patient's core temperature is below 89.6° F (32° C), use internal and external warming methods to raise the patient's body core and surface temperatures 1° to 2° F (0.6° to 1.1° C) per hour.

◆ If the patient's temperature is 86° F to 93° F (30° C to 33.9° C), limit active rewarming to the neck, axilla, or groin areas. Using these techniques in peripheral areas can contribute to a continued drop in core temperature as cold blood from the periphery is mobilized.

◆ If using a hyperthermia blanket, discontinue the warming when core body temperature is within 1° to 2° F of the desired temperature. The patient's temperature will continue to rise even with the device turned off.

◆ If the patient has been hypothermic for longer than 45 to 60 minutes, administer additional fluids to compensate for the expansion of vascular space that occurs during vasodilation in rewarming. Monitor heart rate and hemodynamic parameters closely to evaluate fluid needs and response to treatment.

◆ Monitor serum electrolyte levels closely, especially potassium. Be alert for signs and symptoms of hyperkalemia.

◆ If hyperkalemia occurs, administer calcium chloride, sodium bicarbonate, glucose, and insulin. Anticipate the need for sodium polystyrene sulfonate enemas. If potassium levels are extremely elevated, prepare the patient for dialysis or exchange transfusion.

◆ Offer warm oral fluids if the patient is alert and has an intact gag reflex. Otherwise, administer warmed I.V. fluids.

■ Rapid, slow, or absent pulse
■ Shallow, gasping, or absent respirations
■ Possible hypothermia if the patient was exposed to cold temperatures
■ Cyanosis or pink, frothy sputum (indicating pulmonary edema)
■ Abdominal distention
■ Crackles, rhonchi, wheezing, or apnea

- Tachycardia, an irregular heartbeat (arrhythmia), or cardiac arrest
- Hypotension

Diagnostic test results

- *Arterial blood gas (ABG) analysis* identifies degree of hypoxia, intrapulmonary shunt, and acid-base imbalance and whether hypoxemia, hypercapnia, and combined respiratory and metabolic acidosis are present.
- *Serum electrolyte levels* may reveal hyperkalemia secondary to acidosis or red blood cell hemolysis.
- *Complete blood count* aids in identifying hemolysis if the patient aspirated large amounts of fluid; it also reveals an elevated white blood cell (WBC) count secondary to alveolar inflammation or a decreased WBC count if the patient is hypothermic.
- *Blood urea nitrogen, creatinine levels,* and *urinalysis* indicate adequacy of renal function.
- *Cervical spine X-ray* helps rule out fracture.
- *Serial chest X-rays* reveal inflammation, fluid accumulation, excess air accumulation, fractures, foreign objects, or pulmonary infiltrates suggestive of pulmonary edema.
- *Electrocardiography* reveals myocardial ischemia.

COLLABORATIVE MANAGEMENT

Caring for the patient who has experienced near drowning requires a multidisciplinary approach. Medical and nursing care focuses on maintaining all body functions. A pulmonologist and a respiratory therapist may be involved to manage the patient's ventilatory needs. As other systems become involved, specialists for those systems may be consulted. Social services may be involved to assist with emotional support for the patient and his family as well as assisting with follow-up care issues.

TREATMENT AND CARE

- Assess airway, breathing, and circulation. Initiate cardiopulmonary resuscitation and advanced cardiac life support, as indicated.

RED FLAG Hypothermia decreases a patient's ability to metabolize drugs. Therefore, intervals between doses of I.V. medications should be lengthened for the patient with hypothermia. Be alert for a bolus-like effect that can occur with drug administration, which can result from the vasodilation that occurs during rewarming.

- Administer supplemental oxygen as ordered. If the patient is hypothermic, use warm humidified oxygen to prevent additional cooling.
- Monitor oxygen saturation for evidence of hypoxemia with continuous pulse oximetry and serial ABG analyses.
- Anticipate the need for endotracheal intubation and mechanical ventilation should the patient's respiratory status deteriorate.
- Anticipate using positive end-expiratory pressure (PEEP) if the patient continues to demonstrate hypoxia or pulmonary edema and doesn't respond to increased levels of oxygen. PEEP is especially helpful in freshwater near drowning because alveoli remain open.

RED FLAG The patient may experience low levels of surfactant for 2 to 3 days after aspirating freshwater; therefore, discontinue PEEP carefully and monitor the patient closely for deterioration in respiratory status.

- Auscultate lung sounds every hour for changes such as crackles, rhonchi, or friction rubs. Suction as necessary and send sputum for culture as ordered.
- Place the patient in semi-Fowler's position to maximize chest expansion.
- Keep the patient as quiet and comfortable as possible to minimize oxygen demands.
- Assess for signs of worsening hypoxemia, including use of accessory muscles, stridor, nasal flaring, grunting retractions, tachypnea, tachycardia, and cyanosis. Obtain serial ABG analyses as ordered and monitor for changes.
- Monitor vital signs continuously for changes. Observe skin color and check capillary refill. Notify the physician if capillary refill is greater than 2 seconds. Continuously monitor the patient's core temperature.
- Assist with insertion of a central venous or pulmonary artery catheter and monitor hemodynamic parameters, including central venous pressure, pulmonary artery wedge pressure, and cardiac output, frequently — as often as every 15 minutes.
- Institute continuous cardiac monitoring to evaluate for possible arrhythmias, myocardial ischemia, or adverse effects of treatment.

■ Assess LOC frequently — approximately every 30 to 60 minutes for the first 24 hours. Monitor for signs and symptoms of increased intracranial pressure (ICP). Administer osmotic diuretics as ordered to control ICP.

RED FLAG Closely monitor the patient for signs and symptoms of brain herniation, such as bradycardia, hypotension, widening pulse pressure, and altered respiratory rate and pattern.

■ Ensure I.V. access and administer I.V. fluids as ordered.

■ Monitor intake and output closely.

■ Insert an indwelling urinary catheter and assess urine output hourly.

■ Monitor serum electrolyte levels and renal function studies for changes.

■ Assess the abdomen for distention and presence of bowel sounds every 2 to 4 hours.

RED FLAG Bowel ischemia and necrosis may occur from prolonged periods of hypoxemia and hypotension secondary to shunting of blood to other organs.

■ Insert a nasogastric tube, as indicated, to remove swallowed water and reduce the risk of vomiting and aspiration.

■ If the patient is hypothermic, institute rewarming measures as ordered.

■ Administer medications as ordered (for example, sodium bicarbonate if the patient has metabolic acidosis or aerosolized bronchodilators for bronchospasm).

■ Watch for signs of impending coagulopathy, such as petechiae, bruising, bleeding, or oozing from gums or venipuncture sites. Monitor results of coagulation studies.

■ Provide emotional support and reassurance.

P–Q

Paget's disease

Paget's disease, also called *osteitis deformans*, is a slowly progressive metabolic bone disease characterized by accelerated patterns of bone remodeling. Paget's disease can localize in one or more areas of the skeleton, most commonly in the lumbosacral spine, skull, pelvis, femur, and tibia. Occasionally, however, skeletal deformity is widely distributed.

Paget's disease affects about 2.5 million people older than age 40 in the United States — mostly men. The disease can be fatal, particularly when it's associated with heart failure, bone sarcoma, or giant-cell tumors.

ETIOLOGY
Although the exact cause of Paget's disease is unknown, one theory holds that early viral infection causes a dormant skeletal infection that erupts years after the initial infection.

Other possible causes include:
- benign or malignant bone tumors
- vitamin D deficiency during the bone-developing years of childhood
- autoimmune disease
- estrogen deficiency.

PATHOPHYSIOLOGY
An initial phase of excessive bone resorption (osteoclastic phase) is followed by a reactive phase of excessive abnormal bone formation (osteoblastic phase). Chronic accelerated remodeling eventually enlarges and softens the affected bones. The new bone structure, which is chaotic, fragile, and weak, causes painful deformities of both external contour and internal structure. Repeated episodes of accelerated osteoclastic resorption of spongy bone occur.

Cardiovascular system
- The widespread nature of Paget's disease and extreme vascularity of the newly formed bone increase metabolic demand and creates a continuous need for high cardiac output.
- Increased metabolic demand and high cardiac output can eventually lead to heart failure. (See *Disorders affecting management of Paget's disease,* pages 292 to 295.)

Musculoskeletal system
- The trabeculae diminish, and vascular fibrous tissue replaces marrow. This activity is followed by short periods of rapid, abnormal bone formation.
- The collagen fibers in the new bone are disorganized, and glycoprotein levels in the matrix decrease.
- The partially resorbed trabeculae thicken and enlarge because of excessive bone formation, and the bone becomes soft and weak.
- Impingement of abnormal bone on the spinal cord or sensory nerve root leads to pain and impaired mobility. Pain may also result from the constant inflammation accompanying cell breakdown.
- Pelvic softening may occur, leading to a waddling gait.
- The legs may bow if the femurs or tibias are affected.
- Occasionally, malignant osteosarcoma can occur in the deformed bone.

Neurologic system
- In skull involvement, characteristic cranial enlargement over the frontal and occipital areas can produce headaches, sensory abnormalities, and impaired motor function, depending on the sensory areas affected. For example, blindness and hearing loss with tinnitus and vertigo may result from bony impingement on the cranial nerves.

■ Kyphosis, a spinal curvature, may develop as a result of compression fractures of the vertebrae.
■ Permanent paralysis can occur if the soft bone of the vertebrae fractures and puts pressure on the spinal cord.

Renal system
■ Because of the constant osteoclastic and osteoblastic activity, phosphates and calcium are released and reabsorbed.
■ Phosphates and calcium may then accumulate in the renal pelvis, resulting in renal calculi.
■ Hypercalcemia and gout may also occur.

Respiratory system
■ Chronic accelerated remodeling eventually enlarges and softens the affected bones.
■ Thoracic deformities may impair respiration, eventually leading to respiratory failure.

ASSESSMENT
The effects of Paget's disease vary. The patient may be asymptomatic in the early stages.

Clinical findings
■ Complaints of severe and persistent pain intensifying with weight bearing
■ Headaches if the head is involved; reports of hat size increasing
■ Cranial enlargement over frontal and occipital areas, sensory abnormalities, and impaired motor function (with skull involvement)
■ Kyphosis
■ Barrel chest
■ Asymmetric bowing of the tibia and femur (commonly reduces height)
■ Waddling gait
■ Warm and tender disease sites that are susceptible to pathologic fractures after minor trauma
■ Slow, incomplete healing if a fracture has occurred
■ Anemia

Diagnostic test results
■ *X-rays, computed tomography scan,* and *magnetic resonance imaging* obtained before overt symptoms develop show increased bone expansion and density.

■ *Radionuclide bone scan* shows early Paget's lesions. (Radioisotopes concentrate in areas of active disease.)
■ *Bone biopsy* shows characteristic mosaic pattern.
■ *Serum alkaline phosphatase level* is elevated.
■ *24-hour urine levels* of hydroxyproline (an amino acid excreted by the kidneys and an indicator of osteoclastic hyperactivity) are elevated.
■ *Serum calcium level* is normal or elevated.

COLLABORATIVE MANAGEMENT
Caring for the patient with Paget's disease requires a multidisciplinary approach. An orthopedic specialist can provide medical and surgical treatment of pathologic fractures, correct secondary deformities, and replace joints. A neurosurgical specialist may be involved if the head or spinal cord is affected. He may collaborate with the orthopedic surgeon to relieve pressure of the nerves, reducing sensory deficits and pain. A cardiologist may be consulted if heart failure occurs. A physical therapist and an occupational therapist may assist with optimizing range-of-motion of joints and bone structure. Community support resources may be needed, such as a visiting nurse or home health agency.

TREATMENT AND CARE
■ Bisphosphonates (alendronate [Fosamax], etidronate [Didronel]) may be administered to inhibit osteoclast-mediated bone resorption.
■ Calcitonin (Calcimar), a hormone, and etidronate may be administered to retard bone resorption, reduce serum alkaline phosphate and urinary hydroxyproline secretion, and reduce bone pain. (Calcitonin requires long-term maintenance therapy, but improvement is noticeable after the first few weeks of treatment; etidronate produces improvement after 1 to 3 months.)
■ Mithramycin (Mithracin), a cytotoxic antibiotic, may be administered to decrease serum calcium, urinary hydroxyproline, and serum alkaline phosphatase levels.

DRUG ALERT *Mithramycin produces symptom remission within 2 weeks and biochemical improvement in 1 to 2 months, but may destroy platelets or compromise renal function.*

(Text continues on page 294.)

DISORDERS AFFECTING MANAGEMENT OF PAGET'S DISEASE

This chart highlights disorders that affect the management of Paget's disease.

DISORDER	SIGNS AND SYMPTOMS	DIAGNOSTIC TEST RESULTS
Heart failure (complication)	*Left-sided heart failure* ♦ Dyspnea ♦ Orthopnea ♦ Paroxysmal nocturnal dyspnea ♦ Fatigue ♦ Nonproductive cough ♦ Crackles ♦ Hemoptysis ♦ Tachycardia ♦ Third and fourth heart sounds ♦ Cool, pale skin ♦ Restlessness and confusion *Right-sided heart failure* ♦ Jugular vein distention ♦ Positive hepatojugular reflux ♦ Right-upper-quadrant pain ♦ Anorexia ♦ Nausea ♦ Nocturia ♦ Weight gain ♦ Edema ♦ Ascites or anasarca	♦ Chest X-ray shows increased pulmonary vascular markings, interstitial edema, or pleural effusions and cardiomegaly. ♦ Electrocardiography (ECG) may reveal hypertrophy, ischemic changes or infarction, tachycardia, and extrasystoles. ♦ Liver function test may be abnormal; blood urea nitrogen (BUN) and creatinine levels may be elevated. ♦ Prothrombin time may be prolonged. ♦ B-type natriuretic peptide immunoassay is elevated. ♦ Echocardiography may reveal left ventricular hypertrophy, dilation, and abnormal contractility. ♦ Pulmonary artery pressure, pulmonary artery wedge pressure, and left ventricular end-diastolic pressure are elevated in the presence of left-sided heart failure; right atrial or central venous pressure is elevated in right-sided heart failure. ♦ Radionuclide ventriculography may reveal ejection fraction less than 40% in diastolic dysfunction.
Hypertension (complication)	♦ Typically asymptomatic ♦ Elevated blood pressure readings on at least two consecutive occasions ♦ Occipital headache ♦ Epistaxis ♦ Bruits ♦ Dizziness ♦ Confusion ♦ Fatigue ♦ Blurred vision ♦ Nocturia ♦ Edema	♦ Urinalysis may show protein, casts, red blood cells, or white blood cells. ♦ Elevated BUN and serum creatinine suggest renal disease. ♦ Complete blood count may reveal polycythemia or anemia. ♦ Excretory urography may reveal renal atrophy. ♦ ECG may show left ventricular hypertrophy or ischemia. ♦ Chest X-rays may show cardiomegaly. ♦ Echocardiography may reveal left ventricular hypertrophy.
Osteoarthritis (complication)	♦ Deep, aching joint pain ♦ Stiffness in the morning and after exercise ♦ Crepitus or grating of the joint during motion ♦ Herberden's nodes (bony enlargements of the distal interphalangeal joints) ♦ Altered gait from contractures ♦ Decreased range of motion	♦ Absence of systemic symptoms rules out an inflammatory joint disorder. ♦ Arthroscopy shows bone spurs and narrowing of joint space. ♦ Erythrocyte sedimentation rate is increased. ♦ X-rays may confirm diagnosis by showing narrowing of joint space or margin, cystlike bony deposits in joint spaces, sclerosis of the subchondral space, joint deformity, bony growths, and joint fusion.

TREATMENT AND CARE

- Place the patient in Fowler's position and give supplemental oxygen.
- Weigh the patient daily, and check for peripheral edema.
- Monitor intake and output, vital signs, and mental status.
- Auscultate for third and fourth heart sounds and adventitious lung sounds such as crackles or rhonchi.
- Monitor BUN, creatinine, and serum potassium, sodium, chloride, and magnesium.
- Institute continuous cardiac monitoring to identify and treat arrhythmias promptly.
- Administer angiotensin-converting enzyme (ACE) inhibitors, digoxin, diuretics, beta-adrenergic blockers, human B-type natriuretic peptides, nitrates, and morphine.
- Prepare the patient for possible coronary artery bypass surgery or angioplasty, as appropriate.
- Encourage lifestyle modifications to reduce symptoms.

- Monitor blood pressure and the patient's response to antihypertensive medications.
- Evaluate results of laboratory studies.
- Maintain a reduced-sodium diet.
- Monitor for complications of hypertension such as signs of stroke, myocardial infarction, and renal disease.
- Administer thiazide diuretics, ACE inhibitors, angiotensin-receptor blockers, beta-adrenergic blockers, and calcium-channel blockers.

- Promote adequate rest, particularly after activity. Plan rest periods during the day. Teach the patient to pace activities and avoid overexertion.
- Assist with physical therapy and encourage the patient to perform gentle, isometric range-of-motion exercises.
- If the patient needs surgery, provide appropriate preoperative and postoperative care.
- Provide emotional support and reassurance.
- Assist with care for arthritic joints, such as hot soaks, paraffin dips for the hands, and cervical collar application.
- Ensure proper functioning of supportive devices such as canes, braces, crutches, or walkers, and provide instruction for their use.
- Instruct the patient to take medications, such as aspirin, and nonsteroidal anti-inflammatory drugs, such as ibuprofen (Motrin), exactly as prescribed.

(continued)

DISORDERS AFFECTING
MANAGEMENT OF PAGET'S DISEASE *(continued)*

DISORDER	SIGNS AND SYMPTOMS	DIAGNOSTIC TEST RESULTS
Osteoarthritis *(continued)*	◆ Joint enlargement ◆ Localized headaches	
Renal calculi (complication)	◆ Severe pain ◆ Nausea and vomiting ◆ Fever ◆ Chills ◆ Hematuria ◆ Abdominal distention ◆ Anuria	◆ Kidney-ureter-bladder radiography shows most recent calculi. ◆ Excretory urography confirms diagnosis and determines size and location of calculi. ◆ Kidney ultrasonography helps detect obstructive changes. ◆ Urine culture identifies possible urinary tract infection. ◆ A 24-hour collection of urine reveals calcium oxalate, phosphorus, or uric acid excretion levels; serum calcium and phosphorus levels may be increased.

■ Surgery may be performed to reduce or prevent pathologic fractures, correct secondary deformities, and relieve neurologic impairment; however, drug therapy with calcitonin and etidronate or mithramycin must precede surgery to decrease the risk of excessive bleeding from hypervascular bone.

■ Joint replacement may be necessary; however, it may be difficult because bonding material (polymethacrylate) doesn't set properly on pagetic bone.

■ Assess for pain. Watch for new areas of pain or restricted movements, which may indicate new fracture sites, and sensory or motor disturbances, such as difficulty in hearing, seeing, or walking.

■ Evaluate serum calcium and alkaline phosphatase levels.

■ If the patient is confined to prolonged bed rest, perform skin care measures such as repositioning and use of a flotation mattress, if indicated.

■ Assess fluid status. Monitor intake and output and encourage adequate fluid intake to minimize renal calculi formation.

■ Provide patient teaching about calcitonin administration (self-injection or nasal inhalation), lifestyle changes, and safety measures.

■ Refer the patient to community support agencies and Paget's Foundation.

Peritonitis

An acute or chronic disorder, peritonitis is an inflammation of the peritoneum, the membrane that lines the abdominal cavity and covers the visceral organs. Such inflammation may extend throughout the peritoneum or may be localized as an abscess.

Peritonitis commonly decreases intestinal motility and causes intestinal distention due to gas. Mortality is about 10%, with bowel obstruction and septic shock as the usual cause of death.

ETIOLOGY

Peritonitis typically results from inflammation and perforation of the GI tract following bacterial invasion of the peritoneum. Such invasion may result from appendicitis, diverticulitis, peptic ulcer, ulcerative colitis, acute hemorrhagic pancreatitis, volvulus, strangulated obstruction, abdominal neoplasm, or abdominal trauma. Peritonitis can also result from chemical inflammation due to perforation of a gastric ulcer, release of pancreatic enzymes, or rupture of a fallopian tube, an ovarian cyst, or the bladder.

PATHOPHYSIOLOGY

In peritonitis, bacterial or chemical inflammation of the peritoneum (which is normally sterile), results in accumulation of fluid

TREATMENT AND CARE

- Maintain 24- to 48-hour record of urine pH.
- Encourage the patient to walk, if possible, to aid passage of the stone.
- Promote sufficient intake of fluids to maintain a urine output of 2 to 4 qt/day (2 to 4 L).
- Record intake and output and strain urine.
- Stress the importance of proper diet.
- If surgery is required, maintain patency of tubes and monitor for drainage; never irrigate a nephrostomy tube without a physician's order. Check dressings and monitor vital signs. Notify physician of changes.
- Monitor for signs of infection.

containing protein and electrolytes within the peritoneal cavity. The transparent peritoneum becomes opaque, red, inflamed, and edematous.

Because the peritoneal cavity is resistant to contamination, the infection is typically localized as an abscess. In some cases, however, such as when the peritoneum becomes weakened or injured, the inflammation and infection spread throughout the peritoneal cavity. The resulting inflammatory response can affect multiple body systems. (See *Disorders affecting management of peritonitis,* pages 296 and 297.)

Cardiovascular system

■ Large amounts of fluid from the intravascular space move into the peritoneal cavity, causing hypovolemia and hemoconcentration, as indicated by cool, clammy skin and pallor.

■ If the patient loses excessive fluid, electrolytes, and proteins into the abdominal cavity, dehydration may occur. Hypotension and tachycardia result as the body tries to conserve fluid.

Gastrointestinal system

■ An inflammatory process causes the release of histamine from the peritonitis.

■ Peristaltic action decreases.

■ Fibrin formation occurs around the damage, eventually causing adhesions.

■ If the inflammation is severe or prolonged, adhesions continue to form, ultimately leading to bowel obstruction.

■ The shift in fluid or third-spacing exudate into the peritoneal cavity leads to abdominal distention.

■ The increased secretion in the bowel increases intraluminal pressure, commonly resulting in paralytic ileus.

Neurologic system

■ The shift in fluid out of the vascular space leads to volume depletion. Impaired blood flow and diminished perfusion of cerebral cells cause changes in the patient's level of consciousness.

■ Initial anxiety and restlessness may progress to confusion and lethargy.

Renal system

■ The loss of fluid from the intravascular space leads to a drop in blood pressure and, ultimately, decreased perfusion to the kidneys.

Respiratory system

■ Fluid accumulation in the peritoneal cavity may cause elevation of the diaphragm, leading to an increased respiratory rate.

■ Inflammation of the peritoneum can irritate the nerve fibers in the peritoneum and diaphragm. The resulting pain on inspiration may lead to a decrease in the depth of respirations.

(*Text continues on page 298.*)

DISORDERS AFFECTING
MANAGEMENT OF PERITONITIS

This chart highlights disorders that affect the management of peritonitis.

DISORDER	SIGNS AND SYMPTOMS	DIAGNOSTIC TEST RESULTS
Hypovolemic shock (complication)	◆ Depend on the amount of fluid loss *Minimal volume loss (10% to 15%)* ◆ Slight tachycardia ◆ Normal supine blood pressure ◆ Positive postural vital signs, including a decrease in systolic blood pressure greater than 10 mm Hg or an increase in pulse rate greater than 20 beats/minute ◆ Increased capillary refill time (longer than 3 seconds) ◆ Urine output more than 30 ml/hour ◆ Cool, pale skin on arms and legs ◆ Anxiety *Moderate volume loss (about 25%)* ◆ Rapid, thready pulse ◆ Supine hypotension ◆ Cool truncal skin ◆ Urine output of 10 to 30 ml/hour ◆ Severe thirst ◆ Restlessness, confusion, or irritability *Severe volume loss (40% or more)* ◆ Marked tachycardia ◆ Marked hypotension ◆ Weak or absent peripheral pulses ◆ Cold, mottled, or cyanotic skin ◆ Urine output less than 10 ml/hour ◆ Unconsciousness	◆ Complete blood count reveals low hematocrit and decreased hemoglobin level, red blood cell (RBC) count, and platelet counts. ◆ Metabolic studies reveal elevated serum potassium, sodium, lactate dehydrogenase, creatinine, and blood urea nitrogen (BUN) levels. ◆ Urine studies reveal increased urine specific gravity (greater than 1.020) and urine osmolality and urine sodium levels less than 50 mEq/L. ◆ Urine creatinine levels may be decreased. ◆ Arterial blood gas (ABG) studies may reveal decreased pH and partial pressure of arterial oxygen and increased partial pressure of arterial carbon dioxide. ◆ Gastroscopy, X-rays, and aspiration of gastric contents through a nasogastric tube may reveal evidence of frank or occult bleeding. ◆ Coagulation studies may show evidence of coagulopathy.
Sepsis or septic shock (complication)	◆ Tachycardia and bounding pulse ◆ Restlessness, irritability, and hypoxia ◆ Shallow respirations, tachypnea ◆ Reduced urinary output ◆ Warm, dry skin ◆ Hypotension as compensatory mechanisms fail ◆ Narrowed pulse pressure ◆ Weak, rapid, thready pulse ◆ Reduced urinary output ◆ Cyanosis ◆ Unconsciousness and absent reflexes (in irreversible stages) ◆ Rapidly falling blood pressure with decompensation ◆ Anuria	◆ Blood, urine, or sputum cultures may identify the causative organism. ◆ Coagulation studies may detect coagulopathy from disseminated intravascular coagulation. ◆ White blood cell count and erythrocyte sedimentation rate may be increased. ◆ BUN and creatinine are elevated. ◆ Serum lactate may be increased secondary to anaerobic metabolism. ◆ Serum glucose may be elevated in early stages. ◆ ABG analysis may reveal respiratory alkalosis in early shock or respiratory acidosis in later stages. ◆ Urine specific gravity may be high. ◆ Chest X-rays may be normal in early stages; pulmonary congestion may be seen in later stages. ◆ Hemodynamic monitoring may reveal characteristic patterns of intracardiac pressures and cardiac output.

TREATMENT AND CARE

- Assess the patient for the extent of blood loss and begin fluid replacement.
- Obtain a blood type and crossmatch for blood component therapy; administer.
- Assess airway, breathing, and circulation and institute emergency resuscitative measures as needed.
- Administer supplemental oxygen as ordered and monitor oxygen saturation.
- Monitor vital signs and hemodynamic status continuously for changes. Observe skin color and check capillary refill.
- Institute continuous cardiac monitoring to evaluate for possible arrhythmias, myocardial ischemia, or adverse effects of treatment.
- Assess neurologic status frequently – about every 30 minutes until the patient stabilizes, and then every 2 to 4 hours.
- Monitor urine output at least hourly.
- Administer dopamine or norepinephrine I.V. as ordered to increase cardiac contractility and renal perfusion.
- During therapy, assess skin color and temperature and note changes.
- Watch for signs of impending coagulopathy (such as petechiae, bruising, and bleeding or oozing from gums or venipuncture sites).
- Prepare the patient for surgery as appropriate.

- Assist in identifying and treating underlying cause.
- Maintain a patent airway; prepare for intubation and mechanical ventilation if respiratory distress develops.
- Administer supplemental oxygen to increase oxygenation.
- Perform continuous cardiac monitoring to detect changes in heart rate and rhythm; administer antiarrhythmics as needed.
- Monitor blood pressure, pulse rate, peripheral pulses and other vital signs every 15 minutes; report changes.
- Monitor central venous pressure, pulmonary artery wedge pressure, and cardiac output, as ordered, and report changes.
- Initiate and maintain at least two I.V. lines with large-gauge needles for fluid and drug administration.
- Administer I.V. fluids, crystalloids, colloids, or blood products, as necessary, to maintain intravascular volume.
- Administer antibiotic therapy to eradicate the causative organism.
- Administer inotropic drugs, such as dopamine, dobutamine, and epinephrine to increase heart contractility and cardiac output; monitor blood pressure, cardiac output, peripheral pulses, and circulation; report changes.
- Monitor temperature and institute cooling measures, such as hyperthermia blankets and decreasing room temperature.

ASSESSMENT

The patient's signs and symptoms depend on whether the disorder is assessed early or late in its course.

Clinical findings

■ Complaints of vague, generalized, diffuse abdominal pain or pain over a specific area of inflammation, if the site is localized (early on)
■ With progression, complaints of increasingly severe and unremitting abdominal pain that usually increases with movement and respirations; pain may be referred to the shoulder or the thoracic area; anorexia, nausea, and vomiting; increased anxiety
■ Lying still in bed on back or side with knees flexed to try to alleviate abdominal pain
■ Fever
■ Tachycardia
■ Hypotension
■ Slow, shallow breathing because patient tends move as little as possible to minimize pain
■ Diaphoresis with pale, cool, clammy skin
■ Signs of dehydration, such as dry mucous membranes and poor skin turgor
■ Abdominal distention
■ Bowel sounds initially present but then disappear
■ Abdominal rigidity
■ General tenderness if peritonitis spreads throughout the abdomen; local or point tenderness if peritonitis stays in a specific area
■ Rebound tenderness of abdomen

Diagnostic test results

■ *White blood cell (WBC) count* shows leukocytosis (commonly more than 20,000/µl.
■ *Serum electrolyte levels* may be abnormal; albumin levels may be decreased suggesting bacterial peritonitis.
■ *Abdominal X-rays* demonstrate edematous and gaseous distention of the small and large bowel. With perforation of a visceral organ, the X-ray shows air in the abdominal cavity.
■ *Chest X-rays* may reveal elevation of the diaphragm.
■ *Abdominal ultrasound* may reveal fluid collections.
■ *Paracentesis* discloses the nature of the exudate and permits bacterial culture so appropriate antibiotic therapy can be instituted.

COLLABORATIVE MANAGEMENT

Caring for the patient with peritonitis requires a multidisciplinary approach. Respiratory, renal, cardiac, GI, and infectious disease specialists may be consulted, depending on the underlying disorder. Social services may be necessary to assist with discharge plans, follow-up care, and home care referrals.

TREATMENT AND CARE

■ Administer antibiotics, as indicated; this may include I.V. cefoxitin with an aminoglycoside, or penicillin G and clindamycin with an aminoglycoside, depending on the infecting organisms. Other drugs used include cephalosporins and quinolones.
■ Maintain the patient on nothing-by-mouth status to decrease peristalsis and prevent perforation; administer parenteral fluids and electrolytes, as indicated.
■ Monitor vital signs, fluid intake and output, and the amount of nasogastric (NG) drainage or vomitus.
■ Place the patient in semi-Fowler's position to facilitate deep breathing, reduce pain, and prevent pulmonary complications.
■ Apply antiembolism stockings or use intermittent pneumatic compression devices, as indicated, to prevent deep vein thrombosis.
■ Be prepared to administer supplementary treatment measures, such as preoperative and postoperative analgesics, NG intubation to decompress the bowel and, possibly, a rectal tube to facilitate passage of flatus.
■ If necessary, assist with surgical evacuation of spilled contents and insertion of drains. Be prepared to perform irrigation of the abdominal cavity with antibiotic solutions during surgery, if ordered.
■ Be prepared to assist with paracentesis, as indicated, to remove accumulated fluid.
    If surgery is performed to evacuate the peritoneum:
■ Watch for signs and symptoms of dehiscence (the patient may complain that "something gave way") and abscess formation (continued abdominal tenderness and fever).

- Frequently assess peristaltic activity by listening for bowel sounds and checking for gas, bowel movements, and a soft abdomen.
- When peristalsis returns and temperature and pulse rate are normal, gradually decrease parenteral fluids and increase oral fluids. If the patient has an NG tube in place, clamp it for short intervals. If neither nausea nor vomiting results, begin oral fluids as ordered and tolerated.
- Assess for fluid and electrolyte balance, temperature and WBC count, presence of bowel obstruction or other complications, and normal oral intake and bowel elimination patterns.

Pulmonary embolism

An obstruction of the pulmonary arterial bed, pulmonary embolism (PE) occurs when a mass such as a dislodged thrombus lodges in a pulmonary artery branch, partially or completely obstructing it. This causes a ventilation-perfusion (V̇/Q̇) mismatch, resulting in hypoxemia and intrapulmonary shunting.

The prognosis varies with PE. The pulmonary infarction that results from embolism may be so mild the patient may be asymptomatic. However, massive embolism (more than 50% obstruction of pulmonary arterial circulation) and infarction can cause rapid death.

ETIOLOGY

PE typically results from a dislodged thrombus that originated in the deep veins of the leg veins. Other, less common sources of thrombi include the upper extremities, the right side of the heart, and the pelvic, renal, and hepatic veins.

Although rare, PE can also result from obstruction by bone, air, fat, amniotic fluid, or tumor cells. A foreign object, such as a needle or catheter part, may cause PE. Obstruction may also result from injection of a drug intended for oral administration.

The risk of PE increases with long-term immobility, chronic pulmonary disease, heart failure or atrial fibrillation, thrombophlebitis, polycythemia vera, thrombocytosis, cardiac arrest, defibrillation, cardioversion, autoimmune hemolytic anemia, sickle cell disease, varicose veins, recent surgery, age older than 40, osteomyelitis, pregnancy, lower extremity fractures or surgery, burns, obesity, vascular injury, cancer, and hormonal contraceptive use.

PATHOPHYSIOLOGY

Thrombus formation results from vascular wall damage, venous stasis, or hypercoagulability of the blood. Trauma, clot dissolution, sudden muscle spasm, intravascular pressure changes, or a change in peripheral blood flow can cause the thrombus to loosen or fragment. The thrombus, now called an *embolus,* floats to the heart's right side and enters the lung through the pulmonary artery. There the embolus may dissolve, continue to fragment, or grow. If the embolus is large enough, obstruction to the pulmonary blood flow can occur.

Cardiovascular system
- Initially, hypoxia leads to tachycardia and hypertension.
- Right ventricular failure occurs due to the obstruction in outflow. This, in turn, reduces the output from the left ventricle, ultimately leading to hypotension.

Respiratory system
- Occlusion of the pulmonary artery limits alveolar surfactant production, leading to alveolar collapse and subsequent atelectasis.
- Inadequate tissue oxygenation leads to an initial increase in the respiratory rate, which may progress to respiratory distress.
- If the pulmonary artery becomes completely occluded, respiratory failure may result. (See *Disorders affecting management of pulmonary embolism,* pages 300 and 301.)
- If the embolus enlarges and obstructs most or all pulmonary vessels, death may result.

ASSESSMENT

The signs and symptoms produced by small or fragmented emboli depend on their size, number, and location. If the embolus totally occludes the main pulmonary artery, the patient will have severe signs and symptoms. Assessment may also reveal a predisposing condition.

DISORDERS AFFECTING
MANAGEMENT OF PULMONARY EMBOLISM

This chart highlights disorders that affect the management of pulmonary embolism.

DISORDER	SIGNS AND SYMPTOMS	DIAGNOSTIC TEST RESULTS
Heart failure (complication)	*Left-sided heart failure* ◆ Dyspnea ◆ Orthopnea ◆ Paroxysmal nocturnal dyspnea ◆ Fatigue ◆ Nonproductive cough ◆ Crackles ◆ Hemoptysis ◆ Tachycardia ◆ Third and fourth heart sounds ◆ Cool, pale skin ◆ Restlessness and confusion *Right-sided heart failure* ◆ Jugular vein distention ◆ Positive hepatojugular reflux ◆ Right-upper-quadrant pain ◆ Anorexia, nausea ◆ Nocturia ◆ Weight gain, edema ◆ Ascites or anasarca	◆ Chest X-ray shows increased pulmonary vascular markings, interstitial edema, or pleural effusions and cardiomegaly. ◆ Electrocardiography (ECG) may reveal hypertrophy, ischemic changes or infarction, tachycardia, and extrasystoles. ◆ Liver function test may be abnormal; blood urea nitrogen (BUN) and creatinine levels may be elevated. ◆ Prothrombin time may be prolonged. ◆ B-type natriuretic peptide immunoassay is elevated. ◆ Echocardiography may reveal left ventricular hypertrophy, dilation, and abnormal contractility. ◆ Pulmonary artery pressure, pulmonary artery wedge pressure, and left ventricular end-diastolic pressure are elevated in the presence of left-sided heart failure; right atrial or central venous pressure is elevated in right-sided heart failure. ◆ Radionuclide ventriculography may reveal ejection fraction less than 40% in diastolic dysfunction.
Respiratory failure or acute respiratory distress (complication)	◆ Increased respiratory rate, decreased rate, or normal rate (depending on the cause) ◆ Cyanosis ◆ Crackles, rhonchi, wheezing, and diminished breath sounds ◆ Restlessness, confusion, loss of concentration ◆ Irritability ◆ Coma ◆ Tachycardia ◆ Elevated blood pressure ◆ Arrhythmias	◆ Arterial blood gas (ABG) analysis reveals deteriorating values and a pH below 7.35. ◆ Chest X-rays identify characteristic pulmonary diseases or conditions. ◆ ECG can demonstrate ventricular arrhythmias or right ventricular hypertrophy. ◆ Pulse oximetry reveals decreased arterial oxygen saturation. ◆ White blood cell count detects underlying infection.

Clinical findings

■ Shortness of breath, commonly occurring suddenly and for no apparent reason
■ Pleuritic or anginal pain, which is often sudden and severe
■ Sense of impending doom
■ Low-grade fever
■ Weak, rapid, pulse
■ Hypotension

■ Productive cough, possibly producing blood-tinged sputum
■ Chest splinting
■ Massive hemoptysis
■ Leg edema
■ Cyanosis, syncope, and distended neck veins (with large embolus)
■ Warm, tender area in the extremities, indicating a possible thrombus site

TREATMENT AND CARE

◆ Place the patient in Fowler's position and give supplemental oxygen.
◆ Weigh the patient daily, and check for peripheral edema.
◆ Monitor intake and output, vital signs, and mental status.
◆ Auscultate for third and fourth heart sounds and adventitious lung sounds such as crackles or rhonchi.
◆ Monitor BUN, creatinine, and serum potassium, sodium, chloride, and magnesium.
◆ Institute continuous cardiac monitoring to identify and treat arrhythmias promptly.
◆ Administer angiotensin-converting enzyme (ACE) inhibitors, digoxin, diuretics, beta-adrenergic blockers, human B-type natriuretic peptides, nitrates, and morphine.
◆ Prepare the patient for possible coronary artery bypass surgery or angioplasty, as appropriate.
◆ Encourage lifestyle modifications to reduce symptoms.

◆ Administer oxygen therapy as ordered and monitor for its effectiveness.
◆ Maintain a patent airway, Prepare for endotracheal intubation, if indicated.
◆ In the intubated patient, suction as needed after hyperoxygenation. Observe for changes in quantity, consistency, and color of sputum. Provide humidification to liquefy secretions.
◆ Observe closely for respiratory arrest. Auscultate for chest sounds.
◆ Monitor ABG levels and report changes immediately.
◆ Monitor serum electrolyte levels and correct imbalances.
◆ Monitor fluid balance by recording intake and output or daily weight.
◆ Check the cardiac monitor for arrhythmias.

■ Transient pleural friction rub and crackles at the embolus site
■ Third and fourth heart sound gallops with increased intensity of the pulmonic component of second heart sound
■ Pleural friction rub (if pleural infarction has occurred)
■ Crackles
■ Sudden change in mental status

Diagnostic test results

■ *V/Q scan* demonstrates a mismatch evidenced as decreased or absent perfusion in normally ventilated areas of the lung.
■ *Pulmonary angiography* may show a pulmonary vessel filling defect or an abrupt vessel ending, both of which indicate PE. Although the most definitive test, it's only used if the diagnosis can't be confirmed another

way and if anticoagulant therapy would put the patient at significant risk.

■ *12-lead electrocardiogram (ECG)* helps distinguish PE from myocardial infarction. If the patient has an extensive embolism, the ECG shows right axis deviation; right bundle-branch block; tall, peaked P waves; depressed ST segments; T-wave inversions (a sign of right-sided heart failure); and supraventricular tachyarrhythmias.

■ *Chest X-ray* helps rule out other pulmonary diseases, although it's inconclusive in the 1 to 2 hours after embolism. It may also show areas of atelectasis, an elevated diaphragm, pleural effusion, a prominent pulmonary artery and, occasionally, the characteristic wedge-shaped infiltrate that suggests pulmonary infarction.

■ *Arterial blood gas (ABG)* analysis sometimes reveals decreased partial pressure of arterial oxygen and partial pressure of arterial carbon dioxide levels from tachypnea.

■ *Hemodynamic studies* reveal an elevated pulmonary artery pressure if a thrombotic emboli is present and acutely elevated systolic, diastolic, and mean arterial pressure if a venous air emboli is present.

■ *Magnetic resonance imaging* can identify blood flow changes that point to an embolus or identify the embolus itself.

COLLABORATIVE MANAGEMENT

The patient with PE requires a multidisciplinary approach to care, including maximizing oxygenation, maintaining cardiopulmonary function and hemodynamic status, and reducing oxygen demand with rest and limitation of activity. A surgeon may be consulted if embolectomy is indicated (for example, if other therapies have been ineffective and the patient is experiencing severe hemodynamic compromise). A surgeon may insert a vena caval filter if the patient has had recurrent emboli. A physical therapist and an occupational therapist may assist the patient in adjusting to activity limitations and teach him methods of energy conservation.

TREATMENT AND CARE

■ Provide oxygen therapy, as needed.
■ Administer heparin by I.V. push or continuous drip, as ordered, and monitor partial thromboplastin time (PTT) daily.

　　RED FLAG Effective heparin therapy raises the PTT to more than $1\frac{1}{2}$

times the normal rate. Watch the patient closely for nosebleed, petechiae, and other signs of abnormal bleeding. Check stools for occult blood. Institute bleeding precautions to reduce the risk of hemorrhage.

■ Administer fibrinolytic therapy with urokinase, streptokinase, or alteplase, as ordered, to enhance fibrinolysis of the pulmonary emboli and remaining thrombi.
■ If necessary, administer vasopressors to treat hypotension due to emboli.
■ Be prepared to administer antibiotics for septic emboli and to obtain tests to determine the infection's source.
■ If ordered, give a combination of heparin and dihydroergotamine to prevent postoperative venous thromboembolism.
■ Give oxygen by nasal cannula or mask; assess ABG levels if the patient develops fresh emboli or worsening dyspnea. Be prepared to provide endotracheal intubation with assisted ventilation if breathing is severely compromised.
■ Encourage activity within the patient's limits, including ambulation, isometric exercises, and range of motion, after the patient has stabilized.
■ Continue with oral anticoagulant therapy such as warfarin (Coumadin) for 3 to 6 months after PE.
■ Provide patient teaching about oral anticoagulant therapy, including possible adverse effects and the need for follow-up laboratory testing to monitor therapy.

R

Respiratory acidosis

Respiratory acidosis is an acid-base disturbance characterized by reduced alveolar ventilation. Impaired carbon dioxide clearance leads to hypercapnia (partial pressure of arterial carbon dioxide [$Paco_2$] greater than 45 mm Hg) and acidosis (pH less than 7.35). Respiratory acidosis can be acute (due to a sudden failure in ventilation) or chronic (in long-term pulmonary disease).

ETIOLOGY

Respiratory acidosis can result from neuromuscular problems, depression of the respiratory center in the brain, lung disease, or an airway obstruction. Specific factors that can lead to respiratory acidosis include:
■ drugs (opioids, general anesthetics, hypnotics, alcohol, and sedatives, including such drugs as MCMA or "ecstasy" decrease the sensitivity of the respiratory center)
■ central nervous system (CNS) trauma (injury to the medulla may impair ventilatory drive)
■ cardiac arrest
■ sleep apnea
■ chronic metabolic alkalosis as respiratory compensatory mechanisms try to normalize pH by decreasing alveolar ventilation
■ ventilation therapy
- high-flow oxygen in patients with chronic respiratory disorders suppresses the hypoxic drive to breathe
- high positive end-expiratory pressure in the presence of reduced cardiac output may cause hypercapnia due to increases in dead space
■ neuromuscular diseases, such as myasthenia gravis, Guillain-Barré syndrome, and poliomyelitis (respiratory muscles can't respond properly to respiratory drive)

■ parenchymal lung disease (interferes with alveolar ventilation)
■ chronic obstructive pulmonary disease, respiratory infections, or asthma (decreases the amount of pulmonary surface area available for gas exchange)
■ severe acute respiratory distress syndrome (reduced pulmonary blood flow and poor exchange of carbon dioxide and oxygen between the lungs and blood)
■ chronic bronchitis
■ large pneumothorax
■ extensive pneumonia
■ pulmonary edema.
Prognosis depends on the severity of the underlying disturbance as well as the patient's general clinical condition. The prognosis is least optimistic for patients with debilitating disorders.

PATHOPHYSIOLOGY

A compromise in any of the three essential parts of breathing — ventilation, perfusion, and diffusion — may result in respiratory acidosis. (See *What happens in respiratory acidosis,* pages 304 and 305.) Although it initially affects the respiratory system, respiratory acidosis can affect other body systems, placing the patient at risk for numerous complications.

Cardiovascular system
■ Cardiovascular deterioration occurs when blood pH is less than 7.15.
■ The movement of hydrogen ions into cells overwhelms compensatory mechanisms.
■ Changes in electrolyte concentrations affect cardiac contractility.
■ Anaerobic metabolism produces lactic acid, which depresses the myocardium, leading to shock and cardiac arrest. (See *Disorders affecting management of respiratory acidosis,* pages 306 to 309.)

WHAT HAPPENS IN RESPIRATORY ACIDOSIS

This series of illustrations shows how respiratory acidosis develops at the cellular level.

When pulmonary ventilation decreases, retained carbon dioxide (CO_2) combines with water (H_2O) to form carbonic acid (H_2CO_3) in larger-than-normal amounts. The carbonic acid dissociates to release free hydrogen ions (H^+) and bicarbonate ions (HCO_3^-). The excessive carbonic acid causes a drop in pH. *Look for a partial pressure of arterial carbon dioxide ($Paco_2$) level above 45 mm Hg and a pH level below 7.35.*

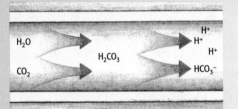

As the pH level falls, 2,3-diphosphoglycerate (2,3-DPG) increases in the red blood cells and causes a change in hemoglobin (Hb) that makes Hb release oxygen (O_2). The altered Hb, now strongly alkaline, picks up H^+ and CO_2, thus eliminating some of the free H^+ and excess CO_2. *Look for decreased arterial oxygen saturation.*

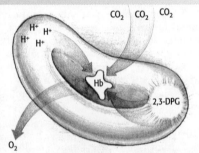

Whenever $Paco_2$ increases, CO_2 builds up in all tissues and fluids, including cerebrospinal fluid and the respiratory center in the medulla. The CO_2 reacts with water to form carbonic acid, which then breaks into free H^+ and bicarbonate ions. The increased amount of CO_2 and free H^+ stimulate the respiratory center to increase the respiratory rate. An increased respiratory rate expels more CO_2 and helps to reduce the CO_2 level in blood and tissues. *Look for rapid, shallow respirations and a decreasing $Paco_2$.*

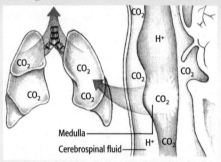

Eventually, CO_2 and H^+ cause cerebral blood vessels to dilate, which increases blood flow to the brain. That increased flow can cause cerebral edema and depress central nervous system activity. *Look for headache, confusion, lethargy, nausea, and vomiting.*

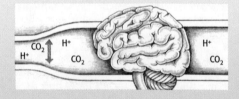

Neurologic system

■ Carbon dioxide and hydrogen ions dilate cerebral blood vessels and increase blood flow to the brain, causing cerebral edema and depressing CNS activity.

■ Profound CNS deterioration occurs as a result of a dangerously low blood pH (less than 7.15).

Renal system

■ As respiratory mechanisms fail, rising $Paco_2$ stimulates the kidneys to retain bicarbonate and sodium ions and excrete hydrogen ions, leading to greater availability of sodium bicarbonate ($NaHCO_3$) to buffer free hydrogen ions.

dissociates to release free hydrogen and bicarbonate (HCO_3^-) ions.

■ Increased $Paco_2$ and free hydrogen ions stimulate the medulla to increase respiratory drive and expel carbon dioxide.

■ As pH falls, 2,3-diphosphoglycerate (2,3-DPG) accumulates in red blood cells, where it alters hemoglobin and releases oxygen. This activity reduces hemoglobin, which is strongly alkaline; picks up hydrogen ions and carbon dioxide; and removes them from the serum.

ASSESSMENT
Clinical features vary according to the underlying disease, the presence of hypoxemia, and the cause, severity, and duration of respiratory acidosis.

Clinical findings
■ Headache
■ Altered level of consciousness, ranging from restlessness, confusion, and apprehension to somnolence and coma
■ Dyspnea
■ Diaphoresis
■ Nausea and vomiting
■ Warm, flushed skin
■ Papilledema
■ Depressed reflexes
■ Fine or flapping tremor (asterixis)
■ Hypoxemia, unless the patient is receiving oxygen
■ Tachycardia
■ Hypertension
■ Atrial and ventricular arrhythmias
■ Hypotension with vasodilation
■ Rapid, shallow respirations
■ Diminished or absent breath sounds over the affected area
■ Greatly decreased respiratory rate if acidosis stems from CNS trauma or lesions or drug overdose
■ Cyanosis (late sign)

Diagnostic test results
■ *Arterial blood gas (ABG) analysis* shows $Paco_2$ greater than 45 mmHg, pH less than 7.35, and normal HCO_3^- in the acute stage (confirms the diagnosis).
■ *Chest X-ray* commonly shows causes such as heart failure, pneumonia, chronic obstructive pulmonary disease (COPD), and pneumothorax.

As respiratory mechanisms fail, the increasing $Paco_2$ stimulates the kidneys to conserve bicarbonate and sodium ions and to excrete H^+, some in the form of ammonium (NH_4). The additional HCO_3^- and sodium combine to form extra sodium bicarbonate ($NaHCO_3$), which is then able to buffer more free H^+. *Look for increased acid content in the urine, increased serum pH and HCO_3^- levels, and shallow, depressed respirations.*

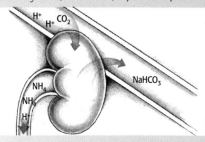

As the concentration of H^+ overwhelms the body's compensatory mechanisms, the H^+ moves into the cells, and potassium (K) ions move out. A concurrent lack of oxygen causes an increase in the anaerobic production of lactic acid, which further skews the acid-base balance and critically depresses neurologic and cardiac functions. *Look for hyperkalemia, arrhythmias, increased $Paco_2$, decreased partial pressure of arterial oxygen (Pao_2), decreased pH, and decreased level of consciousness.*

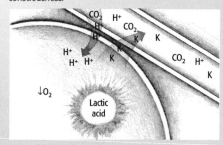

Respiratory system
■ Decreased pulmonary ventilation leads to increased $Paco_2$, and the carbon dioxide level rises in all tissues (including the medulla) and in all fluids (including cerebrospinal fluid).
■ Retained carbon dioxide combines with water to form carbonic acid (H_2CO_3), which

(Text continues on page 308.)

DISORDERS AFFECTING MANAGEMENT OF RESPIRATORY ACIDOSIS

This chart highlights disorders that affect the management of respiratory acidosis.

DISORDER	SIGNS AND SYMPTOMS	DIAGNOSTIC TEST RESULTS
Cardiac arrhythmias (complication)	◆ May be asymptomatic ◆ Dizziness ◆ Hypotension ◆ Syncope ◆ Weakness ◆ Cool, clammy skin ◆ Altered level of consciousness ◆ Reduced urine output ◆ Shortness of breath ◆ Chest pain	◆ Electrocardiography (ECG) detects arrhythmias as well as ischemia and infarction that may result in arrhythmias. ◆ Laboratory testing may reveal electrolyte abnormalities, acid-base abnormalities, or drug toxicities that may cause arrhythmias.
Hyperkalemia (complication)	◆ Abdominal cramping ◆ Diarrhea ◆ Hypotension ◆ Irregular pulse rate; tachycardia changing to bradycardia ◆ Irritability ◆ Muscle weakness, especially of the lower extremities ◆ Nausea ◆ Paresthesia	◆ Serum potassium level is greater than 5 mEq/L. ◆ ECG reveals changes (first noted as a tall, tented T wave; widened QRS complex; prolonged PR interval; flattened or absent P wave; and depressed ST-segment). ◆ Arterial blood gas (ABG) analysis reveals decreased pH and metabolic acidosis.
Shock (coexisting)	◆ Tachycardia and bounding pulse ◆ Restlessness and hypoxia ◆ Restlessness and irritability ◆ Tachypnea ◆ Reduced urinary output or anuria ◆ Cool, pale skin ◆ Hypotension ◆ Narrowed pulse pressure ◆ Reduced stroke volume ◆ Weak, rapid, thready pulse ◆ Shallow respirations	◆ Coagulation studies may detect coagulopathy from disseminated intravascular coagulation. ◆ White blood cell count and erythrocyte sedimentation rate may be increased. ◆ Blood urea nitrogen and creatinine are elevated. ◆ Serum lactate may be increased. ◆ Serum glucose may be elevated in early stages. ◆ Cardiac enzymes and proteins may be elevated. ◆ ABG analysis may reveal respiratory alkalosis in early shock or respiratory acidosis in later stages. ◆ Urine specific gravity may be high. ◆ Chest X-rays may be normal in early stages; pulmonary congestion may be seen in later stages. ◆ Hemodynamic monitoring may reveal characteristic patterns of intracardiac pressures and cardiac output.

TREATMENT AND CARE

- When life-threatening arrhythmias develop, rapidly assess level of consciousness, respirations, and pulse rate.
- Initiate cardiopulmonary resuscitation if indicated.
- Evaluate cardiac output resulting from arrhythmias.
- If the patient develops heart block, prepare for cardiac pacing.
- Administer antiarrhythmic agents as ordered.
- Prepare to assist with medical procedures if indicated.
- Assess intake and output every hour; insert an indwelling urinary catheter as indicated to ensure accurate urine measurement.
- Document arrhythmias in a monitored patient and assess for possible causes and effects.
- If the patient's pulse is abnormally rapid, slow, or irregular, watch for signs of hypoperfusion, such as hypotension and diminished urine output.
- Monitor for predisposing factors, such as fluid and electrolyte imbalance or possible drug toxicity.

- Assess vital signs. Anticipate cardiac monitoring if the patient's serum potassium level exceeds 6 mEq/L.
- Monitor the patient's intake and output and report an output of less than 30 ml/hour.
- Administer a slow calcium gluconate I.V. infusion to counteract the myocardial depressant effects of hyperkalemia.
- For a patient receiving repeated insulin and glucose treatments, check for signs and symptoms of hypoglycemia, including muscle weakness, syncope, hunger, and diaphoresis.
- Administer sodium polystyrene sulfonate and monitor serum sodium levels which may rise; assess for signs of heart failure. Encourage the patient to retain sodium polystyrene sulfonate enemas for 30 to 60 minutes. Monitor the patient for hypokalemia when administering the drug on 2 or more consecutive days.
- Monitor bowel sounds and the number and character of bowel movements.
- Monitor serum potassium level and related laboratory test results.
- Begin continuous cardiac monitoring if serum potassium level exceeds 6 mEq/L.
- If the patient has acute hyperkalemia that doesn't respond to other treatments, prepare for dialysis.
- If the patient has muscle weakness, implement safety measures.
- Assess for signs of hypokalemia after treatment.

- Assist in identifying and treating the underlying cause.
- Maintain a patent airway; prepare for intubation and mechanical ventilation if respiratory distress develops.
- Administer supplemental oxygen.
- Use continuous cardiac monitoring to detect changes in heart rate and rhythm; administer antiarrhythmics as necessary.
- Monitor blood pressure, pulse rate, peripheral pulses, and other vital signs every 15 minutes; report changes.
- Monitor central venous pressure, pulmonary artery wedge pressure, and cardiac output, as ordered, and report changes.
- Initiate and maintain at least two I.V. lines with large-gauge needles for fluid and drug administration.
- Administer I.V. fluids, crystalloids, colloids, or blood products, as necessary, to maintain intravascular volume.
- Administer inotropic drugs, such as dopamine, dobutamine, and epinephrine, to increase heart contractility and cardiac output.
- Administer vasodilators, such as nitroglycerin or nitroprusside, with a vasopressor to reduce the left ventricle's workload.
- Monitor intake, output, and daily weight. Administer diuretics to reduce preload if patient has fluid volume overload.
- Initiate intra-aortic balloon pump therapy to reduce the work of the left ventricle by decreasing systemic vascular resistance. Monitor the patient carefully.
- Monitor the patient receiving thrombolytic therapy or coronary artery revascularization per facility protocol.

(continued)

DISORDERS AFFECTING
MANAGEMENT OF RESPIRATORY ACIDOSIS *(continued)*

DISORDER	SIGNS AND SYMPTOMS	DIAGNOSTIC TEST RESULTS
Shock *(continued)*	◆ Cyanosis ◆ Unconsciousness and absent reflexes in irreversible stages	◆ ECG determines heart rate and detects arrhythmias, ischemic changes, and MI. ◆ Echocardiography determines left ventricular function and reveals valvular abnormalities.

■ *Serum potassium level* is usually greater than 5 mEq/L.

■ *Serum chloride level* is low.

■ *Urine pH* is acidic as the kidneys excrete hydrogen ions to return blood pH to normal.

■ *Drug screening* may confirm suspected drug overdose.

COLLABORATIVE MANAGEMENT
Caring for the patient with respiratory acidosis requires a multidisciplinary approach. A pulmonologist and a respiratory therapist collaborate to manage the patient's ventilatory efforts and restore normal ABG values. A cardiologist may be consulted if a heart condition is the underlying cause or if the patient develops an arrhythmia or cardiac arrest. A renal care specialist may assist in managing the patient's pH and ABG status to help normalize values. A neurologist may be consulted if the underlying cause is related to the CNS or if the patient develops CNS sequelae.

TREATMENT AND CARE
■ Be prepared to perform or assist with:
– removal of a foreign body from the airway
– providing an artificial airway through endotracheal intubation or tracheotomy and mechanical ventilation (if the patient can't breathe spontaneously)
– measures to increase partial pressure of arterial oxygen to at least 60 mm Hg and pH greater than 7.2 to prevent cardiac arrhythmias

– administration of aerosolized or I.V. bronchodilators to open constricted airways
– administration of antibiotics to treat pneumonia
– insertion of chest tubes to correct pneumothorax
– administration of positive end-expiratory pressure to prevent alveolar collapse
– administration of thrombolytic or anticoagulant therapy for massive pulmonary emboli
– bronchoscopy to remove excessive retained secretions.

■ If the underlying cause is a chronic respiratory disorder such as COPD, expect to:
– administer bronchodilators, corticosteroids, and oxygen at low flow rates
– perform gradual reduction in $Paco_2$ to baseline to provide sufficient chloride and potassium ions to enhance renal excretion of bicarbonate (in chronic respiratory acidosis).

RED FLAG *The patient with COPD generally receives lower concentrations of oxygen because his medulla is accustomed to high carbon dioxide levels. Lack of oxygen or hypoxic drive stimulates breathing; excessive oxygen diminishes that drive and depresses the respiratory effort, further reducing alveolar ventilation.*

■ Administer appropriate drug therapy for underlying conditions such as myasthenia gravis.

■ Be prepared to assist with dialysis or administer charcoal to remove toxic drugs.

■ Correct associated metabolic alkalosis.

◆ Prepare for emergency surgery if repair of a ruptured papillary muscle is required or if a ventricular septal defect is present.
◆ Monitor the patient with a ventricular assist device.

■ Carefully administer I.V. sodium bicarbonate.
■ Monitor vital signs, and assess cardiac rate and rhythm.
■ Continually assess respiratory patterns, including rate and depth of respirations and breath sounds.
■ Frequently monitor the patient's neurologic status for changes.
■ Evaluate results of ABG studies, pulse oximetry, or serum electrolyte studies.
■ Perform tracheal suctioning, incentive spirometry, and postural drainage.
■ Encourage coughing and deep breathing exercises as indicated.
■ Ensure adequate fluid intake and monitor intake and output.

Respiratory alkalosis

Respiratory alkalosis is an acid-base disturbance characterized by a partial pressure of arterial carbon dioxide ($Paco_2$) less than 35 mm Hg and blood pH greater than 7.45. Hypocapnia (below normal $Paco_2$) occurs when the lungs eliminate more carbon dioxide (CO_2) than the cells produce.

Respiratory alkalosis is the most common acid-base disturbance in patients who are critically ill and, when severe, has a poor prognosis.

ETIOLOGY
Any condition that increases the respiratory rate or depth can cause the lungs to eliminate CO_2. Eliminating CO_2 causes a decrease in $Paco_2$ as well as an increase in pH.

Causes of respiratory alkalosis fall into two categories:
■ Pulmonary causes include severe hypoxemia, pneumonia, interstitial lung disease, pulmonary vascular disease, acute asthma, and mechanical overventilation.
■ Nonpulmonary causes include anxiety, fever, aspirin toxicity, metabolic acidosis, central nervous system inflammation or tumor, sepsis, hepatic failure, and pregnancy.

Acute hypoxia secondary to high altitude, pulmonary disease, severe anemia, pulmonary embolus, or hypotension can also lead to respiratory alkalosis.

PATHOPHYSIOLOGY
Increased pulmonary ventilation leads to excessive exhalation of CO_2, resulting in hypocapnia. Chemical reduction of carbonic acid occurs, along with excretion of hydrogen and bicarbonate ions, and elevated pH. (See *What happens in respiratory alkalosis,* pages 310 and 311.)

Although it begins in the respiratory system, respiratory alkalosis can affect other body systems, placing the patient at risk for numerous complications. (See *Disorders affecting management of respiratory alkalosis,* pages 312 and 313.)

Cardiovascular system
■ Hypocapnia stimulates the carotid and aortic bodies and the medulla, increasing the heart rate (which hypokalemia can further aggravate) without increasing blood pressure. Stimulation can also alter the excitabil-

WHAT HAPPENS IN RESPIRATORY ALKALOSIS

This series of illustrations shows how respiratory alkalosis develops at the cellular level. When pulmonary ventilation increases above the amount needed to maintain normal carbon dioxide (CO_2) levels, excessive amounts of CO_2 are exhaled. This causes hypocapnia (a fall in $Paco_2$), which leads to a reduction in carbonic acid (H_2CO_3) production, a loss of hydrogen (H^+) ions and bicarbonate (HCO_3^-) ions, and a subsequent rise in pH. *Look for a pH level above 7.45, a $Paco_2$ level below 35 mm Hg, and an HCD_3^- level below 22 mEq/L.*

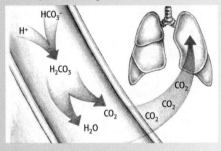

In defense against the rising pH, H^+ ions are pulled out of the cells and into the blood in exchange for potassium (K) ions. The H^+ ions entering the blood combine with HCO_3^- ions to form carbonic acid, which lowers pH. *Look for a further decrease in HCO_3^- levels, a fall in pH, and a fall in serum potassium levels (hypokalemia).*

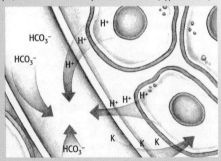

Hypocapnia stimulates the carotid and aortic bodies and the medulla, which causes an increase in heart rate without an increase in blood pressure. *Look for angina, electrocardiogram changes, restlessness, and anxiety.*

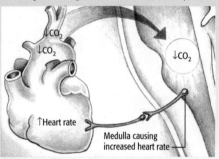

$\downarrow CO_2$
$\downarrow CO_2$
$\downarrow CO_2$
↑Heart rate
Medulla causing increased heart rate

Simultaneously, hypocapnia produces cerebral vasoconstriction, which prompts a reduction in cerebral blood flow. Hypocapnia also overexcites the medulla, pons, and other parts of the autonomic nervous system. *Look for increasing anxiety, diaphoresis, dyspnea, alternating periods of apnea and hyperventilation, dizziness, and tingling in the fingers or toes.*

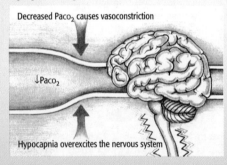

Decreased $Paco_2$ causes vasoconstriction

$\downarrow Paco_2$

Hypocapnia overexcites the nervous system

ity of the myocardium, leading to arrhythmias.

■ The risk for arrhythmias is further compounded by the shift of potassium into the cells, which can lead to hypokalemia and the

inhibition of calcium ionization, ultimately leading to hypocalcemia.

■ Continued low $Paco_2$ increases vasoconstriction, ultimately impairing blood flow to the peripheral tissues.

blood flow. It also overexcites the medulla, pons, and other parts of the autonomic nervous system, resulting in anxiety and dizziness.

■ Continued low $Paco_2$ and the resulting vasoconstriction increases cerebral and peripheral hypoxia.

■ Severe alkalosis inhibits calcium ionization, thus nerves and muscles become progressively more excitable. Hypocalcemia can occur.

■ Eventually, alkalosis overwhelms the CNS, resulting in a decreased level of consciousness, hyperreflexia, carpopedal spasms, tetany, seizures, and coma.

Renal system
■ If hypocapnia lasts more than 6 hours, the kidneys increase secretion of bicarbonate and reduce secretion of hydrogen, leading to low pH.

Respiratory system
■ Hypocapnia occurs in respiratory alkalosis regardless of the underlying cause. The rate and depth of respirations increase in an attempt to retain CO_2 and decrease pH.

■ Increasing serum pH causes hydrogen ions to shift from cells to the blood in exchange for potassium ions. The hydrogen ions combine with available bicarbonate ions in the blood to form carbonic acid, resulting in decreased pH.

ASSESSMENT
An increase in the rate and depth of respirations is a primary sign of respiratory alkalosis. Other signs and symptoms vary, depending on the severity of the condition.

Clinical findings
■ Complaints of muscle weakness or difficulty breathing
■ Deep, rapid breathing (possibly more than 40 breaths/minute and much like the Kussmaul's respirations that characterize diabetic acidosis)
■ CNS and neuromuscular disturbances (cardinal sign) including anxiety, restlessness, confusion or syncope, tingling in fingers and toes, progressive decrease in LOC, seizures, and coma
■ Diaphoresis
■ Agitation
■ Light-headedness or dizziness

(Text continues on page 314.)

When hypocapnia lasts more than 6 hours, the kidneys increase secretion of HCO_3^- and reduce excretion of H^+. Periods of apnea may result if the pH remains high and the $Paco_2$ remains low. *Look for slowed respiratory rate, hypoventilation, and Cheyne-Stokes respirations.*

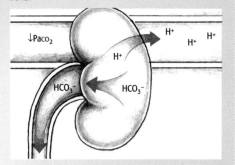

Continued low $Paco_2$ increases cerebral and peripheral hypoxia from vasoconstriction. Severe alkalosis inhibits calcium (Ca) ionization, which in turn causes increased nerve excitability and muscle contractions. Eventually, the alkalosis overwhelms the central nervous system and the heart. *Look for decreasing level of consciousness, hyperreflexia, carpopedal spasm, tetany, arrhythmias, seizures, and coma.*

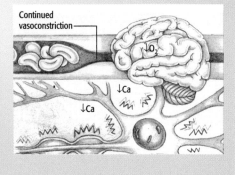

■ Eventually, alkalosis overwhelms the heart's ability to function.

Neurologic system
■ Hypocapnia causes cerebral vasoconstriction, which prompts a reduction in cerebral

DISORDERS AFFECTING
MANAGEMENT OF RESPIRATORY ALKALOSIS

This chart highlights disorders that affect the management of respiratory alkalosis.

DISORDER	SIGNS AND SYMPTOMS	DIAGNOSTIC TEST RESULTS
Cardiac arrhythmias (complication)	◆ Palpitations ◆ Chest pain ◆ Dizziness ◆ Weakness, fatigue ◆ Irregular heart rhythm ◆ Hypotension ◆ Syncope ◆ Altered level of consciousness ◆ Diaphoresis ◆ Pallor ◆ Cold, clammy skin	◆ 12-lead electrocardiography (ECG) identifies waveform changes associated with the arrhythmia. ◆ Laboratory testing reveals hyperkalemia, electrolyte abnormalities, hypoxemia, or acid-base abnormalities.
Hypocalcemia (complication)	◆ Anxiety ◆ Irritability ◆ Twitching around the mouth ◆ Laryngospasm ◆ Seizures ◆ Muscle cramps ◆ Paresthesias of the face, fingers, or toes ◆ Tetany ◆ Positive Chvostek's and Trousseau's signs ◆ Hypotension ◆ Arrhythmias ◆ Hyperactive deep tendon reflexes	◆ Serum calcium level is less than 8.5 mg/dl. ◆ Ionized calcium level is usually below 4.5 mg/dl. ◆ Platelet count is decreased. ◆ EGG shows lengthened QT interval, prolonged ST segment, and arrhythmias. ◆ Serum protein levels may reveal changes because half of serum calcium is bound to albumin.
Hypokalemia (complication)	◆ Dizziness ◆ Hypotension ◆ Arrhythmias ◆ Cardiac arrest ◆ Nausea, vomiting ◆ Anorexia ◆ Diarrhea ◆ Decreased peristalsis ◆ Abdominal distention ◆ Muscle weakness ◆ Fatigue ◆ Leg cramps	◆ Serum potassium is less than 3.5 mEq/L. ◆ Arterial blood gas analysis reveals metabolic alkalosis. ◆ EGG changes include flattened T waves, elevated U waves, and a depressed ST segment.

TREATMENT AND CARE

◆ Evaluate the monitored patient's ECG regularly for arrhythmias and assess hemodynamic parameters as indicated. Document arrhythmias and notify the physician immediately.
◆ Assess an unmonitored patient for rhythm disturbances. If the patient's pulse rate is abnormally rapid, slow, or irregular, watch for signs of hypoperfusion, such as hypotension and diminished urine output.
◆ As ordered, obtain an ECG tracing in an unmonitored patient to confirm and identify the type of arrhythmia present.
◆ Administer medications such as antiarrhythmic agents, as ordered, and monitor the patient for adverse effects.
◆ If a life-threatening arrhythmia develops, rapidly assess the patient's level of consciousness, pulse and respiratory rates, and hemodynamic parameters. Be alert for trends. Monitor EGG continuously. Be prepared to initiate cardiopulmonary resuscitation or cardioversion if indicated.

◆ Assess cardiovascular status and neurologic status for changes; monitor vital signs frequently.
◆ Monitor respiratory status, including rate, depth, and rhythm. Watch for stridor, dyspnea, and crowing.
◆ Keep a tracheotomy tray and a handheld resuscitation bag at the bedside in case laryngospasm occurs.
◆ Institute cardiac monitoring, and evaluate for changes in heart rate and rhythm.
◆ Assess for Chvostek's sign or Trousseau's sign.
◆ Administer I.V. calcium replacement therapy carefully. Check magnesium and phosphate levels because a low magnesium level must be corrected before I.V. calcium can be effective; if the phosphate level is too high, calcium won't be absorbed.
◆ Ensure the patency of the I.V. line because infiltration can cause tissue necrosis and sloughing; give oral replacements as ordered. Give calcium supplements 1 to 1½ hours after meals. If GI upset occurs, give the supplement with milk.
◆ Monitor pertinent laboratory test results, including calcium, albumin, and magnesium levels and those of other electrolytes. Remember to check the ionized calcium level after every 4 units of blood transfused.
◆ Institute seizure precautions and safety measures to prevent injury.

◆ Monitor vital signs, especially pulse and blood pressure; check heart rate and rhythm and ECG tracings in patients with a serum potassium level less than 3 mEq/L (severe hypokalemia).
◆ Assess the patient's respiratory rate, depth, and pattern. Keep a manual resuscitation bag at the bedside of a patient with severe hypokalemia.
◆ Monitor serum potassium levels.
◆ Monitor and document fluid intake and output, especially when administering I.V. potassium replacement. Urine volume should be greater than 30 mL/hour to prevent rebound hyperkalemia.
◆ Check for signs of hypokalemia-related metabolic alkalosis, including irritability and paresthesia.
◆ Insert and maintain patent I.V. access.
◆ Administer I.V. potassium replacement solutions as prescribed. Administer I.V. potassium infusions cautiously. Make sure that infusions are diluted and mixed thoroughly in adequate amounts of fluid. Use premixed potassium solutions when possible.
◆ Continuously monitor heart rate and rhythm and ECG tracings of patients receiving potassium infusions of more than 5 mEq/hour or a concentration of more than 40 mEq/L of fluid.
◆ Never give potassium by I.V. push or as a bolus.
◆ Monitor the patient for signs and symptoms of hyperkalemia that may result due to potassium replacement.
◆ To prevent gastric irritation, administer oral supplements in at least 4 oz (118 ml) of fluid or with food; Never crush slow-release oral potassium supplement tablets. The patient could experience a rapid rise in potassium levels.
◆ Check for signs of constipation, such as abdominal distention and decreased bowel sounds. Although medication may be prescribed to combat constipation, avoid laxatives that promote potassium loss.

- Tachycardia
- Alternating periods of apnea and hyperventilation
- Hyperreflexia
- Carpopedal spasm
- Tetany
- Arrhythmias

Diagnostic test results

- *Arterial blood gas (ABG)* analysis shows $Paco_2$ less than 35 mm Hg, elevated pH in proportion to the decrease in $Paco_2$ in the acute stage that decreases toward normal in the chronic stage, and normal bicarbonate in the acute stage but less than normal in the chronic stage (confirms respiratory alkalosis, rules out respiratory compensation for metabolic acidosis).
- *Serum electrolyte studies* detect metabolic disorders causing compensatory respiratory alkalosis; serum chloride levels may be low in severe respiratory alkalosis.
- *Electrocardiography* reveals changes that may indicate cardiac arrhythmias.
- *Toxicology screening* reveals possible salicylate poisoning.
- *Urine pH* is basic as kidneys excrete bicarbonate to raise blood pH.

COLLABORATIVE MANAGEMENT

Respiratory alkalosis requires a multidisciplinary approach to care. A pulmonologist and a respiratory therapist will manage ventilatory interventions and care aimed at restoring normal ABG values. A cardiologist may be consulted if the patient develops an arrhythmia. A renal care specialist may be consulted to assist in normalizing the patient's pH and ABG values. A neurologist may be involved if the underlying cause involves the CNS or if the patient develops CNS sequelae. The patient may also need referrals to community or home care assistive services.

TREATMENT AND CARE

- Treatment focuses on correcting the underlying condition. Be prepared to perform or assist with:
- removal of ingested toxins, such as salicylates, by inducing emesis or performing gastric lavage
- treatment of fever or sepsis
- oxygen administration for acute hypoxemia

- treatment of CNS disease
- anxiety-reduction measures such as sedatives or antianxiety agents
- adjustment of tidal volume and minute ventilation in patients on mechanical ventilation to prevent hyperventilation.

RED FLAG *For hyperventilation caused by severe anxiety, have the patient breathe into a paper bag, which forces him to breathe exhaled carbon dioxide, thereby raising the carbon dioxide level.*

- Frequently monitor vital signs and neurologic, neuromuscular, and cardiovascular functioning. If the patient is receiving mechanical ventilation, frequently check ventilator settings.
- Evaluate ABG and serum electrolyte levels and report variations immediately. Remember that twitching and cardiac arrhythmias may be associated with alkalosis and electrolyte imbalances.
- Reassure the patient and maintain a quiet, calm environment.
- Institute seizure precautions and safety measures.

Rheumatoid arthritis

Rheumatoid arthritis (RA) is a chronic, systemic inflammatory disease that primarily attacks peripheral joints and the surrounding muscles, tendons, ligaments, and blood vessels. Partial remissions and unpredictable exacerbations mark the course of this potentially crippling disease.

RA occurs worldwide, affecting more than 6.5 million people in the United States alone. The disease occurs in women three times more often than men. RA can occur at any age, but the peak onset period for women is between ages 30 and 60. In most patients, RA follows an intermittent course and allows normal activity between exacerbations. However, 10% of patients experience total disability from severe joint deformity, associated extra-articular symptoms such as vasculitis, or both.

RA usually requires lifelong treatment, which may include surgery. The prognosis worsens with the development of nodules, vasculitis, and high titers of rheumatoid factor.

ETIOLOGY

Although the cause of RA is unknown, several theories have been proposed.

■ Individuals with genetic predisposition may experience abnormal immune activation leading to inflammation, complement activation, and cell proliferation within joints and tendon sheaths.

■ Onset of RA may be linked to hormone action, lifestyle factors, or viral or bacterial infection.

■ RA may develop as an autoimmune response causing formation of an immunoglobulin (Ig) M antibody against IgG (also called *rheumatoid factor [RF]*). RF aggregates into complexes and causes inflammation that leads to cartilage damage and triggers other immune responses.

PATHOPHYSIOLOGY

In RA, an autoimmune response causes inflammation in one or more joints. The resulting cartilage damage triggers additional immune responses, including complement activation. Polymorphonuclear leukocytes, macrophages, and lymphocytes are attracted to the area of inflammation. The immune complexes formed by the RF aggregation are destroyed or disintegrated by the leukocytes and macrophages. Subsequently, lysosomal enzymes are released, which cause destruction of the joint cartilage. This destruction sets up an inflammatory response, which draws more lymphocytes and plasma cells to the area, ultimately causing a continuous cycle of events. Continued inflammation results in hyperplasia of the cells in the synovial space and tissues. Increased capillary permeability secondary to the inflammatory response leads to swelling; vasodilation and resultant increased blood flow lead to redness and warmth.

Although typically thought of as a disorder of the musculoskeletal system, the inflammatory response can extend beyond the joints, affecting other body systems.

Cardiovascular system

■ Vasculitis results from an inflammatory response in the small and medium arterioles. Ischemia and necrosis of the affected areas can occur, ultimately leading to skin breakdown or myocardial tissue ischemia and necrosis.

■ Immune complex invasion and subsequent ischemia and necrosis of the myocardial tissue can lead to pericarditis.

Musculoskeletal system

■ If not arrested, the inflammatory process in the joints occurs in four stages: synovitis, pannus, fibrous ankylosis, and calcification.

– Synovitis develops from congestion and edema of the synovial membrane and joint capsule. Infiltration by lymphocytes, macrophages, and neutrophils continues the local inflammatory response. These cells as well as fibroblast-like synovial cells, produce enzymes that help to degrade bone and cartilage.

– Pannus — thickened layers of granulation tissue — covers and invades cartilage and eventually destroys the joint capsule and bone.

– Fibrous ankylosis — fibrous invasion of the pannus and scar formation — occludes the joint space; bone atrophy and misalignment causes visible deformities and disrupts the articulation of opposing bones, leading to muscle atrophy and imbalance and, possibly, partial dislocations (subluxations) or compression fractures. (See *Visualizing joint changes,* pages 316 and 317.)

– Fibrous tissue calcifies, resulting in bony ankylosis and total immobility.

■ As the disease progresses, the inflammation and destruction occurs to joints of the body, resulting in decreased joint mobility and pain.

■ Osteoporosis and compression fractures can occur secondary to weakening of the joint.

■ Disorders such as Sjögren's syndrome can develop because of the underlying autoimmune processes. (See *Disorders affecting management of rheumatoid arthritis,* pages 318 and 319.)

Neurologic system

■ Immune complex invasion can affect the tissue of the eyes and peripheral nerves.

■ Scleritis and peripheral neuropathy may occur, leading to numbness or tingling in the feet and loss of sensation in the fingers.

Respiratory system

■ Immune complex formation and the resultant inflammatory response can cause pulmonary tissue damage and necrosis, lead-

VISUALIZING JOINT CHANGES

Inflammatory changes in the joint are characteristic of rheumatoid arthritis. The joint inflammation progresses through four stages: synovitis, pannus formation, fibrous ankylosis and joint fixation. These illustrations highlight the inflammatory changes of the knee, hand and wrist, and hip joints.

Knee

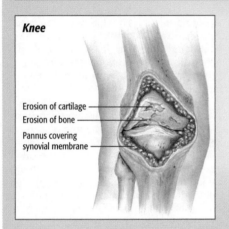

Erosion of cartilage
Erosion of bone
Pannus covering synovial membrane

Hand and wrist

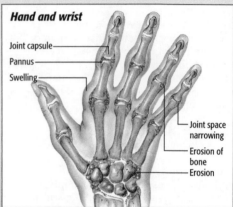

Joint capsule
Pannus
Swelling

Joint space narrowing
Erosion of bone
Erosion

ing to pulmonary nodules or fibrosis and pleuritis.

ASSESSMENT

RA usually develops insidiously; initial signs and symptoms are nonspecific. Early findings are most likely related to the initial inflammatory reactions that occur before the synovium becomes inflamed.

Clinical findings

Initially, manifestations may include:
- fatigue
- malaise
- anorexia and weight loss
- persistent low-grade fever
- lymphadenopathy
- vague articular symptoms.

As the disease progresses the patient may develop:
- specific localized, bilateral, and symmetrical articular symptoms, frequently in the fingers at the proximal interphalangeal, metacarpophalangeal, and metatarsophalangeal joints, possibly extending to the wrists, knees, elbows, and ankles from inflammation of the synovium

- stiffening of affected joints after inactivity, especially on arising in the morning due to progressive synovial inflammation and destruction
- joint pain and tenderness.

Additional signs and symptoms include:
- spindle-shaped fingers from marked edema and congestion in the joints
- redness and warmth at the joint
- diminished joint function and deformities as synovial destruction continues
- flexion deformities or hyperextension of metacarpophalangeal joints, subluxation of the wrist, and stretching of tendons pulling the fingers to the ulnar side (ulnar drift or characteristic swan-neck or boutonnière deformity from joint swelling and loss of joint space)
- carpal tunnel syndrome from synovial pressure on the median nerve causing paresthesia in the fingers
- gradual appearance of rheumatoid nodules on elbows, hands, or Achilles tendon
- vasculitis, possibly leading to skin lesions, leg ulcers, and multiple systemic complications

■ *Complete blood count* usually shows moderate anemia, slight leukocytosis, and slight thrombocytosis.

COLLABORATIVE MANAGEMENT

Caring for the patient with RA requires a multidisciplinary approach. A rheumatoid specialist will guide the management. A surgeon may be involved if the patient requires a synovectomy or other surgery. A physical therapist will provide strategies to help the patient maintain range of motion. An occupational therapist will provide training to facilitate the patient's ability to perform activities of daily living. Cardiovascular and respiratory specialists may be needed if the patient develops cardiovascular or respiratory complications. A home-care specialist may be consulted to provide support in the home environment.

TREATMENT AND CARE

■ Salicylates, particularly aspirin (mainstay of therapy), decrease inflammation and relieve joint pain.
■ Nonsteroidal anti-inflammatory drugs, such as fenoprofen (Nalfon), ibuprofen (Motrin), and indomethacin (Indocin), relieve inflammation and pain.
■ Cycloogenase-2 (COX-2) inhibitors, such as celecoxib (Celebrex), inhibit the COX-2 enzyme involved in the inflammatory response while sparing the COX-1 enzyme involved in prostaglandin synthesis.
■ Antimalarials, such as hydroxychloroquine sulfate (Plaquenil), sulfasalazine (Azulfidine), gold salts, and penicillamine (Cuprimine) reduce acute and chronic inflammation.
■ Corticosteroids, such as prednisone, may be administered in low doses for anti-inflammatory effects or higher doses for an immunosuppressive effect on T cells.
■ Azathioprine (Imuran), cyclosporine (Neoral), and methotrexate (Folex) may be administered early in the disease process to suppress the T- and B-lymphocyte proliferation that causes destruction of the synovium.
■ If indicated, prepare the patient for surgery, which may include:
– synovectomy (removal of destructive, proliferating synovium, usually in the wrists, knees, and fingers) to possibly halt or delay the course of the disease

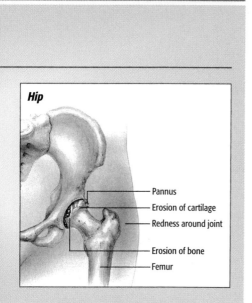

Hip

— Pannus
— Erosion of cartilage
— Redness around joint
— Erosion of bone
— Femur

■ pericarditis, pulmonary nodules of fibrosis, pleuritis, or inflammation of the sclera and overlying tissues of the eye
■ peripheral neuropathy with numbness or tingling in the feet or weakness and loss of sensation in the fingers
■ stiff, weak, or painful muscles secondary to limited mobility and decreased use.

Diagnostic test results

■ *X-rays* show bone demineralization and soft-tissue swelling (early stages), cartilage loss and narrowed joint spaces, and cartilage and bone destruction and erosion, subluxations, and deformities (later stages).
■ *RF titer* is positive (1:160 or higher) in 75% to 80% of patients.
■ *Synovial fluid analysis* shows increased volume and turbidity but decreased viscosity and elevated white blood cell count (usually greater than 10,000/μl).
■ *Serum protein electrophoresis* possibly shows elevated serum globulin levels.
■ *Erythrocyte sedimentation rate* and *C-reactive protein levels* reveal elevations in 85% to 90% of patients.

DISORDERS AFFECTING
MANAGEMENT OF RHEUMATOID ARTHRITIS

This chart highlights disorders that affect the management of rheumatoid arthritis.

DISORDER	SIGNS AND SYMPTOMS	DIAGNOSTIC TEST RESULTS
Osteoporosis (complication)	◆ Vertebral collapse ◆ Backache with pain that radiates around the trunk ◆ Increased deformity of the spine ◆ Kyphosis ◆ Loss of height ◆ Markedly aged appearance	◆ X-rays show typical degeneration in the lower thoracic and lumbar vertebrae. The vertebral bodies may appear flattened and may look denser than normal. ◆ Bone mineral density shows demineralization. Loss of bone mineral becomes evident in later stages. ◆ Dual- or single-photon absorptiometry allows measurement of bone mass, which helps to assess the extremities, hips, and spine. ◆ Serum calcium, phosphorus, and alkaline phosphatase levels are all within normal limits, but parathyroid hormone level may be elevated. ◆ Bone biopsy shows thin, porous, but otherwise normal-looking bone.
Sjögren's syndrome (complication)	◆ Confirmed rheumatoid arthritis and a history of slowly developing sicca complex (in about 50% of patients) ◆ Oral dryness, redness, burning, difficulty swallowing, ulcers, dental caries ◆ Difficulty talking ◆ Abnormal sense of taste or smell (or both) ◆ Photosensitivity, eye fatigue, itching and mucoid discharge ◆ Dyspareunia and pruritus ◆ Generalized itching ◆ Fatigue ◆ Recurrent low-grade fever ◆ Arthralgia or myalgia and extraglandular findings, such as pneumonitis, nephritis, arthritis, neuropathy, and vasculitis	◆ A patient with Sjögren's syndrome has at least two of these conditions: xerophthalmia, xerostomia, and an associated autoimmune or lymphoproliferative disorder. ◆ Antinuclear antibody testing is positive.
Spinal compression fractures (complication)	◆ Muscle spasms and back pain that worsens with movement ◆ Point tenderness with cervical fractures ◆ Pain radiating to other body areas with dorsal and lumbar fractures ◆ Mild paresthesia to quadriplegia and shock (if injury involves the spinal cord)	◆ Computed tomography scan, magnetic resonance imaging, and X-rays locate fracture.

– osteotomy (cutting of bone or excision of a wedge of bone) to realign joint surfaces and redistribute stress
– tendon transfers to prevent deformities or relieve contractures

– joint reconstruction or total joint arthroplasty, such as metatarsal head and distal ulnar resectional arthroplasty or insertion of a Silastic prosthesis between metacarpophalangeal and proximal interphalangeal joints (severe disease)

TREATMENT AND CARE

◆ Carefully position the patient.
◆ Assist in ambulation and prescribed exercises.
◆ Check skin for redness, warmth, and new sites of pain, which may indicate new fracture.
◆ Perform passive range-of-motion exercises, or encourage the patient to perform active exercise.
◆ Institute safety precautions and help prevent fractures.
◆ Provide a balanced diet high in nutrients that support skeletal metabolism, such as vitamin D, calcium, and protein.
◆ Administer an analgesic and use heat to relieve pain.
◆ Teach the patient about the drug regimen, bracing (if indicated), and proper body mechanics

◆ Advise the patient to avoid drugs that decrease saliva production, such as atropine derivatives, antihistamines, anitcholinergics, and antidepressants.
◆ Suggest high-protein, high-calorie liquid supplements to prevent malnutrition when mouth ulcers are painful.
◆ Encourage good oral hygiene.
◆ Suggest use of sunglasses to protect eyes.
◆ Encourage humidification in the home to prevent dryness of nasal passages.
◆ Advise to avoid prolonged hot showers and baths and to use moisturizing lotions to help ease dry skin.

◆ Suspect cord damage until proven otherwise.
◆ Immobilize the patient on a firm surface.
◆ Prepare for surgical correction as necessary.
◆ Institute traction, as ordered, and assess circulation and effects of traction.
◆ Assist the patient with turning, log rolling, deep breathing, and coughing to prevent complications.
◆ Monitor vital signs and neurologic status; report changes.
◆ Assess respiratory function and effort.

– arthrodesis (joint fusion) for stability and relief from pain (sacrifices joint mobility).
■ Prepare the patient for possible diaphoresis to remove IgG and IgG-circulating immune complexes from the plasma (for patients with severe RA who haven't responded to drug therapy).
■ Carefully assess all joints for deformities, contractures, immobility, and inability to perform activities of daily living.

■ Administer analgesics and use heat to manage pain.

■ Provide meticulous skin care, including checking for rheumatoid nodules, pressure ulcers, and breakdowns due to immobility, vascular impairment, drug therapy, or improper splinting.

■ Monitor the duration as well as the intensity of morning stiffness; duration is a more accurate reflection of the severity of the disease.

■ Use splints and assistive devices to promote self-care and independence as indicated.

■ Provide patient teaching related to living with a chronic condition and using measures to promote maximum independence and minimize complications.

S

Scoliosis

Scoliosis is a lateral curvature of the thoracic, lumbar, or thoracolumbar spine. The curve may be convex to the right (more common in thoracic curves) or to the left (more common in lumbar curves). Scoliosis is commonly associated with kyphosis (hump back) and lordosis (swayback).

ETIOLOGY

Scoliosis may be either functional or structural. Functional, or postural, scoliosis results from poor posture or a discrepancy in leg lengths rather than from fixed deformity of the spinal column.

Structural scoliosis involves deformity of the vertebral bodies and may occur in the following forms.

■ Congenital scoliosis may occur as wedge vertebrae, fused ribs or vertebrae, or hemivertebrae.

■ Paralytic or musculoskeletal scoliosis develops several months after asymmetric paralysis of the trunk muscles from polio, cerebral palsy, muscular dystrophy, or certain spinal cord injuries.

■ Idiopathic scoliosis, the most common type, may be transmitted as an autosomal dominant or multifactorial trait. It appears in a previously straight spine during adolescence.

Idiopathic scoliosis can be further classified according to age at onset.

■ Infantile — affects mostly male infants between birth and age 3 and causes left thoracic and right lumbar curves

■ Juvenile — affects both sexes between ages 4 and 10 and causes varying types of curvature

■ Adolescent — generally affects girls from age 10 until skeletal maturity and causes varying types of curvature

■ Adult — generally the result of untreated adolescent scoliosis or asymmetric degeneration of spinal elements (osteoporosis).

About 2% to 3% of adolescents have scoliosis. In general, the greater the magnitude of the curve and the younger the child at the time of diagnosis, the greater the risk of spinal abnormality progression. Favorable outcomes are usually achieved with optimal treatment.

PATHOPHYSIOLOGY

The underlying pathophysiology of scoliosis involves the vertebral bones; however, other systems can be affected, such as the cardiovascular and respiratory systems, as the curvature increases.

Cardiovascular system

■ Restricted lung capacity due to rib cage deformity leads to constriction of pulmonary blood vessels and obstruction of pulmonary blood flow.

■ Obstructed pulmonary blood flow increases pulmonary vascular resistance, leading to pulmonary hypertension, right ventricular hypertrophy, and, possibly, cor pulmonale.

Musculoskeletal system

■ The vertebrae rotate, forming the convex part of the curve, causing rib prominence along the thoracic spin and waistline asymmetry in the lumbar spine.

■ Differential stresses on vertebral bone causes an imbalance of osteoblastic activity, leading to rapid progression of the curve during the adolescent growth spurt.

Respiratory system

■ Rib cage deformity due to rotation of the vertebral column may lead to chest wall abnormalities that impair respiratory function.

■ Restriction of chest wall motion decreases lung capacity, leading to respiratory insuf-

DISORDERS AFFECTING MANAGEMENT OF SCOLIOSIS

This chart highlights disorders that affect the management of scoliosis.

DISORDER	SIGNS AND SYMPTOMS	DIAGNOSTIC TEST RESULTS
Respiratory insufficiency (complication)	◆ Dyspnea on exertion ◆ Diminished chest movement ◆ Restlessness, irritability, and confusion ◆ Tachypnea, tachycardia ◆ Diminished breath sounds; possible adventitious breath sounds ◆ Possibly fever (if pneumonia is present)	◆ Arterial blood gas (ABG) analysis may indicate early respiratory failure if partial pressure of arterial oxygen is low (usually less than 70 mm Hg), partial pressure of arterial carbon dioxide is greater than 45 mm Hg, and the bicarbonate level is normal. ◆ Pulmonary function studies reveal a decrease in vital capacity, total lung capacity, and inspiratory capacity. ◆ Pulse oximetry may reveal a decreased oxygen saturation level.
Vertebral disk disease (complication)	◆ Back pain ◆ Sciatica ◆ Muscle spasm	◆ Magnetic resonance imaging reveals degenerative changes or disk herniation. ◆ Lumbosacral X-rays rule out tumors

ficiency and, ultimately, respiratory failure (if left untreated). (See *Disorders affecting management of scoliosis.*)

ASSESSMENT

The most common curve in functional or structural scoliosis occurs in the thoracic segment, with convexity to the right and compensatory curves (S curves) in the cervical and lumbar segments, both with convexity to the left. As the spine curves laterally, compensatory curves develop to maintain body balance. Scoliosis rarely produces subjective symptoms until it's well established.

Clinical findings

■ Complaints of backache, fatigue, and dyspnea
■ One hip that appears higher than the other (uneven appearance of pants legs or hemlines)
■ Unequal shoulder heights, elbow levels, and heights of iliac crests

■ Asymmetrical thoracic cage and misalignment of the spinal vertebrae when the patient bends over
■ Asymmetrical paraspinal muscles, rounded on the convex side of the curve and flattened on the concave side
■ Asymmetrical gait (see *Screening for scoliosis,* page 324)

Diagnostic test results

■ *Anterior, posterior* and *lateral spinal X-rays* taken with the patient standing upright and bending confirm scoliosis and determine the degree of curvature and flexibility of the spine.
■ *Scoliometer* measures the angle of trunk rotation.
■ *Bone growth studies* may help determine skeletal maturity.
■ *Bone mineral density studies* may help determine bone strength, especially in older patients.

TREATMENT AND CARE

- ◆ Institute oxygen therapy.
- ◆ Assess the patient's respiratory status at least every 2 hours, or more often as indicated. Observe for a positive response to oxygen therapy, such as improved breathing, color, and oximetry and ABG values.
- ◆ Position the patient for optimal breathing effort.
- ◆ Maintain a normothermic environment to reduce the patient's oxygen demand.
- ◆ Monitor vital signs, heart rhythm, and fluid intake and output.
- ◆ Encourage use of incentive spirometry and deep-breathing exercises every 2 hours.

- ◆ Initiate heat applications.
- ◆ Administer nonsteroidal anti-inflammatory drugs.
- ◆ Apply transcutaneous electrical nerve stimulation.
- ◆ Monitor neurovascular status.
- ◆ Prepare for surgery, if necessary.
- ◆ Encourage an exercise program.
- ◆ Refer the patient to a physical therapist.

COLLABORATIVE MANAGEMENT

Scoliosis can affect numerous body systems, thereby necessitating a multidisciplinary approach to care. Orthopedic specialists, including surgeons, may be consulted to provide casting, bracing, or surgery. A physical therapist may assist with exercises to maximize mobility and prevent complications related to treatments. A respiratory therapist may provide measures to ensure adequate lung expansion if rib cage deformities are present. Social services may be needed to provide referrals for follow-up and information about community support services.

TREATMENT AND CARE

The severity of the deformity and potential spine growth determine appropriate treatment, which may include close observation, a brace and appropriate exercise program, surgery, or a combination of these. To be most effective, treatment should begin early, when spinal deformity is still subtle.

- ■ For a curve less than 25 degrees, or mild scoliosis, treatment includes:
- – X-rays to monitor curve
- – examination every 3 months.
- ■ For a curve of 30 to 50 degrees, treatment includes:
- – spinal exercises and a brace (may halt progression but doesn't reverse the established curvature; braces can be adjusted as the patient grows and worn until bone growth is complete)
- – transcutaneous electrical stimulation (alternative therapy, although effectiveness hasn't been proven).
- ■ For a curve of 40 degrees or more, treatment includes:
- – surgery (supportive instrumentation with spinal fusion; newer techniques allow for curvature correction while maintaining spinal flexibility)
- – periodic postoperative checkups for several months to monitor stability of the correction.
- ■ Provide emotional support, especially if the patient is an adolescent. Young patients with scoliosis are likely to be distressed by limitations on activities and by the need to wear orthopedic appliances.
- ■ Give meticulous skin and cast care.

The patient who needs a brace will require the following measures in addition to those described above.

- ■ Collaborate with a physical therapist, a social worker, and an orthotist to teach the patient about the care and use of the brace. Explain that he'll need to wear it for 23 hours per day, removing it only for bathing and exercise. Teach the patient how to care for the brace and suggest wearing loose-fitting, oversized clothes for greater comfort.
- ■ Teach the patient measures for skin care; suggest wearing a snug-fitting T-shirt under the brace. Counsel him to keep the skin clean and dry and to avoid using lotions, ointments, or powders on areas where the brace touches the skin.
- ■ Explain that he'll need to avoid vigorous sports and suggest appropriate activities and exercise.

If the patient needs traction or a cast before surgery:
- ■ Explain to the patient and his family why a cast or traction is being used. Teach them

SCREENING FOR SCOLIOSIS

When assessing the patient for an abnormal spinal curve, tell her to remove her shirt and stand as straight as she can with her back to you. Instruct her to distribute her weight evenly on each foot. While she does this, observe both sides of her back from neck to buttocks. Look for these signs:

♦ uneven shoulder height and shoulder blade prominence
♦ unequal distance between the arms and the body
♦ asymmetrical waistline
♦ uneven hip height
♦ a sideways lean.

With the patient's back still facing you, ask her to do the "forward-bend" test. In this test, she places her palms together and slowly bends forward, keeping her head down. Look for these signs:

♦ asymmetrical thoracic spine or prominent rib cage (rib hump) on either side
♦ asymmetrical waistline.

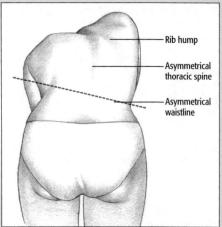

skin, cast, and traction care, as well as pain management techniques.

■ After corrective surgery, assess sensation, movement, color, and blood supply in all extremities every hour for the first 48 hours and then several times per day, noting signs of neurovascular deficit.

■ Assist with active range-of-motion (ROM) arm exercises to help maintain muscle strength and quadriceps-setting, calf-pumping, and active ROM exercises of the ankles and feet.

■ Monitor for complications such as skin breakdown, and for signs of cast syndrome, such as nausea, vomiting, abdominal pressure, and abdominal pain.

Septic shock

Low systemic vascular resistance and elevated cardiac output characterize septic shock, a type of distributive shock in which vasodilation causes hypovolemia. Septic shock can affect virtually every body system, and, if left untreated, can be fatal.

ETIOLOGY

Any pathogenic organism can cause septic shock. Gram-negative bacteria, such as *Escherichia coli, Klebsiella pneumoniae, Serratia, Enterobacter,* and *Pseudomonas* rank as the most common causes and account for up to 70% of all cases. Opportunistic fungi cause about 3% of cases. Rare causative organisms include mycobacteria and some viruses and protozoa.

Normal flora—organisms whose presence on the skin or in the intestines is harmless or even beneficial—can cause overwhelming infection if they infiltrate the blood. Alteration in the body's defenses may permit such infiltration; it may also result from penetration by such devices as I.V. or intra-arterial lines, urinary catheters, or knife or bullet wounds.

🚩 **RED FLAG** *Septic shock can occur in anyone with impaired immunity, but elderly people are at greatest risk.*

About two-thirds of septic shock cases occur in hospitalized patients, most of whom have underlying diseases. Those at high risk for septic shock include patients with burns, diabetes mellitus, immunosuppression, malnutrition, stress, and chronic cardiac, hepatic, or renal disorders. Also at risk are patients who have undergone invasive diagnostic or therapeutic procedures, surgery, traumatic wounds, or excessive antibiotic therapy.

PATHOPHYSIOLOGY

Endotoxins released by bacteria trigger an immune response in which macrophages secrete immune mediators such as tumor necrosis factor (TNF) or interleukin-1. The immune mediators cause increased release of platelet-activating factor (PAF), prostaglandins, leukotrienes, thromboxane A_2, kinins, and complement.

Cardiovascular system

■ As the body's defense system activates chemical mediators, low systemic vascular resistance and increased cardiac output results. Blood flow is unevenly distributed in the microcirculation and plasma leaks from the capillaries, causing functional hypovolemia. Eventually, the hypovolemia leads to decreased cardiac output and poor tissue perfusion and hypotension, causing multisystem organ dysfunction syndrome, and, ultimately, death.

Hematologic system

■ The release of TNF and endotoxins activates the clotting cascade, damaging tissue.
■ The mediators involved in the inflammatory process upset the balance of coagulation and fibrinolysis, which may lead to disseminated intravascular coagulation. (See *Disorders affecting management of septic shock,* pages 326 to 329.)

Integumentary system

■ Vasodilation of peripheral vessels and decreased systemic vascular resistance cause the patient's skin to appear flushed.
■ Later, peripheral vasoconstriction occurs and systemic vascular resistance increases, leading to pallor and cyanosis.

Neurologic system

■ Vasodilation and vasoconstriction affect the cerebral blood vessels, leading to changes in levels of consciousness (LOC).

Respiratory system

■ Increased capillary permeability in the pulmonary vasculature affects gas exchange.
■ Fluid shifting leads to pulmonary edema, alveolar damage, and alveolar collapse.
■ The release of histamine from endotoxins further damages the alveolar capillary membrane, leading to increased fluid shifting.
■ Continued pulmonary edema and inflammation can lead to fibrosis and acute respiratory distress syndrome (ARDS).

Urinary system

■ Endotoxin production promotes vasoconstriction, impairing blood flow to the kidneys.
■ Glomerular membrane damage and increased capillary permeability can lead to renal failure.

ASSESSMENT

The patient's history may include a disorder or a treatment that causes immunosuppression, or a history of invasive tests or treatments, surgery, or trauma. At onset, the patient may have fever and chills, although 20% of patients may be hypothermic.

Clinical findings

The hyperdynamic phase of septic shock occurs early and progresses to the hypodynamic phase if treatment is delayed. Because improved monitoring allows for early detection of signs and symptoms, most patients exhibit findings associated with the hyperdynamic phase.

Hyperdynamic (warm) phase

■ Increased cardiac output
■ Peripheral vasodilation
■ Decreased systemic vascular resistance
■ Flushed skin that may feel warm and dry
■ Altered LOC (agitation, anxiety, irritability, and shortened attention span)
■ Rapid, shallow respirations
■ Urine output below normal
■ Rapid, full, bounding pulse
■ Normal or slightly elevated blood pressure

(*Text continues on page 330.*)

DISORDERS AFFECTING
MANAGEMENT OF SEPTIC SHOCK

This chart highlights disorders that affect the management of septic shock.

DISORDER	SIGNS AND SYMPTOMS	DIAGNOSTIC TEST RESULTS
Acute renal failure (complication)	◆ Oliguria, azotemia and, rarely, anuria ◆ Electrolyte imbalance, metabolic acidosis ◆ Anorexia, nausea, vomiting, diarrhea or constipation, stomatitis, bleeding, hematemesis, dry mucous membranes, and uremic breath ◆ Headache, drowsiness, irritability, confusion, peripheral neuropathy, seizures, and coma ◆ Skin dryness, pruritus, pallor, purpura and, rarely, uremic frost ◆ Hypotension (early), hypertension, arrhythmias, fluid overload, heart failure, systemic edema, anemia, and altered clotting mechanisms (later) ◆ Pulmonary edema ◆ Kussmaul's respirations	◆ Blood studies show elevated blood urea nitrogen (BUN), serum creatinine, and potassium levels; decreased bicarbonate level, hematocrit, and hemoglobin levels; and low blood pH. ◆ Urine studies show casts, cellular debris, and decreased specific gravity. ◆ Creatinine clearance test measures glomerular filtration rate and reflects the number of remaining functioning nephrons. ◆ Electrocardiography shows tall, peaked T waves; widening QRS complex; and disappearing P waves if hyperkalemia is present.
Acute respiratory distress syndrome (ARDS) (complication)	◆ Dyspnea on exertion ◆ Diminished breath sounds ◆ Tachypnea, tachycardia ◆ Increased respiratory distress with use of accessory muscles ◆ Restlessness, apprehension ◆ Dry cough or frothy sputum ◆ Cool, clammy skin that progresses to pallor and cyanosis ◆ Basilar crackles, rhonchi ◆ Decreased mental status ◆ Arrhythmias such as premature ventricular contractions ◆ Labile hypotension	◆ Arterial blood gas (ABG) analysis initially shows decreased partial pressure of arterial oxygen despite oxygen supplementation; partial pressure of arterial carbon dioxide ($Paco_2$) is decreased, causing an increase in blood pH; as ARDS worsens, $Paco_2$ increases and pH decreases as the patient becomes acidotic. ◆ Initially, chest X-rays may be normal. Basilar infiltrates begin to appear in about 24 hours. In later stages, lung fields have a ground-glass appearance; and, as fluid fills the alveoli, white patches appear. ◆ Pulmonary artery wedge pressure is 18 mm Hg or lower.
Disseminated intravascular coagulation (DIC) (complication)	◆ Abnormal bleeding without a history of a hemorrhagic disorder ◆ Bleeding into the skin, such as cutaneous oozing, petechiae, ecchymoses, and hematomas. ◆ Bleeding from surgical or invasive procedure sites such as incisions or venipuncture sites ◆ Nausea, vomiting ◆ Severe muscle, back, and abdominal pain or chest pain ◆ Hemoptysis, epistaxis ◆ Seizures ◆ Oliguria	◆ Platelet count is decreased. ◆ Fibrinogen level is less than 150 mg/dl. ◆ Prothrombin time is more than 15 seconds. ◆ Partial thromboplastin time is more than 60 seconds. ◆ Fibrin degradation products are increased, commonly greater than 45 mcg/ml. ◆ D-dimer test is positive at less than 1:8 dilution. ◆ Fibrin monomers are positive; levels of factors V and VIII are diminished with fragmentation of red blood cells. ◆ Hemoglobin is less than 10 g/dl. ◆ Urine studies reveal BUN greater than 25 mg/dl. ◆ Serum creatinine level is greater than 1.3 mg/dl.

TREATMENT AND CARE

◆ Measure and record intake and output, including body fluids. Weigh the patient daily.
◆ Anticipate fluid restriction to minimize edema.
◆ Assess hemoglobin levels and hematocrit and replace blood components.
◆ Monitor vital signs. Watch for and report signs of pericarditis (pleuritic chest pain, tachycardia pericardial friction rub), inadequate renal perfusion (hypotension) and acidosis.
◆ Maintain proper electrolyte balance. Strictly monitor potassium levels.
◆ Administer medications as ordered.
◆ Prepare for hemodialysis or peritoneal dialysis to correct electrolyte and fluid imbalances.
◆ Assess the patient frequently, especially during emergency treatment to lower potassium levels. If the patient receives hypertonic glucose and insulin infusions, monitor potassium and glucose levels. If sodium polystyrene sulfonate is used rectally, make sure the patient doesn't retain it and become constipated. Doing so prevents bowel perforation.
◆ Maintain nutritional status. Provide a high-calorie, low-protein, low-sodium diet with vitamin supplements. Give the anorexic patient small, frequent meals.
◆ Encourage frequent coughing and deep breathing and perform passive range-of-motion exercises.
◆ Provide good mouth care frequently.

◆ Assess the patient's respiratory status, including lung sounds, heart rate, and blood pressure at least every 2 hours, or more often if indicated. Note respiratory rate, rhythm, and depth, reporting dyspnea and accessory muscle use. Be alert for inspiratory retractions. If the patient has injuries that affect his lungs, watch for adverse respiratory changes, especially in the first few days after the injury, when his condition may appear to be improving.
◆ Administer oxygen as ordered; assess oxygen saturation continuously; and monitor serial ABG levels.
◆ Check ventilator settings frequently. Assess hemodynamic parameters if a pulmonary catheter is inserted.
◆ Institute continuous cardiac monitoring and watch for arrhythmias.
◆ Monitor the patient's level of consciousness, noting confusion or mental sluggishness.
◆ Be alert for signs of treatment-induced complications, including arrhythmias, DIC, GI bleeding, infection, malnutrition, paralytic ileus, pneumothorax, pulmonary fibrosis, renal failure, thrombocytopenia, and tracheal stenosis.
◆ Give sedatives, as ordered, to reduce restlessness. Administer sedatives and analgesics at regular intervals if the patient is receiving neuromuscular blocking agents.
◆ Administer anti-infective agents, as ordered, if the underlying cause is sepsis or an infection.
◆ Place the patient in a comfortable position that maximizes air exchange such as semi-Fowler's or high-Fowler's position.
◆ Evaluate the patient's serum electrolyte levels frequently.
◆ Monitor urine output hourly to ensure adequate renal function. Weigh the patient daily.
◆ Record caloric intake. Administer tube feedings and parenteral nutrition.

◆ Ensure a patent airway and assess breathing and circulation. Monitor vital signs, cardiac and respiratory status closely, at least every 30 minutes – or more frequently – depending on the patient's condition.
◆ Observe skin color and check peripheral circulation, including color, temperature, and capillary refill.
◆ Administer supplemental oxygen and monitor oxygen saturation with continuous pulse oximetry and serial ABG studies; anticipate the need for endotracheal intubation and mechanical ventilation should the patient's respiratory status deteriorate.
◆ Assess neurologic status at least every hour – or more often, if indicated – for changes.
◆ Assess extent of blood loss and begin fluid replacement as ordered. Obtain a type and crossmatch for blood component therapy, and administer.
◆ If hypotension occurs, administer vasoactive drugs, such as amrinone, dobutamine, dopamine, epinephrine, and nitroprusside.
◆ Assess hemodynaic parameters, as indicated.
◆ Institute continuous cardiac monitoring to evaluate for possible arrhythmias, myocardial ischemia, or adverse effects of treatment.

(continued)

DISORDERS AFFECTING
MANAGEMENT OF SEPTIC SHOCK *(continued)*

DISORDER	SIGNS AND SYMPTOMS	DIAGNOSTIC TEST RESULTS
Disseminated intravascular coagulation (DIC) *(continued)*	◆ Diminished peripheral pulses ◆ Hypotension ◆ Mental status changes, including confusion	
Multiple organ dysfunction syndrome (complication)	◆ Tachycardia ◆ Increased respiratory rate; hyperventilation ◆ Oliguria or anuria ◆ Petechiae and purpura (with skin infection) ◆ Jaundice ◆ Confusion ◆ Coma ◆ Profound depression in mental status ◆ Poor distal perfusion, cool skin, cool extremities, delayed capillary refill ◆ Inflamed or swollen tympanic membranes, sinus tenderness, pharyngeal exudates, stridor, cervical lymphadenopathy (if patient has head and neck infection) ◆ Tenderness, guarding or rebound, rectal tenderness or swelling (if GI infection present) ◆ Costovertebral angle tenderness, pelvic tenderness, cervical motion pain, adnexal tenderness (with pelvic and genitourinary infections) ◆ Localized crackles or evidence of consolidation (if chest and pulmonary infection present) ◆ Regurgitant valvular murmur (with cardiac infection) ◆ Diminished bowel sounds	◆ Microbiologic studies show occult bacterial infection or bacteremia in sepsis and can indicate the specific microbial etiology. ◆ Platelet count decreases at onset of serious stress and falls with persistent sepsis; DIC may develop. ◆ White blood cell count is greater than 15,000 cells/μl or neutrophil band count is greater than 1,500 cells/μl, indicating bacterial infection. ◆ Serum creatinine and BUN are elevated if renal system is involved. ◆ Serum transaminase and bilirubin levels are increased. ◆ Alkaline phosphate and alanine aminotransferase are altered, indicating hepatic involvement. ◆ ABG analysis may show elevated serum lactate levels – evidence of tissue hypoperfusion. Higher serum lactate indicates a worse degree of shock and higher mortality. ◆ Altered prothrombin time and partial thromboplastin time show evidence of coagulopathy, as in DIC. ◆ Urinalysis and urine culture may show infecting organism in urinary tract infection. ◆ Tissue stain and culture from sites of potential infection may be positive for the causative organism. ◆ Chest X-ray may show infiltrates. ◆ Abdominal X-rays (supine and upright or lateral decubitus) may show source of intra-abdominal sepsis. ◆ Computed tomography (CT) scan may help diagnosis intra-abdominal abscess or retroperitoneal source of infection. CT scan of the head in patients with increased intracranial pressure or in patients undergoing lumbar puncture may show focal defects, sinusitis, or otitis (if meningitis is suspected). ◆ X-ray of the area of suspected involvement may show presence of soft tissue gas and spread of infection beyond disease site; surgical exploration may be required. ◆ Lumbar puncture may show evidence of meningitis. ◆ Pulmonary artery catheterization shows evidence of altered cardiac output and tissue oxygenation.

TREATMENT AND CARE

◆ Administer medications including I.V. heparin in low doses, antifibrinolytic agents, vitamin K, and folate.
◆ Assess urine output hourly.
◆ Check all stools and drainage for occult blood.
◆ Inspect skin and mucous membranes for signs of bleeding; assess all invasive insertion sites and dressings for evidence of frank bleeding or oozing. Weigh the dressings that are wet or saturated to aid in determining extent of blood loss. Watch for bleeding from the GI and genitourinary tracts.
◆ Institute bleeding precautions. Limit all invasive procedures, such as venipunctures and intramuscular injections, as much as possible. Apply pressure for 3 to 5 minutes over venous insertion sites and 10 to 15 minutes over arterial sites.
◆ Institute safety precautions to minimize the risk of injury.

◆ Support respiratory and circulatory function with mechanical ventilation, supplemental oxygen, hemodynamic monitoring, and fluid volume therapy.
◆ Closely monitor renal function, including hourly urine output measurements and serial laboratory tests, for trends indicating renal failure.
◆ Prepare the patient for dialysis if indicated.
◆ Administer pharmacologic therapy, such as antimicrobial agents, vasopressors (such as dopamine and norepinephrine), isotonic crystalloid solutions (such as normal saline and lactated Ringer's solution), and colloids (such as albumin).

Hypodynamic (cold) phase
- Decreased cardiac output
- Peripheral vasoconstriction
- Increased systemic vascular resistance
- Inadequate tissue perfusion
- Pale and possibly cyanotic skin with possible mottled peripheral areas
- Decreased LOC (Obtundation and coma may be present.)
- Rapid, shallow respirations
- Urine output less than 25 mL/hour or absent

Diagnostic test results
- *Blood cultures* are positive for the offending organism.
- *Complete blood count* shows the presence or absence of anemia and leukopenia, severe or absent neutropenia and, usually, the presence of thrombocytopenia.
- *Arterial blood gas studies* may reveal metabolic acidosis, hypoxemia, and low partial pressure of arterial carbon dioxide ($Paco_2$) early on that progresses to increased $Paco_2$ (thereby indicating respiratory acidosis).
- *Blood urea nitrogen* and *creatinine levels* are increased and *creatinine clearance* is decreased.
- *Prothrombin time, partial thromboplastin time,* and *bleeding time* are increased; *platelets* are decreased and *fibrin split* products are decreased.
- *Electrocardiography* shows ST-depression, inverted T waves, and arrhythmias resembling myocardial infarction.
- *Amylase* and *lipase levels* may show pancreatic insufficiency.
- *Hepatic enzyme levels* are elevated due to liver ischemia.
- *Blood glucose levels* are initially elevated, and then decrease.
- *Chest X-rays* reveal evidence of pneumonia (as the underlying infection) or adult respiratory distress syndrome (indicating progression of septic shock).

COLLABORATIVE MANAGEMENT
Caring for a patient with septic shock requires a multidisciplinary approach. An infectious disease specialist may be involved to identify the causative organism and determine and coordinate antimicrobial treatment. A dietitian may assist in managing the patient's metabolic needs and direct the ad-

ministration of parenteral nutrition. A renal care specialist may be required if the patient requires dialysis or develops kidney failure. A pulmonary specialist may be required to maintain a patent airway on ventilatory support. A cardiologist may assist with hemodynamic management. A physical therapist may assist if the patient requires splinting and range-of-motion exercises to maintain mobility. The patient and his family may benefit from social services or spiritual counseling.

TREATMENT AND CARE
- Locate and treat the underlying infection. Remove I.V., intra-arterial, or urinary drainage catheters.
- Initiate aggressive antimicrobial therapy appropriate for the causative organism. Culture and sensitivity tests help determine the most effective antimicrobial drug.
- Anticipate surgery if the infection was caused by bowel perforation, an abscess, or a wound.
- Be prepared to reduce or discontinue immunosuppressive drug therapy.
- Expect to administer granulocyte transfusions if the patient has severe neutropenia.
- Initiate oxygen therapy to maintain arterial oxygen saturation greater than 95%.
- Anticipate the need for mechanical ventilation if respiratory failure occurs.
- Administer colloid or crystalloid infusions to increase intravascular volume and raise blood pressure.

RED FLAG *Be alert for signs and symptoms of possible fluid overload, such as dyspnea, tachypnea, crackles, peripheral edema, jugular vein distention, and increased pulmonary artery pressures.*
- After sufficient fluid volume has been replaced, diuretics such as furosemide can be given to maintain urine output above 20 ml/hour. If fluid replacement fails to increase blood pressure, a vasopressor such as dopamine can be started.
- Prepare to administer blood transfusions if anemia is present.
- Assess cardiopulmonary status, including oxygen saturation levels, for evidence of hypoxemia.

RED FLAG *Suspect ARDS in the patient receiving mechanical ventilation if he needs increasing fraction of inspired oxy-*

gen in conjunction with increasing levels of positive end-expiratory pressure to maintain partial pressure of arterial oxygen above 60 mm Hg.
- Frequently monitor vital signs, including temperature and blood pressure.

RED FLAG Temperature is usually elevated in the early stages of septic shock, and the patient commonly experiences shaking chills. As shock progresses, temperature typically drops and the patient experiences diaphoresis. If the patient's systolic blood pressure drops below 80 mm Hg, increase the oxygen flow rate, and notify the physician immediately. Systolic blood pressure below 80 mm Hg usually results in inadequate coronary artery blood flow, cardiac ischemia, arrhythmias, and further complications of low cardiac output. A progressive drop in blood pressure accompanied by a thready pulse usually signals inadequate cardiac output from reduced intravascular volume.

- Use continuous cardiac monitoring to evaluate for possible arrhythmias, myocardial ischemia, or adverse effects of treatment.
- Assess neurologic status every 30 minutes until the patient stabilizes, and then every 2 to 4 hours, as indicated by the patient's status.
- Assess urine output hourly.
- Use strict aseptic technique for all invasive procedures to control infection.

Sickle cell anemia

Sickle cell anemia is a congenital hemolytic anemia resulting from defective hemoglobin molecules. Approximately one in 10 blacks carries the abnormal gene, and one in every 400 to 600 black children has sickle cell anemia. The prognosis varies, but most individuals live into their fourth or fifth decade.

ETIOLOGY
Sickle cell anemia is an autosomal recessive disorder resulting from a mutation of the hemoglobin (Hb) S gene, which is located on chromosome 11. A person who is heterozygous for the gene has the sickle cell trait

(carrier) but remains asymptomatic. If two carriers have offspring, each child has a one in four chance of developing the disease.

PATHOPHYSIOLOGY
Sickle cell anemia results from substitution of the amino acid, valine, for glutamic acid in the Hb S gene encoding the beta chain of Hb. Abnormal Hb S in the red blood cells (RBCs) becomes insoluble during hypoxia. As a result, these cells become rigid, rough, and elongated, forming a crescent or sickle shape. (See *Characteristics of sickled cells*, page 332.)

The sickling produces hemolysis. The altered cells accumulate in the capillaries and smaller blood vessels, increasing the viscosity of the blood. Normal circulation is impaired, causing pain, tissue infarctions, and swelling.

Each patient with sickle cell anemia has a different hypoxic threshold and particular factors that trigger a sickle cell crisis. Illness, exposure to cold, stress, acidotic states, or a pathophysiologic process that pulls water out of the sickle cells can precipitate sickle cell crisis. (See *Sickle cell crisis*, page 333.) The obstructions lead to anoxic changes that cause additional sickling and blockage.

Cardiovascular system
- Sickled cells accumulate in the heart and blood vessels, obstructing blood flow.
- Oxygen delivery to the heart and organs supplied by the blood vessels is diminished, causing ischemia and, possibly, necrosis.
- Obstruction and ischemia, when coupled with the already sluggish blood flow and chronic anemia, can lead to heart failure, cardiomegaly, and systolic murmurs. (See *Disorders affecting management of sickle cell anemia*, pages 334 to 337.)

Genitourinary system
- The blood vessels supplying the kidneys can become obstructed by sickle cells, which can lead to decreased renal perfusion that, in turn, affects the capillary permeability of the glomerulus and may lead to renal failure.
- Plasma proteins, such as albumin, can be lost, leading to hyperproteinuria and hypoalbuminemia, which may progress to nephrotic syndrome.

CHARACTERISTICS OF SICKLED CELLS

Normal red blood cells (RBCs) and sickled cells vary in shape, life span, oxygen-carrying capacity, and the rate at which they're destroyed. These illustrations show normal and sickled cells and list their major differences.

Normal RBCs
◆ 120-day life span
◆ Hemoglobin (Hb) has normal oxygen-carrying capacity
◆ 12 to 14 g/ml of Hb
◆ RBCs destroyed at normal rate

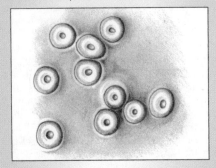

Sickled cells
◆ 30- to 40-day life span
◆ Hb has decreased oxygen-carrying capacity
◆ 6 to 9 g/ml of Hb
◆ RBCs destroyed at accelerated rate

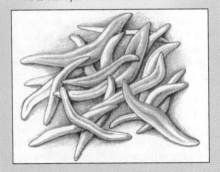

Immune system
■ Obstruction of blood flow to the spleen by sickled cells leads to ischemia, impairing the spleen's filtering capability. Functioning cells are gradually replaced with fibrotic tissue.
■ Impaired splenic function places the patient at high risk for infections.

Neurologic system
■ Sickle cells accumulate in cerebral vessels, obstructing the blood flow to the brain and leading to decreased cerebral perfusion and cerebral ischemia. Stroke may occur.

ASSESSMENT
Symptoms of sickle cell anemia typically develop after age 4 months because fetal hemoglobin inhibits sickling.

The patient who presents with lethargy, listlessness, sleepiness, irritability, severe pain, fever, and paleness of the lips, tongue, palms, or nail beds may be experiencing any of the following crises.
■ *Aplastic (or megaloblastic) crisis* occurs due to bone marrow depression associated with infection — usually human parvovirus — and is characterized by pallor, lethargy, sleepiness, dyspnea, possible coma, markedly decreased bone marrow activity, and RBC hemolysis.
■ *Acute sequestration crisis* (rare) results from sudden massive entrapment of cells in the spleen and liver. It affects children ages 8 months to 2 years and may cause lethargy, pallor, and hypovolemic shock.
■ *Hemolytic crisis* (rare) typically affects patients who also have glucose-6-phosphate dehydrogenase deficiency. In this crisis, degenerative changes cause liver congestion and enlargement and worsening chronic jaundice.

Clinical findings
■ Family history of the mutated Hb S gene
■ Chronic fatigue
■ Unexplained dyspnea or dyspnea on exertion
■ Joint swelling, aching bones
■ Severe localized and generalized pain
■ Leg ulcers (especially on the ankles)
■ Frequent infections
■ Priapism
■ Hepatomegaly
■ Dark urine
■ Low-grade fever
■ Jaundice

SICKLE CELL CRISIS

Infection, exposure to cold, high altitudes, overexertion, or other situations that cause cellular oxygen deprivation may trigger a sickle cell crisis. The deoxygenated, sickle-shaped red blood cells stick to the capillary wall and each other, blocking blood flow and causing cellular hypoxia. The crisis worsens as tissue hypoxia and acidic waste products cause more sickling and cell damage. With each new crisis, organs and tissues are slowly destroyed; the spleen and kidneys are particularly prone to damage.

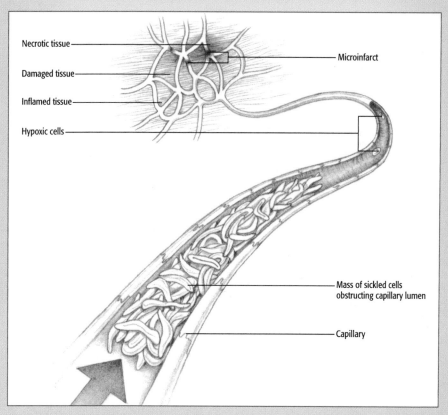

In sickle cell crisis:
- Severe pain
- Hematuria
- Lethargy
- Irritability
- Pale lips, tongue, palms, and nail beds

Diagnostic test results
- *Hb electrophoresis* shows abnormal Hb S.
- *Electrophoresis* of the umbilical cord blood provides screening for all neonates at risk.
- *Stained blood smear* shows sickle cells.
- *Blood studies* reveal low RBC counts, elevated white blood cell and platelet counts, decreased erythrocyte sedimentation rate, increased serum iron levels, decreased RBC survival, and reticulocytosis. Hb levels may be low or normal.
- *Lateral chest X-ray* shows "Lincoln log" deformity in the vertebrae of many adults and some adolescents.

(*Text continues on page 336.*)

DISORDERS AFFECTING
MANAGEMENT OF SICKLE CELL ANEMIA

This chart highlights disorders that affect the management of sickle cell anemia.

DISORDER	SIGNS AND SYMPTOMS	DIAGNOSTIC TEST RESULTS
Acute renal failure (complication)	◆ Oliguria, azotemia and, rarely, anuria ◆ Electrolyte imbalance, metabolic acidosis ◆ Anorexia, nausea, vomiting, diarrhea or constipation, stomatitis, bleeding, hematemesis, dry mucous membranes, and uremic breath ◆ Headache, drowsiness, irritability, confusion, peripheral neuropathy, seizures, and coma ◆ Skin dryness, pruritus, pallor, purpura and, rarely, uremic frost ◆ Hypotension (early); hypertension, arrhythmias, fluid overload, heart failure, systemic edema, anemia, and altered clotting mechanisms (later) ◆ Pulmonary edema ◆ Kussmaul's respirations	◆ Blood studies show elevated BUN, serum creatinine, and potassium levels; decreased bicarbonate level, hematocrit, and hemoglobin levels; and low blood pH. ◆ Urine studies show casts, cellular debris, and decreased specific gravity; urine sodium level is more than 40 mEq/L. ◆ Creatinine clearance test measures glomerular filtration rate and reflects the number of remaining functioning nephrons. ◆ ECG shows tall, peaked T waves; widening QRS complex; and disappearing P waves if hyperkalemia is present.
Heart failure (complication)	*Left-sided heart failure* ◆ Dyspnea ◆ Orthopnea ◆ Paroxysmal nocturnal dyspnea ◆ Fatigue ◆ Nonproductive cough ◆ Crackles ◆ Hemoptysis ◆ Tachycardia ◆ Third and fourth heart sounds ◆ Cool, pale skin ◆ Restlessness and confusion *Right-sided heart failure* ◆ Jugular vein distention ◆ Positive hepatojugular reflux ◆ Right-upper-quadrant pain ◆ Anorexia, nausea ◆ Nocturia ◆ Weight gain, edema ◆ Ascites or anasarca	◆ Chest X-ray shows increased pulmonary vascular markings, interstitial edema, or pleural effusions and cardiomegaly. ◆ Electrocardiography (ECG) may reveal hypertrophy, ischemic changes or infarction, tachycardia, and extrasystoles. ◆ Liver function test may be abnormal; blood urea nitrogen (BUN) and creatinine levels may be elevated. ◆ Prothrombin time may be prolonged. ◆ B-type natriuretic peptide immunoassay is elevated. ◆ Echocardiography may reveal left ventricular hypertrophy, dilation, and abnormal contractility. ◆ Pulmonary artery pressure, pulmonary artery wedge pressure, and left ventricular end-diastolic pressure are elevated in the presence of left-sided heart failure; right atrial or central venous pressure is elevated in right-sided heart failure. ◆ Radionuclide ventriculography may reveal ejection fraction less than 40% in diastolic dysfunction.
Stroke (complication)	◆ Headache with no known cause ◆ Numbness or weakness of the face, arm, or leg, especially on one side of the body ◆ Confusion, trouble speaking or understanding ◆ Trouble seeing or walking, dizziness, and loss of coordination	◆ Magnetic resonance imaging or a computed tomography scan shows evidence of thrombosis or hemorrhage. ◆ Brain scan reveals ischemia (may not be positive for up to 2 weeks after the stroke). ◆ Lumbar puncture may reveal blood in the cerebrospinal fluid (if hemorrhagic). ◆ Carotid ultrasound may detect a blockage, stenosis, or reduced blood flow.

TREATMENT AND CARE

◆ Measure and record intake and output, including body fluids. Weigh the patient daily.
◆ Anticipate fluid restriction to minimize edema.
◆ Assess hemoglobin levels and hematocrit and replace blood components.
◆ Monitor vital signs. Watch for and report signs of pericarditis (pleuritic chest pain, tachycardia, pericardial friction rub), inadequate renal perfusion (hypotension) and acidosis.
◆ Maintain proper electrolyte balance. Strictly monitor potassium levels.
◆ Administer medications such as diuretic therapy to treat oliguric phase; sodium polystyrene sulfonate by mouth or enema to reverse hyperkalemia; and hypertonic glucose, insulin, and sodium bicarbonate I.V. for more severe hyperkalemic symptoms.
◆ Prepare for hemodialysis or peritoneal dialysis to correct electrolyte and fluid imbalances.
◆ Assess the patient frequently, especially during emergency treatment to lower potassium levels. If the patient receives hypertonic glucose and insulin infusions, monitor potassium and glucose levels. If sodium polystyrene sulfonate is used rectally, make sure the patient doesn't retain it and become constipated. Doing so prevents bowel perforation.
◆ Maintain nutritional status. Give the anorexic patient small, frequent meals.
◆ Encourage frequent coughing and deep breathing and perform passive range-of-motion exercises.
◆ Provide frequent mouth care.

◆ Place the patient in Fowler's position and give supplemental oxygen.
◆ Weigh the patient daily, and check for peripheral edema.
◆ Monitor intake and output, vital signs, and mental status.
◆ Auscultate for third and fourth heart sounds and adventitious lung sounds such as crackles or rhonchi.
◆ Monitor BUN, creatinine, and serum potassium, sodium, chloride, and magnesium.
◆ Institute continuous cardiac monitoring to identify and treat arrhythmias promptly.
◆ Administer angiotensin-converting enzyme inhibitors, digoxin, diuretics, beta-adrenergic blockers, human B-type natriuretic peptides, nitrates, and morphine.
◆ Encourage lifestyle modifications, as appropriate.

◆ Administer medications such as antiplatelet agents to prevent recurrent stroke (but not in hemorrhagic stroke); benzodiazepines to treat seizures; anticonvulsants to treat or prevent seizures after the patient's condition has stabilized; thrombolytics, such as alteplase, for emergency treatment of embolic stroke (typically within 3 hours of onset), aspirin or heparin for patients with embolic or thrombotic stroke who aren't candidates for alteplase, stool softeners to prevent straining; antihypertensives and antiarrhythmics to reduce risks associated with recurrent stroke; corticosteroids to minimize associated cerebral edema, and analgesics to relieve headache following a hemorrhagic stroke.
◆ Maintain a patent airway and provide oxygen. If unconscious, the patient may aspirate saliva. Place the patient in lateral position to promote drainage, or suction as needed.
◆ Insert an artificial airway and start mechanical ventilation or supplemental oxygen if needed.

(continued)

DISORDERS AFFECTING
MANAGEMENT OF SICKLE CELL ANEMIA *(continued)*

DISORDER	SIGNS AND SYMPTOMS	DIAGNOSTIC TEST RESULTS
Stroke *(continued)*		◆ Angiography can help pinpoint the site of occlusion or rupture. ◆ Electroencephalography may help localize the area of damage.

COLLABORATIVE MANAGEMENT

Sickle cell anemia requires a multidisciplinary approach to care. Specialists in hematology, cardiology, and immunology may be involved depending on the patient's status and whether the patient is experiencing a sickle cell crisis. A pain management specialist may assist with pain control measures during an acute crisis. A dietitian may assist with meal planning and measures to ensure adequate hydration.

TREATMENT AND CARE

■ Give large amounts of oral or I.V. fluids to correct hypovolemia and prevent dehydration and vessel occlusion.
■ Administer packed RBC transfusion as ordered to correct hypovolemia or anemia.
■ Administer sedation and analgesics for pain.
■ Administer oxygen to correct hypoxia. Keep in mind that short-term, prolonged administration of oxygen can depress bone marrow functioning and lead to more severe anemia.
■ In neonates, administer hydroxyurea to reduce painful episodes by increasing the production of fetal Hb, which seems to alleviate symptoms.
■ Administer iron and folic acid supplements to prevent anemia.
■ Anticipate the use of vaccines to prevent illness and anti-infectives, such as low-dose penicillin, possibly to prevent complications in patients with sickle cell anemia.
■ Provide supportive measures during crises and precautions for prevention of crisis, including avoiding dehydration, strenuous exercise, vasoconstricting medications or clothing, and cold temperatures.

■ Discuss infection prevention measures with the patient, such as avoiding crowds or individuals with known infections, maintaining proper nutrition, and proper hand washing.
■ Refer the patient to genetic counseling and community support.

Spinal cord injury

Usually the result of trauma to the head or neck, spinal cord injuries (SCIs) include fractures, contusions, and compressions of the vertebral column. Spinal cord injuries most commonly occur in the 12th thoracic, first lumbar, and 5th, 6th, and 7th cervical areas.

The prognosis for a patient with an SCI depends on the degree of injury. Most patients with SCIs eventually regain some degree of independence. However, morbidity is high, most commonly arising from pulmonary or renal complications such as infection.

ETIOLOGY

Most serious SCIs result from motor vehicle accidents, falls, diving into shallow water, and gunshot wounds. Less serious injuries result from lifting heavy objects and minor falls. Approximately 10,000 people suffer SCIs each year; most are males between ages 18 to 25. Spinal cord injury may also result from hyperparathyroidism and neoplastic lesions.

PATHOPHYSIOLOGY

Spinal cord injury results from acceleration, deceleration, or other deforming forces, usually applied from a distance. Mechanisms involved with spinal cord injury include:
■ hyperextension from acceleration-deceleration forces and sudden reduction in the anteroposterior diameter of the spinal cord
■ hyperflexion from sudden and excessive force, propelling the neck forward or causing an exaggerated movement to one side
■ vertical compression from force applied from the top of the cranium along the vertical axis through the vertebra
■ rotational forces from twisting, which adds shearing forces.

The spinal cord is an important neurologic structure that plays a major role in nerve impulse transmission. Depending on the severity and location of the injury, effects can be widespread.

Neurologic system
■ Injury causes microscopic hemorrhages in the gray matter and pia arachnoid.
■ The hemorrhages gradually increase in size until all of the gray matter is filled with blood, which causes necrosis.
■ From the gray matter, the blood enters the white matter, where it impedes the circulation within the spinal cord.
■ Ensuing edema causes compression and decreases the blood supply; thus, the spinal cord loses perfusion and becomes ischemic; edema and hemorrhage are greatest approximately two segments above and below the injury.
■ Edema temporarily adds to the patient's dysfunction by increasing pressure and compressing the nerves. (See *Disorders affecting management of spinal cord injury,* pages 338 and 339.)
■ In the gray matter, an inflammatory reaction prevents restoration of circulation. Phagocytes appear at the injury site within 36 to 48 hours after the injury, macrophages engulf degenerating axons, and collagen replaces the normal tissue. Scarring and meningeal thickening leaves the nerves in the area blocked or tangled.

Respiratory system
■ Edema and hemorrhage, if near the 3rd to 5th cervical vertebrae, may interfere with phrenic nerve impulse transmission to the diaphragm, inhibiting respiratory function.

ASSESSMENT

Assessment (including a neurologic assessment) helps locate the level of injury and detect cord damage. Clinical manifestations vary depending on the type and degree of injury. (See *Types of spinal cord injury,* pages 340 and 341.)

Clinical findings
■ History of trauma, a neoplastic lesion, an infection that could produce a spinal abscess, or an endocrine disorder
■ Muscle spasm and back or neck pain that worsens with movement; in cervical fractures, pain that causes point tenderness; in dorsal and lumbar fractures, pain that may radiate to other areas, such as the legs
■ Mild paresthesia to tetraplegia and shock; in milder injury, symptoms that may be delayed several days or weeks
■ Surface wounds that occurred with the spinal injury
■ Pain
■ Loss of sensation

DISORDERS AFFECTING
MANAGEMENT OF SPINAL CORD INJURY

This chart highlights disorders that affect the management of spinal cord injury.

DISORDER	SIGNS AND SYMPTOMS	DIAGNOSTIC TEST RESULTS
Autonomic dysreflexia (complication)	◆ Bradycardia ◆ Hypertension ◆ Severe, pounding headache ◆ Cold or goose-fleshed skin below the lesion ◆ Diaphoresiss, flushed feeling, and flushing of skin above the level of the lesion ◆ Pallor below the level of the lesion ◆ Chills	◆ None; diagnosis is primarily based on signs and symptoms. ◆ Tests support evidence of spinal cord trauma above level T6.
Neurogenic shock (complication)	◆ Orthostatic hypotension ◆ Bradycardia ◆ Inability to sweat below the level of the injury	◆ None; diagnosis is primarily based on signs and symptoms. ◆ Tests support evidence of spinal cord trauma.
Respiratory failure (complication)	◆ Diminished chest movement ◆ Restlessness, irritability, and confusion ◆ Decreased level of consciousness ◆ Pallor, possible cyanosis of skin and mucous membranes ◆ Tachypnea, tachycardia (strong and rapid initially, but thready and irregular in later stages) ◆ Cold, clammy skin and frank diaphoresis, especially around the forehead and face ◆ Diminished breath sounds; possible adventitious breath sounds ◆ Possible cardiac arrhythmias	◆ Arterial blood gas (ABG) analysis indicates early respiratory failure when partial pressure of arterial oxygen is low (usually less than 70 mm Hg), partial pressure of arterial carbon dioxide is greater than 45 mm Hg, and the bicarbonate level is normal. ◆ Serial vital capacity reveals readings less than 800 ml. ◆ Electrocardiography may indicate arrhythmias. ◆ Pulse oximetry reveals a decreased oxygen saturation level. Levels less than 50% indicate impaired tissue oxygenation.

Diagnostic test results

■ *Spinal X-rays* (the most important diagnostic measure) detect the fracture.

■ *Myelography, magnetic resonance imaging (MRI),* and *computed tomography (CT) scans* locate the fracture and site of the compression. CT or MRI scans also reveal spinal cord edema and may reveal a spinal mass.

■ *Neurologic evaluation* locates the level of injury and detects cord damage.

■ *Lumbar puncture* may show increased cerebrospinal fluid pressure from a lesion or trauma in spinal compression.

COLLABORATIVE MANAGEMENT
Acute SCI affects many body systems, thereby necessitating a multidisciplinary ap-

TREATMENT AND CARE

◆ Elevate the head of the bed.
◆ Monitor blood pressure and heart rate every 3 to 5 minutes.
◆ Determine the underlying stimulus for the event, such as a blocked catheter, fecal impaction, or urinary tract infection; remove or correct it.
◆ Administer antihypertensives.

◆ Minimize abrupt changes in position.
◆ Monitor blood pressure frequently when the patient is lying, sitting, and standing, if appropriate.
◆ Assess heart rate frequently; administer medications to promote cardiac function.
◆ Avoid excessive bed covers and extremes in room temperature

◆ Institute oxygen therapy immediately to optimize oxygenation of pulmonary blood.
◆ Prepare for endotracheal (ET) intubation and mechanical ventilation if necessary; anticipate the need for high-frequency or pressure ventilation to force airways open.
◆ Administer drug therapy, such as bronchodilators, to open airways, corticosteroids to reduce inflammation, continuous I.V. solutions of positive inotropic agents (which increase cardiac output) and vasopressors (which induce vasoconstriction) to maintain blood pressure, and diuretics to reduce fluid overload and edema.
◆ Assess the patient's respiratory status at least every 2 hours, or more often as indicated. Observe for a positive response to oxygen therapy, such as improved breathing, color, and oximetry and ABG values. Provide assisted coughing.
◆ Position the patient for optimal breathing effort.
◆ Maintain a normothermic environment to reduce the patient's oxygen demand.
◆ Monitor vital signs, heart rhythm, and fluid intake and output.
◆ If the patient is intubated, auscultate the lungs to check for accidental intubation of the esophagus or the mainstem bronchus. Be alert for aspiration, broken teeth, nosebleeds, and vagal reflexes causing bradycardia, arrhythmias, and hypotension. Perform suctioning using strict aseptic technique.
◆ Monitor oximetry and capnography values to detect changes in the patient's condition.
◆ Note the amount and quality of lung secretions and look for changes in the patient's status.
◆ Check cuff pressure on the ET tube to prevent erosion from an overinflated cuff. Normal cuff pressure is about 20 mm Hg.
◆ Implement measures to prevent nasal tissue necrosis. Position and maintain the nasotracheal tube midline in the nostrils and reposition daily. Tape the tube securely but use skin protection measures and nonirritating tape to prevent skin breakdown.
◆ Provide a means of communication for patients who are intubated and alert.

proach to care. Emergency medical service personnel typically provide care before the patient arrives at the facility, ensuring the patient's airway, breathing, and circulation and immobilizing him to stabilize his spine and prevent cord damage. A respiratory therapist may assist with pulmonary hygiene and care of the ventilator-dependent patient. A neurosurgeon may be needed to relieve the pressure due to compression of the spinal column. If the cause of compression is a neoplastic lesion, a chemotherapy and radiation specialist may direct this aspect of treatment. A physical therapist can provide training to help the patient maintain joint range of motion (ROM) and mobility. An occupational therapist can assist with devel-

(Text continues on page 342.)

TYPES OF SPINAL CORD INJURY

Injury to the spinal cord can be classified as complete or incomplete. An incomplete spinal injury may be an anterior cord syndrome, central cord syndrome, or Brown-Séquard's syndrome, depending on the area of the cord affected. This chart highlights the characteristic signs and symptoms of each.

TYPE	DESCRIPTION	SIGNS AND SYMPTOMS
Complete transsection 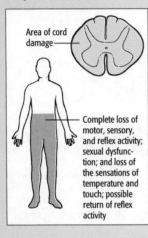	◆ All tracts of the spinal cord completely disrupted ◆ All functions involving the spinal cord below the level of transsection lost ◆ Complete and permanent loss	◆ Loss of motor function (quadriplegia) with cervical cord transsection; paraplegia with thoracic cord transsection ◆ Muscle flaccidity ◆ Loss of all reflexes and sensory function below the level of the injury ◆ Bladder and bowel atony ◆ Paralytic ileus ◆ Loss of vasomotor tone in lower body parts with low and unstable blood pressure ◆ Loss of perspiration below the level of the injury ◆ Dry, pale skin ◆ Respiratory impairment
Incomplete transsection: Central cord syndrome 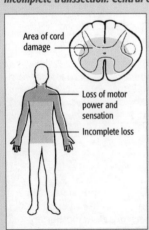	◆ Center portion of cord affected ◆ Typically from hyperextension injury	◆ Motor deficits greater in upper than lower extremities ◆ Variable degree of bladder dysfunction

Image labels for Complete transsection: "Area of cord damage"; "Complete loss of motor, sensory, and reflex activity; sexual dysfunction; and loss of the sensations of temperature and touch; possible return of reflex activity"

Image labels for Central cord syndrome: "Area of cord damage"; "Loss of motor power and sensation"; "Incomplete loss"

TYPE	DESCRIPTION	SIGNS AND SYMPTOMS

Incomplete transsection: Anterior cord syndrome

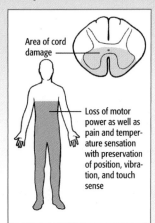

Area of cord damage

Loss of motor power as well as pain and temperature sensation with preservation of position, vibration, and touch sense

♦ Occlusion of anterior spinal artery
♦ Occlusion from pressure of bone fragments

♦ Loss of motor function below the level of the injury
♦ Loss of pain and temperature sensations below the level of the injury
♦ Intact touch, pressure, position, and vibration senses

Incomplete transsection: Brown-Séquard's syndrome

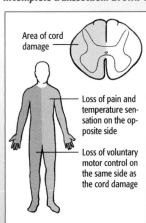

Area of cord damage

Loss of pain and temperature sensation on the opposite side

Loss of voluntary motor control on the same side as the cord damage

♦ Hemisection of cord affected
♦ Most common in stabbing and gunshot wounds
♦ Damage to cord on only one side

♦ Ipsilateral paralysis or paresis below the level of the injury
♦ Ipsilateral loss of touch, pressure, vibration, and position sense below the level of the injury
♦ Contralateral loss of pain and temperature sensations below the level of the injury

Adapted with permission from Hickey, J. V. *The Clinical Practice of Neurological and Neurosurgical Nursing*, 5th ed. Philadelphia: Lippincott Williams & Wilkins, 2003, pp 419-421.

oping assistive devices and retraining the patient to perform activities of daily living. A speech therapist can teach the patient exercises to swallow more effectively. Social services may be contacted to assist with rehabilitative services and home care.

TREATMENT AND CARE

■ Perform secondary airway, breathing, circulation, and defibrillation survey, including vital signs, level of consciousness (LOC), and oxygen saturation. If the patient hasn't been immobilized, do so immediately to prevent further injury.

RED FLAG Suspect cord damage in all spinal injuries until diagnosis is established.

■ Cervical injuries require immobilization using a hard cervical collar, skeletal traction with skull tongs, or a halo device.

■ Anticipate administering I.V. methylprednisolone to reduce inflammation (doses in the first 3 hours appear to be most effective).

■ Expect to treat an unstable dorsal or lumbar fracture with a plaster cast, a turning frame and, in severe fracture, laminectomy and spinal fusion.

■ Provide wound care and tetanus prophylaxis unless the patient has recently been immunized for surface wounds that accompany the SCI.

■ Perform a neurologic assessment to establish a baseline, including LOC and motor and sensory function. Continually assess the patient's LOC for changes, such as increasing restlessness or anxiety.

■ Frequently assess respiratory status — at least every hour, initially. Establish baseline parameters for tidal volume, vital capacity, negative inspiratory forces, and minute volume. Auscultate lung sounds, and monitor oxygen saturation levels.

■ Partial pressure of arterial oxygen less than 60 mm Hg and partial pressure of arterial carbon dioxide greater than 50 mm Hg accompanied by a decreasing pH suggest the need for mechanical ventilation secondary to atelectasis, pneumonia, or respiratory muscle fatigue.

RED FLAG If the patient isn't intubated when admitted to the emergency department, hemorrhage and edema at the injury site can increase cord damage and lead to

a higher level of dysfunction and altered respiratory function, necessitating mechanical ventilation. If the patient requires intubation and a cervical spine injury hasn't been ruled out, hyperextension of his neck is contraindicated. Perform nasal intubation or orotracheal intubation with the cervical spine immobilized manually.

■ Assess cardiac function at least every hour, initially, including continuous cardiac, blood pressure, and hemodynamic monitoring, if indicated.

RED FLAG Loss of vascular motor control below the level of SCI leads to hypotension, causing vasodilation and a relative hypovolemia. Orthostatic hypotension may occur in patients with SCI to the cervical or high thoracic area. This sudden drop in blood pressure could lead to cerebral hypoxia and loss of consciousness. To prevent orthostatic hypotension, change the patient's position slowly and perform ROM exercises every 2 hours.

■ Assess GI functioning for indications of ulceration, bleeding, abdominal distention, or decreased peristalsis. Paralytic ileus is a common problem for patients with SCI, usually occurring within the first 72 hours after the injury.

■ Assess urinary output hourly during the initial period, reporting urine output less than 0.5 ml/kg/hour for 2 consecutive hours.

■ Assess the patient frequently for signs and symptoms of autonomic dysreflexia. Be alert for throbbing headache, cutaneous vasodilation, and sweating above the level of the injury; sudden severe elevation in blood pressure; and piloerection, pallor; chills, and vasoconstriction below the level of injury.

RED FLAG If the patient develops signs and symptoms of autonomic dysreflexia, immediately elevate the head of the bed, monitor blood pressure and heart rate every 3 to 5 minutes, and determine the underlying stimulus for the event (for example, a blocked catheter, fecal impaction, or urinary tract infection) and remove or correct it. Administer antihypertensive agents.

■ Initiate rehabilitation measures as soon as possible.

Stroke

A stroke, also known as a *brain attack,* is a sudden impairment of cerebral circulation in one or more blood vessels supplying the brain. Impaired cerebral circulation interrupts or diminishes oxygen supply, typically causing serious damage and, possibly, necrosis, in brain tissues.

Stroke is the third most common cause of death in the United States and the most common cause of neurologic disability. It strikes more than 500,000 people annually and is fatal in approximately one-half of cases. Although stroke may occur in younger persons, most patients experiencing stroke are older than age 65. In fact, the risk of stroke doubles with each decade of life after age 55.

Blacks have a 60% higher risk of stroke than Whites or Hispanics of the same age, which is believed to be due to the increased prevalence of hypertension in Blacks. In addition, strokes in Blacks usually result from disease in the small cerebral vessels, whereas strokes in whites are typically the result of disease in the large carotid arteries. The mortality rate from stroke for Blacks is twice that for Whites.

Timely restoration of normal circulation improves the prognosis for patients who have experienced a stroke. However, about one-half of the patients who survive a stroke remain permanently disabled and experience a recurrence within weeks, months, or years.

ETIOLOGY
Stroke typically results from one of three causes:
■ Thrombosis of the cerebral arteries supplying the brain or of the intracranial vessels occluding blood flow (see *Types of stroke,* page 344)
■ Embolism from thrombus outside the brain, such as in the heart, aorta, or common carotid artery
■ Hemorrhage (from an intracranial artery or vein), resulting from hypertension, ruptured aneurysm, arteriovenous malformation, trauma, hemorrhagic disorder, or septic embolism

Risk factors include:
■ pre-hypertension
■ hypertension
■ family history of stroke
■ history of transient ischemic attacks (TIAs)
■ cardiac disease, including arrhythmias, coronary artery disease, acute myocardial infarction, dilated cardiomyopathy, and valvular disease
■ diabetes
■ familial hyperlipidemia
■ cigarette smoking and illicit drug use such as cocaine
■ peripheral artery disease
■ blood disorders such as polycythemia or sickle cell anemia
■ increased alcohol intake
■ obesity, sedentary lifestyle
■ sleep apnea
■ use of hormonal contraceptives.

PATHOPHYSIOLOGY
The underlying event in stroke is deprivation of oxygen and nutrients. Normally, if the arteries become blocked, autoregulatory mechanisms help maintain cerebral circulation until collateral circulation develops to deliver blood to the affected area. However, if the compensatory mechanisms become overworked or if cerebral blood flow remains impaired for more than a few minutes, oxygen deprivation leads to infarction of brain tissue. The brain cells cease to function because they can't store glucose or glycogen for use and they can't engage in anaerobic metabolism.

Neurologic system
Pathophysiologic processes vary depending on the type of stroke.

Thrombotic or embolic stroke
■ A thrombotic or embolic stroke causes ischemia. Some of the neurons served by the occluded vessel die from lack of oxygen and nutrients.
■ Neuron death results in cerebral infarction, in which tissue injury triggers an inflammatory response that increases intracranial pressure (ICP).
■ Injury to surrounding cells disrupts metabolism and leads to changes in ionic trans-

TYPES OF STROKE

Strokes are typically classified as ischemic or hemorrhagic depending on the underlying cause. This chart describes the major types of strokes.

TYPE OF STROKE	DESCRIPTION
Ischemic: Thrombotic	◆ Most common type of stroke ◆ Frequently the result of atherosclerosis; also associated with hypertension, smoking, diabetes ◆ Thrombus in extracranial or intracranial vessel blocks blood flow to the cerebral cortex ◆ Carotid artery most commonly affected extracranial vessel ◆ Common intracranial sites include bifurcation of carotid arteries, distal intracranial portion of vertebral arteries, and proximal basilar arteries ◆ May occur during sleep or shortly after awakening, during surgery, or after a myocardial infarction
Ischemic: Embolic	◆ Second most common type of stroke ◆ Embolus from heart or extracranial arteries floats into cerebral bloodstream and lodges in middle cerebral artery or branches ◆ Embolus commonly originates during atrial fibrillation ◆ Typically occurs during activity ◆ Develops rapidly
Ischemic: Lacunar	◆ Subtype of thrombotic stroke ◆ Hypertension creates cavities deep in white matter of the brain, affecting the internal capsule, basal ganglia, thalamus, and pons ◆ Lipid-coated lining of the small penetrating arteries thickens and weakens wall, causing microaneurysms and dissections
Hemorrhagic	◆ Third most common type of stroke ◆ Typically caused by hypertension or rupture of aneurysm ◆ Diminished blood supply to area supplied by ruptured artery and compression by accumulated blood

port, localized acidosis, and free radical formation.

■ Calcium, sodium, and water accumulate in the injured cells, and excitatory neurotransmitters are released.

■ Consequent continued cellular injury and swelling set up a vicious cycle of further damage.

Hemorrhagic stroke

■ Impaired cerebral perfusion causes infarction, and the blood itself acts as a space-occupying mass, exerting pressure on the brain tissues.

■ The brain's regulatory mechanisms attempt to maintain equilibrium by increasing blood pressure to maintain cerebral perfusion pressure.

■ The increased ICP forces cerebrospinal fluid (CSF) out, thus restoring the balance. If the hemorrhage is small, the patient may live with only minimal neurologic deficits. If the bleeding is heavy, ICP increases rapidly and perfusion stops. Even if the pressure returns to normal, many brain cells die.

■ Initially, the ruptured cerebral blood vessels may constrict to limit the blood loss.

■ This vasospasm further compromises blood flow, leading to more ischemia and cellular damage.

■ If a clot forms in the vessel, decreased blood flow promotes ischemia.

■ If the blood enters the subarachnoid space, meningeal irritation occurs.

■ Blood cells that pass through the vessel wall into the surrounding tissue may break down and block the arachnoid villi, causing hydrocephalus. (See *Disorders affecting management of stroke*, pages 346 and 347.)

Cardiovascular system

■ Cerebral ischemia and infarction can ultimately affect the autonomic nervous system, which can alter blood vessel constriction and dilation, heart rate, blood pressure, and cardiac contractility.
■ Cardiovascular effects are increasingly problematic if the patient has an underlying disorder such as heart disease or hypertension.

Musculoskeletal system

■ Cerebral infarction can lead to a disturbance in impulse transmission via the cranial and peripheral nerves, altering motor and sensory function.
■ Changes in sensation or mobility can lead to pressure areas, especially with prolonged bedrest or limited activity. In addition, the ability of the blood vessels to constrict and dilate as necessary may be altered, increasing the risk of impaired blood flow to the area. Subsequently, pressure ulcers may develop.

Respiratory system

■ If infarction resulting from increased ICP and decreased perfusion involves the respiratory center in the medulla, respiration — including the depth and rate — can be affected because nerve impulse transmission via the phrenic nerves to the diaphragm and intercostal nerves to the intercostal muscles is interrupted.
■ If the pons (the location for apneustic and pneumotaxic centers) is affected, breathing patterns become altered and impulse transmission via the cranial nerves may be interrupted.
■ If the glossopharyngeal (CN IX) and vagus nerves(CN X) are affected, impaired swallowing and possible aspiration may occur.

ASSESSMENT

Clinical features of stroke vary with the artery affected (and, consequently, the portion of the brain it supplies), the severity of the damage, and the extent of collateral circulation that develops to help the brain compensate for decreased blood supply. (See *Assessment findings in stroke*, page 348.)

RED FLAG *When assessing a patient who may have experienced a stroke, remember this: If the stroke occurs in the left hemisphere, it produces signs and symptoms on the right side; if it occurs in the right hemisphere, signs and symptoms appear on the left side. However, a stroke that causes cranial nerve damage produces signs of cranial nerve dysfunction on the same side as the hemorrhage or infarct.*

Clinical findings

■ Sudden onset of hemiparesis or hemiplegia or a gradual onset of dizziness, mental disturbances, or seizures possibly accompanied by loss of consciousness or sudden development of aphasia
■ Unconsciousness or changes in level of consciousness such as decreased attention span, difficulties with comprehension, emotional lability, forgetfulness, and a lack of motivation
■ Anxiety
■ Communication and mobility difficulties
■ Possible urinary incontinence
■ Loss of voluntary muscle control and hemiparesis or hemiplegia on one side of the body
■ In the initial phase, flaccid paralysis with decreased deep tendon reflexes
■ After the initial phase, increase in muscle tone and, in some cases, muscle spasticity on the affected side
■ Hemianopsia on the affected side of the body
■ In patients with left-sided hemiplegia, problems with visual-spatial relations
■ Sensory losses, ranging from slight impairment of touch to the inability to perceive the position and motion of body parts
■ Difficulty interpreting visual, tactile, and auditory stimuli

Diagnostic test results

■ *Computed tomography (CT)* scan identifies ischemic stroke within the first 72 hours of symptom onset; and evidence of hemorrhagic stroke (lesions larger than 1 cm) immediately.
■ *Magnetic resonance imaging* assists in identifying areas of ischemia or infarction and cerebral swelling.
■ *Cerebral angiography* reveals disruption or displacement of the cerebral circulation

(*Text continues on page 349.*)

DISORDERS AFFECTING
MANAGEMENT OF STROKE

This chart highlights disorders that affect the management of stroke.

DISORDER	SIGNS AND SYMPTOMS	DIAGNOSTIC TEST RESULTS
Aspiration pneumonia (complication)	◆ Fever ◆ Crackles ◆ Dyspnea ◆ Hypertension initially (as a compensatory mechanism); then hypotension ◆ Tachycardia ◆ Cough with blood-tinged or yellow or green sputum ◆ Cyanosis	◆ Chest X-ray reveals infiltrates. ◆ Sputum for Gram stain and culture and sensitivity may reveal inflammatory cells and possible secondary bacterial infection. ◆ Bronchoscopy or transtracheal aspiration reveals possible secondary bacterial infection.
Hydrocephalus (complication)	◆ Distended scalp veins ◆ Thin, shiny, fragile-looking scalp skin ◆ Projectile vomiting ◆ Decreased level of consciousness ◆ Ataxia ◆ Incontinence ◆ Headache ◆ Blurred vision ◆ Papilledema ◆ Downward deviation of eyes (setting sun sign) ◆ Impaired intellect	◆ Skull X-rays may show thinning of the skull. ◆ Angiography shows vessel abnormalities caused by stretching. ◆ Computed tomography scan and magnetic resonance imaging reveal variations in tissue density and possible fluid in the ventricular system. ◆ Lumbar puncture reveals normal or increased fluid pressure. ◆ Ventriculography shows ventricular dilation with excess fluid.
Pressure ulcers (complication)	◆ Blanching erythema (first clinical sign): varying from pink to bright red depending on the patient's skin color (in dark-skinned people, purple discoloration or a darkening of normal skin color); area whitens with application of pressure, but color returns within 1 to 3 seconds if capillary refill is good ◆ Pain at the site and surrounding area ◆ Localized edema ◆ Increased body temperature (in more severe cases, cool skin due to more severe damage or necrosis) ◆ Nonblanching erythema (more severe cases) ranging from dark red to purple or cyanotic, indicating deeper dermal involvement ◆ Blisters, crusts, or scaling as the skin deteriorates and the ulcer progresses ◆ Dusky-red, possibly mottled, lesion that doesn't bleed easily (in cases of deep ulcer originating at the bony prominence below the skin surface) ◆ Possible foul-smelling, purulent drainage from ulcerated lesion ◆ Eschar tissue on and around the lesion	◆ Physical examination shows presence of the ulcer. ◆ Wound culture with exudate suggests infection. ◆ White blood cell count may be elevated with infection. ◆ Total serum protein and serum albumin levels show severe hypoproteinemia.

TREATMENT AND CARE

◆ Maintain a patent airway and oxygenation. Place the patient in Fowler's position to maximize chest expansion and give supplemental oxygen as ordered. Monitor oxygen saturation and arterial blood gas levels as ordered.
◆ Assess carbon dioxide levels closely to prevent increased intracranial pressure (ICP) and decreased cerebral perfusion pressure.
◆ Assess respiratory status often, at least every 2 hours. Auscultate the lungs for abnormal breath sounds. If respiratory status deteriorates, anticipate the need for intubation and mechanical ventilation.
◆ Encourage coughing and deep breathing.
◆ Adhere to standard precautions and institute appropriate transmission-based precautions, depending on the causative organism associated with secondary bacterial infection.
◆ Institute cardiac monitoring to detect arrhythmias secondary to hypoxemia.
◆ Reposition the patient to maximize chest expansion, allow rest, and reduce discomfort and anxiety.
◆ Administer drug therapy, such as bronchodilators and antimicrobials.

◆ Position the patient on his side to prevent aspiration.
◆ Handle the head gently and pad the area under head.
◆ Prepare for insertion of a shunt, ventriculostomy, or ICP monitoring as indicated.
◆ Administer medications, such as osmotic diuretics and corticosteroids.
◆ Monitor neurologic status for evidence of increasing pressure and deterioration.

◆ Frequently inspect the skin for possible changes in color, turgor, temperature, and sensation. Examine an existing ulcer for changes in size or degree of damage.
◆ Assess the patient for pain.
◆ Reposition the patient at least every 2 hours around the clock.
◆ Perform passive range-of-motion exercises, or encourage the patient to do active exercises, if possible.
◆ Use pressure relief aids on the patient's bed.
◆ Provide meticulous skin care. Keep the skin clean and dry without the use of harsh soaps.
◆ Change bedding frequently as indicated.
◆ Perform wound care using strict aseptic technique.
◆ Assist with debridement as needed.
◆ Encourage adequate nutritional intake; consult with the dietitian to develop a diet to promote granulation of new tissue.

ASSESSMENT FINDINGS IN STROKE

A stroke can leave one patient with mild hand weakness and another with complete unilateral paralysis. In both patients, the functional loss reflects damage to the brain area normally perfused by the occluded or ruptured artery. In general, assessment findings associated with a stroke may include:

◆ unilateral limb weakness
◆ speech difficulties
◆ numbness on one side
◆ headache
◆ vision disturbances (diplopia, hemianopsia, ptosis)
◆ vertigo
◆ anxiety
◆ altered level of consciousness (LOC).

Typical assessment findings based on the artery affected are highlighted in the chart below.

AFFECTED ARTERY	ASSESSMENT FINDINGS
Middle cerebral artery	◆ Aphasia ◆ Dysphasia ◆ Visual field deficits ◆ Hemiparesis of affected side (more severe in the face and arm than in the leg)
Carotid artery	◆ Weakness ◆ Paralysis ◆ Numbness ◆ Sensory changes ◆ Vision disturbances on the affected side ◆ Altered LOC ◆ Bruits ◆ Aphasia ◆ Ptosis
Vertebrobasilar artery	◆ Weakness on the affected side ◆ Numbness around lips and mouth ◆ Visual field deficits ◆ Diplopia ◆ Poor coordination, slurred speech ◆ Dysphagia ◆ Vertigo ◆ Nystagmus ◆ Amnesia ◆ Ataxia
Anterior cerebral artery	◆ Confusion ◆ Weakness ◆ Numbness, especially in the leg on the affected side ◆ Incontinence ◆ Loss of coordination ◆ Impaired motor and sensory functions ◆ Personality changes
Posterior cerebral artery	◆ Visual field deficits (homonymous hemianopsia) ◆ Sensory impairment ◆ Dyslexia ◆ Perseveration (abnormally persistent replies to questions) ◆ Coma ◆ Cortical blindness ◆ Absence of paralysis (usually)

by occlusion such as stenosis or acute thrombus or hemorrhage.

■ *Doppler ultrasound* identifies blockages in carotid artery.

■ *Digital subtraction angiography* shows evidence of occlusion of cerebral vessels, lesions, or vascular abnormalities.

■ *Carotid duplex scan* identifies stenosis greater than 60%.

■ *Brain scan* shows ischemic areas but may not be conclusive for up to 2 weeks after stroke.

■ *Single photon-emission CT* and *positron emission tomography scans* identify areas of altered metabolism surrounding lesions not yet able to be detected by other diagnostic tests.

■ *Noncontrast CT scan* differentiates between ischemic stroke and intracerebral and subarachnoid hemorrhages.

■ *Transesophageal echocardiogram* reveals cardiac disorders, such as atrial thrombi, atrial septal defect, or patent foramen ovale, as causes of thrombotic stroke.

■ *Lumbar puncture* reveals bloody CSF when stroke is hemorrhagic.

■ *Ophthalmoscopy* may identify signs of hypertension and atherosclerotic changes in retinal arteries.

■ *EEG* helps identify damaged areas of the brain.

COLLABORATIVE MANAGEMENT

The patient with an acute stroke requires multidisciplinary care. Typically, emergency services (EMS) personnel are involved in confirming the signs and symptoms of an acute stroke, completing the primary survey, and transporting the patient to the care facility. A speech therapist may assist the patient with defects in swallowing as well as speaking. A physical therapist helps the patient regain mobility and maintain range of motion. An occupational therapist helps the patient relearn basic activities of daily living, such as dressing, bathing, and cooking. The patient and his family may benefit from pastoral or spiritual counseling and support groups. Social services ensures continuity of care after discharge to the patient's home or to a rehabilitation facility and assists with follow-up care and financial and emotional concerns.

TREATMENT AND CARE

■ The essential steps to treating a patient with a stroke can be summarized as the seven D's: detection, dispatch, delivery, door, data, decision, and drug.

– *Detection* involves early identification of signs and symptoms by the patient or family members to ensure the best outcome.

– *Dispatch* involves EMS response and delivery of the patient to the health care facility.

– *Door* involves the patient's arrival at the ED with rapid triage and assessment.

– *Data* refers to all of the information obtained to determine the course of therapy.

– *Decision* involves identifying the most appropriate treatment based on the patient's situation, assessment findings, and the type of injury.

– *Drug* refers to the initiation of appropriate pharmacologic treatment.

■ For ischemic strokes, administer fibrinolytics, the initial drug therapy of choice which is initiated within 60 minutes of the patient arriving in the ED. Criteria for fibrinolytic therapy are:

– acute ischemic stroke associated with significant neurologic deficit

– onset of symptoms less than 3 hours before initiation of treatment. (See *Fibrinolytic therapy contraindications*, page 350.)

■ Manage ICP with monitoring, hyperventilation (to decrease partial pressure of arterial carbon dioxide, which lowers ICP), osmotic diuretics (mannitol, to reduce cerebral edema), and corticosteroids (dexamethasone, to reduce inflammation and cerebral edema).

RED FLAG *If the patient is receiving steroids to relieve cerebral edema, administer histamine-2 receptor antagonists as ordered to minimize the risk of GI bleeding; monitor for GI irritation and check the stool for blood.*

■ Administer stool softeners to prevent straining, which increases ICP, and anticonvulsants to treat or prevent seizures.

■ Surgery for large cerebellar infarction may be necessary to remove infarcted tissue and decompress remaining live tissue.

■ Aneurysm repair may be required to prevent further hemorrhage.

■ Percutaneous transluminal angioplasty or stent insertion may be performed to open occluded vessels.

FIBRINOLYTIC THERAPY CONTRAINDICATIONS

Criteria that exclude a patient from receiving fibrinolytic therapy for treatment of ischemic stroke include:

◆ evidence of intracranial hemorrhage during pretreatment evaluation
◆ suspicion of subarachnoid hemorrhage during pretreatment
◆ history of recent (within 3 months) intracranial or intraspinal surgery, serious head trauma, or previous stroke
◆ history of intracranial bleeding
◆ uncontrolled hypertension at time of treatment
◆ seizure at stroke onset
◆ active internal bleeding
◆ intracranial neoplasm, arteriovenous malformation, or aneurysm
◆ known bleeding diathesis, including but not limited to: current use of an anticoagulant such as warfarin, International Normalized Ratio greater than 1.7, or prothrombin time greater than 15 seconds; use of heparin within 48 hours before the onset of stroke with elevation of partial thromboplastin time or platelet count less than 100,000/µL.

■ Anticoagulant therapy (heparin, warfarin) maintains vessel patency and prevents further clot formation.
■ Antiplatelet agents (aspirin or ticlopidine) reduce the risk of platelet aggregation and subsequent clot formation (for patients with TIAs).
■ Carotid endarterectomy (for TIA) may be performed to open partially occluded carotid arteries.
■ Provide analgesics, such as acetaminophen, to relieve headache associated with hemorrhagic stroke.
■ Secure and maintain the patient's airway, and anticipate the need for endotracheal intubation and mechanical ventilation as necessary; monitor oxygen saturation levels with pulse oximetry and serial arterial blood gas studies as ordered.
■ Administering supplemental oxygen, as ordered, to maintain oxygen saturation greater than 95%.
■ Assess the patient's neurologic status frequently, at least every 15 to 30 minutes initially, then every hour as indicated. Note

LOC and ability to respond to stimuli, pupillary response, motor and sensory function, and reflexes. Observe for signs and symptoms of increased ICP, and monitor ICP as ordered. If the patient develops hydrocephalus, prepare him for a ventriculostomy.
■ Assess hemodynamic status frequently, including central venous pressure and pulmonary artery pressure.
■ Assess vital signs, including heart and respiratory rates, at least every 15 minutes until stabilized. Monitor blood pressure every 15 minutes, possibly with the use of direct intra-arterial blood pressure monitoring. Use continuous cardiac monitoring to detect arrhythmias.

DRUG ALERT *If the patient is receiving fibrinolytic therapy, maintain blood pressure below 185/110 mm Hg to minimize the risk of bleeding complications. If the patient isn't a candidate for fibrinolytic therapy, administer antihypertensive therapy only for markedly elevated blood pressures (diastolic pressure greater than 140 mm Hg, blood pressure greater than 220/120 mm Hg, or mean blood pressure about 130 mm Hg) because inducing lower perfusion pressures may increase ischemia and worsen the stroke. If antihypertensive therapy is indicated, expect to administer labetalol 20 mg I.V. push over 1 to 2 minutes, then 40 to 80 mg every 10 minutes to a maximum dose of 300 mg; or sodium nitroprusside, 0.25 to 0.3 mg/kg/ minute, titrating to maintain blood pressure within acceptable ranges without inducing hypotension.*
■ Monitor temperature for increases.

RED FLAG *If a patient is experiencing a hemorrhagic stroke, blood can accumulate in the subarachnoid space. This blood triggers an inflammatory response in the body, causing the temperature to rise. Institute measures to reduce hyperthermia (such as cooling blankets) and antipyretics (such as acetaminophen).*
■ Institute bleeding precautions for the patient receiving fibrinolytic therapy and assess for signs and symptoms of bleeding every 15 to 30 minutes.
■ Assess for seizures. Administer anticonvulsants, such as phenytoin, lorazepam, or diazepam, as ordered and institute safety precautions to prevent injury.
■ Monitor fluid intake and output and electrolyte balance.

■ Ensure adequate nutrition, enterally or parenterally, as appropriate. Check for gag reflex before offering small oral feedings of semisolid foods (if patient is awake and alert). Position the patient on his side to prevent aspiration if vomiting occurs. Have the patient sit upright with head tilted slightly forward when eating.

■ Position the patient in correct body alignment to promote pulmonary drainage and prevent upper airway obstruction.

■ Encourage coughing and deep breathing and incentive spirometry (if not intubated) to prevent atelectasis.

■ Use specialized pressure-reducing mattresses or overlays to minimize the risk of pressure ulcers.

■ Perform passive range-of-motion exercises for the affected and unaffected sides.

■ Apply antiembolism stockings or intermittent sequential compression devices to prevent deep vein thrombosis.

■ Establish a means of communication and provide psychological support.

RED FLAG After a stroke, a patient may experience emotional lability with mood fluctuations, which may result from brain damage or as a reaction to being dependent. Be sure to provide support and encouragement.

Subarachnoid hemorrhage

Subarachnoid hemorrhage (SAH) occurs when a cerebral, or intracranial, aneurysm ruptures. With cerebral aneurysm, a weakness in the wall of a cerebral artery causes localized dilation. Most cerebral aneurysms are berry (saccular) aneurysms, saclike outpouchings in cerebral arteries. Cerebral aneurysms usually arise at an arterial junction in the circle of Willis, the circular anastomosis forming the major cerebral arteries at the base of the brain.

The incidence of cerebral aneurysm is slightly higher in women than in men, especially in those women in their late 40s or early to mid-50s, but a cerebral aneurysm can occur at any age in either sex.

About 50% of all patients who suffer a subarachnoid hemorrhage die immediately.

Of those who survive untreated, 40% die from the effects of hemorrhage and another 20% die later from recurring hemorrhage. New treatments are improving the prognosis.

ETIOLOGY

A congenital defect, a degenerative process, a combination of the two, or trauma may cause cerebral aneurysm. In most cases, rupture occurs abruptly without a specific cause.

PATHOPHYSIOLOGY

Blood flow exerts pressure against a congenitally weak arterial wall, stretching it and causing a rupture.

Endocrine system

■ Blood spills into brain tissue.

■ Dilation of the third ventricle exerts mechanical pressure on the hypothalamus, causing progressive loss of nerve tissue, ultimately leading to hypothalamic dysfunction.

■ Hypothalamic dysfunction leads to impaired synthesis and transport, or release of antidiuretic hormone (ADH).

■ ADH doesn't respond to changes in plasma osmolarity, and the kidneys are unable to reabsorb water in the distal and collecting tubules, which leads to excretion of large amounts of dilute urine.

Neurologic system

■ An aneurysm can produce neurologic symptoms by exerting pressure on the surrounding structures such as the cranial nerves.

■ With rupture, blood spills into the space normally occupied by cerebrospinal fluid (CSF).

■ Blood may also spill into brain tissue, where a clot can cause potentially fatal increased intracranial pressure (ICP) and brain tissue damage.

■ Clots in the basal cisterns are believed to undergo hemolysis. This process causes a release of substances that initiate spasms of the cerebral blood vessels, causing vasospasm. (See *Disorders affecting management of subarachnoid hemorrhage,* pages 352 and 353.)

(Text continues on page 354.)

DISORDERS AFFECTING MANAGEMENT
OF SUBARACHNOID HEMORRHAGE

This chart highlights disorders that affect the management of subarachnoid hemorrhage.

DISORDER	SIGNS AND SYMPTOMS	DIAGNOSTIC TEST RESULTS
Diabetes insipidus (complication)	◆ Extreme polyuria—usually 4 to 6 L/day of dilute urine but sometimes as much as 30 L/day, with a low specific gravity (less than 1.005) ◆ Polydipsia, particularly for cold, iced drinks ◆ Nocturia ◆ Fatigue (in severe cases) ◆ Dehydration, characterized by weight loss, poor tissue turgor, dry mucous membranes, constipation, muscle weakness, dizziness, tachycardia, and hypotension	◆ Urinalysis reveals almost colorless urine of low osmolality (less than 200 mOsml/kg) and low specific gravity (less than 1.005). ◆ A water deprivation test confirms the diagnosis by demonstrating renal inability to concentrate urine (evidence of ADH deficiency). ◆ If the patient has central diabetes insipidus, subcutaneous injection of 5 units of vasopressin produces decreased urine output with increased specific gravity.
Respiratory failure (complication)	◆ Diminished chest movement ◆ Restlessness, irritability, and confusion ◆ Decreased level of consciousness (LOC) ◆ Pallor, possible cyanosis of skin and mucous membranes ◆ Tachypnea, tachycardia (strong and rapid initially, but thready and irregular in later stages) ◆ Cold, clammy skin and frank diaphoresis ◆ Diminished breath sounds; possible adventitious breath sounds ◆ Possible cardiac arrhythmias	◆ Arterial blood gas (ABG) analysis indicates early respiratory failure when partial pressure of arterial oxygen is low (usually less than 70 mm Hg), partial pressure of arterial carbon dioxide is greater than 45 mm Hg, and the bicarbonate level is normal. ◆ Serial vital capacity reveals readings less than 800 ml. ◆ Electrocardiography (ECG) may indicate arrhythmias. ◆ Pulse oximetry reveals a decreasing oxygen saturation level. Levels less than 50% indicate impaired tissue oxygenation.
Vasospasm (complication)	◆ Intense headache ◆ Decreased LOC; increased confusion ◆ Increased blood pressure ◆ Aphasia ◆ Partial paralysis	◆ Cerebral angiography reveals altered cerebral blood flow, vessel lumen dilation, and differences in arterial filling. ◆ Computed tomography scan identifies evidence of aneurysm and possible hemorrhage; it may also identify hydrocephalus, areas of infarction, and the extent of blood spillage within the cisterns around the brain. ◆ Magnetic resonance imaging may help locate the aneurysm and the bleeding. ◆ Positron-emission tomography shows the chemical activity of the brain and the extent of tissue damage. ◆ ECG commonly shows flattened or depressed T waves. ◆ Lumbar puncture and CSF analysis reveal blood in CSF; elevated CSF pressure, protein, and white blood cell count; and decreased glucose level.

TREATMENT AND CARE

◆ Anticipate using thiazide diuretics to reduce urine volume by creating mild salt depletion.
◆ Record fluid intake and output carefully; monitor daily weights.
◆ Watch for signs of hypovolemic shock, and monitor blood pressure and heart and respiratory rates regularly, especially during the water deprivation test.
◆ Monitor urine specific gravity between doses.
◆ Watch for decreased specific gravity with increased urine output, indicating an inability to concentrate urine and the need for the next dose or a dosage increase.
◆ Provide meticulous skin and mouth care, and apply a lubricant to cracked or sore lips.
◆ Make sure caloric intake is adequate and the meal plan is low in sodium.

◆ Institute oxygen therapy immediately to optimize oxygenation of pulmonary blood.
◆ Prepare for endotracheal (ET) intubation and mechanical ventilation if necessary; anticipate the need for high-frequency or pressure ventilation to force airways open.
◆ Administer drug therapy, such as bronchodilators, to open airways, corticosteroids to reduce inflammation, continuous I.V. solutions of positive inotropic agents (which increase cardiac output) and vasopressors (which induce vasoconstriction) to maintain blood pressure, and diuretics to reduce fluid overload and edema.
◆ Assess the patient's respiratory status at least every 2 hours, or more often as indicated. Observe for a positive response to oxygen therapy, such as improved breathing, color, and oximetry and ABG values.
◆ Position the patient for optimal breathing effort.
◆ Maintain a normothermic environment to reduce the patient's oxygen demand.
◆ Monitor vital signs, heart rhythm, and fluid intake and output.
◆ If the patient is intubated, auscultate the lungs to check for accidental intubation of the esophagus or the mainstem bronchus. Be alert for aspiration, broken teeth, nosebleeds, and vagal reflexes causing bradycardia, arrhythmias, and hypotension. Perform suctioning, as ordered, using strict aseptic technique. Check cuff pressure on the ET tube to prevent erosion from an overinflated cuff. Normal cuff pressure is about 20 mm Hg.
◆ Monitor oximetry and capnography values to detect changes in the patient's condition.
◆ Note the amount and quality of lung secretions and look for changes in the patient's status.
◆ Implement measures to prevent nasal tissue necrosis with a nasotracheal tube.
◆ Provide a means of communication for patients who are intubated and alert.

◆ Anticipate the use of hypervolemic hemodilution therapy, such as administration of normal saline, whole blood, packed red blood cells, albumin, plasma protein fraction (increase circulating volume to reverse or prevent ischemia secondary to vasospasm) and crystalloid solution (to decrease blood viscosity).
◆ Monitor closely for signs and symptoms of increased intracranial pressure (ICP).
◆ Monitor the patient's blood pressure and ICP continuously.
◆ Assess closely for signs and symptoms of fluid overload.
◆ Monitor urine output every hour.
◆ Auscultate lungs for crackles; observe for jugular vein distention; and monitor central venous pressure and pulmonary artery pressure for increases.

Respiratory system
■ Increased ICP caused by blood filling the brain tissue can lead to serious problems with the respiratory system because the major control centers are located in the brain.
■ Pressure on the respiratory center in the medulla interrupts nerve impulse transmission from the phrenic nerves to the diaphragm and from the intercostal nerves to the intercostal muscles, altering both the depth and rate of respirations. If the pons (the location of the apneustic and pneumotaxic centers) is affected, breathing patterns become altered.
■ Interruption in nerve impulse transmission to the diaphragm can lead to respiratory failure.

ASSESSMENT
The patient with a cerebral aneurysm may be asymptomatic. Typically, the aneurysm is found on a routine physical examination.

Clinical findings
The patient at risk for SAH may exhibit premonitory symptoms resulting from oozing of blood into the subarachnoid space. The symptoms, which may persist for several days, include:
■ headache
■ intermittent nausea
■ nuchal rigidity
■ stiff back and legs.

Usually, however, the rupture occurs abruptly and without warning, causing:
■ sudden, severe headache caused by increased pressure from bleeding into closed space
■ nausea and projectile vomiting related to increased pressure
■ altered level of consciousness (LOC), including deep coma, depending on the severity and location of bleeding, from increased pressure caused by increased cerebral blood volume.

Additional findings may include:
■ meningeal irritation, resulting in nuchal rigidity, back and leg pain, fever, restlessness, irritability, occasional seizures, photophobia, blurred vision, secondary to bleeding into the meninges
■ hemiparesis, hemisensory defects, dysphagia, and visual defects from bleeding into the brain tissues

■ diplopia, ptosis, dilated pupil, and inability to rotate the eye from compression on the oculomotor nerve if the aneurysm is near the internal carotid artery.

The severity of SAH is graded according to the patient's signs and symptoms. (See *Hunt-Hess classification for subarachnoid hemorrhage.*)

Diagnostic test results
■ *Cerebral angiography* reveals altered cerebral blood flow, vessel lumen dilation, and differences in arterial filling.
■ *Computed tomography (CT) scan* identifies evidence of aneurysm and possible hemorrhage; it may also identify hydrocephalus, areas of infarction, and the extent of blood spillage within the cisterns around the brain.
■ *Magnetic resonance imaging* may help locate the aneurysm and the bleeding.
■ *Positron-emission tomography* shows the chemical activity of the brain and the extent of tissue damage.
■ *Electrocardiography* commonly shows flattened or depressed T waves.
■ *Lumbar puncture (LP)* and *CSF analysis* reveal blood in CSF; elevated CSF pressure, protein, and white blood cell count; and decreased glucose level.

RED FLAG *Because LP increases the risk for herniation and rebleeding in patients with SAH and increased ICP, the procedure is performed only if the results of the CT scan are inconclusive.*

COLLABORATIVE MANAGEMENT
The patient with a SAH requires a multidisciplinary approach to care. A neurosurgeon may be involved to evaluate the need for surgery and determine the course of treatment. If the patient experiences neurologic deficits, he may require physical rehabilitation, nutritional therapy, occupational therapy, and respiratory therapy.

TREATMENT AND CARE
■ Initial emergency treatment includes oxygenation and ventilation.
■ To reduce the risk of rebleeding, the physician may attempt to repair the aneurysm surgically by clipping, ligating, or wrapping the aneurysm neck with muscle.
■ Newer surgical techniques include interventional radiology in conjunction with

endovascular balloon therapy to occlude the aneurysm or the vessel, and cerebral angioplasty to treat arterial vasospasm.

■ The timing of surgery is controversial; many patients with grade III or higher anterior circulation aneurysms have surgery within 1 to 3 days.

■ After surgical repair, the patient's condition depends on the extent of damage from the initial bleed and the degree of successful treatment of the resulting complications. Surgery can't improve the patient's neurologic condition unless it removes a hematoma or reduces the compression effect.

■ If surgical correction poses too much risk (in very elderly patients and those with heart, lung, or other serious diseases), if the aneurysm is in a particularly dangerous location, or if vasospasm necessitates a delay in surgery, the patient may receive conservative treatment.

■ Ensure bed rest in a quiet, darkened room with head of the bed flat or raised less than 30 degrees; if immediate surgery isn't possible, such bed rest may continue for 4 to 6 weeks.

■ Avoid coffee, other stimulants, and aspirin to reduce the risk of rupture and blood pressure elevation, which increases the risk of rupture.

■ Administer medications, as ordered, such as codeine or another analgesic as needed, to maintain rest and minimize the risk of pressure changes leading to rupture; hydralazine or another antihypertensive, if the patient is hypertensive, to reduce the risk of rupture; a vasoconstrictor to maintain blood pressure at the optimum level (20 to 40 mm Hg above normal), if necessary; corticosteroids to reduce cerebral edema and meningeal irritation; phenytoin or another anticonvulsant to prevent or treat seizures secondary to pressure and tissue irritation from bleeding; phenobarbital or another sedative to prevent agitation leading to hypertension and reduce the risk of rupture; aminocaproic acid, an inhibitor of fibrinolysis, to minimize the risk of rebleeding by delaying blood clot lysis (controversial).

■ Secure and maintain the patient's airway. Anticipate the need for endotracheal intubation and mechanical ventilation, as necessary.

HUNT-HESS CLASSIFICATION FOR SUBARACHNOID HEMORRHAGE

The severity of symptoms accompanying subarachnoid hemorrhage (SAH) varies from patient to patient, depending on the site and the amount of bleeding. The Hunt-Hess classification identifies five grades that characterize an SAH from a ruptured cerebral aneurysm:

◆ *Grade I (minimal bleeding)* – The patient is alert and oriented without symptoms.

◆ *Grade II (mild bleeding)* – The patient is alert and oriented, with a mild to severe headache and nuchal rigidity.

◆ *Grade III (moderate bleeding)* – The patient is lethargic and confused or drowsy, with nuchal rigidity and, possibly, a mild focal deficit such as hemiparesis.

◆ *Grade IV (severe bleeding)* – The patient is stuporous, with nuchal rigidity and, possibly, moderate to severe focal deficits, hemiplegia, early decerebrate rigidity, and vegetative disturbances.

◆ *Grade V (moribund; often fatal)* – If the rupture is nonfatal, the patient is in a deep coma, with such severe neurological deficits as decerebrate rigidity and moribund appearance.

■ Administer supplemental oxygen, as ordered. Use pulse oximetry and serial arterial blood gas studies to guide therapy.

RED FLAG Maintaining adequate oxygenation is crucial because the development of cerebral hypoxia, along with hypoxemia and hypercapnia, can lead to increased cerebral vasodilation, subsequently increasing cerebral edema and ICP.

■ Assess neurologic status at least every hour, or more frequently if indicated. Monitor ICP as ordered.

RED FLAG Decreased LOC, unilaterally enlarged pupil, onset or worsening of hemiparesis or motor deficit, increased blood pressure, decreased heart rate, worsened or sudden headache, renewed or persistent vomiting, and renewed or worsened nuchal rigidity may indicate an enlarging aneurysm, rebleeding, an intracranial clot, vasospasm, or another complication.

ANEURYSM PRECAUTIONS

Aneurysm precautions are measures to help prevent increased intracranial pressure and reduce the risk of rebleeding by minimizing increases in blood pressure. Although the specific precautions may vary among facilities, the following general guidelines are helpful.

♦ Place the patient on immediate and complete bed rest in a dimly lit, quiet, nonstressful environment.

♦ Keep the head of the patient's bed flat or slightly elevated (15 to 30 degrees).

♦ Avoid hyperflexion, hyperextension, or hyperrotation of the neck (minimizes jugular venous compression).

♦ Have the patient avoid activities involving isometric muscle contraction, such as pulling or pushing on the side rails or against the foot of the bed. Provide passive range-of-motion exercises.

♦ Administer stool softeners to prevent straining. Advise the patient to avoid bearing down with bowel movements (Valsalva's maneuver); encourage him to exhale slowly when defecating or voiding.

♦ Avoid rectal temperature measurement, suppositories, enemas, or digital impaction removal.

♦ Urge the patient to avoid coughing; administer antitussives, if ordered.

♦ Administer antiemetics as ordered to prevent or manage vomiting.

♦ Eliminate coffee, tea, or other caffeinated beverages from the patient's intake.

♦ Assist with personal care and activities of daily living to prevent exertion.

♦ Eliminate exposure to external stimuli, such as television, radio, and books.

♦ Restrict visitors to family; encourage visitors to talk quietly with the patient, avoiding stressful topics as much as possible.

■ Administer mannitol as ordered for sudden increases in ICP.

RED FLAG Monitor renal function status, including urine output and electrolytes, before and during mannitol administration. Be alert for a rebound effect of mannitol and a subsequent rebound increase

in ICP due to the increase in circulating volume, which may occur 8 to 12 hours after administration. Assess the patient closely. Anticipate the possible use of furosemide to reduce this effect.

■ Assess hemodynamic status frequently and determine the patient's cerebral perfusion pressure (CPP). Institute cerebral blood flow monitoring as ordered to determine CPP.

■ Assess vital signs, including heart rate, respiratory rate, and blood pressure, at least every 15 minutes until stabilized; monitor temperature for elevation.

RED FLAG If the aneurysm ruptures and blood accumulates in the subarachnoid space, it triggers an inflammatory response in the body that causes the patient's temperature to rise. Institute measures to reduce hyperphrenia, such as cooling blankets and antipyretics.

■ Administer antihypertensives, such as hydralazine, propranolol, labetalol, or sodium nitroprusside, as ordered to maintain blood pressure within the desired range. Anticipate the use of direct intra-arterial blood pressure monitoring.

■ Suction the airway according to facility policy as necessary to prevent hypoxia and vasodilatation from carbon dioxide accumulation. Suction for less than 20 seconds to avoid increased ICP.

■ Institute aneurysm precautions to prevent increased ICP and minimize the risk for rebleeding. (See *Aneurysm precautions.*)

■ Turn the patient frequently and institute measures to prevent skin breakdown.

■ Apply antiembolism stockings or intermittent sequential compression devices to the patient's legs to reduce the risk of deep vein thrombosis.

Syndrome of inappropriate antidiuretic hormone

Syndrome of inappropriate antidiuretic hormone (SIADH) occurs when excessive antidiuretic hormone (ADH) secretion is triggered by stimuli other than increased extracellular fluid osmolarity and decreased extracellular fluid volume. The prognosis varies with the degree of disease and the speed at which it develops; however, SIADH usually resolves within 3 days of effective treatment.

ETIOLOGY

SIADH is a relatively common complication of surgery or critical illness. Usually, SIADH results from oat cell carcinoma of the lung, which secretes excessive ADH or vasopressor-like substances. Other neoplastic diseases (such as pancreatic, duodenal, and prostatic cancers, Hodgkin's disease, lymphomas, and thymoma) may also trigger SIADH.

SIADH may also result from:
■ central nervous system (CNS) disorders, including brain tumor or abscess, stroke, head injury, and Guillain-Barré syndrome
■ pulmonary disorders (such as pneumonia, tuberculosis, lung abscess) and positive-pressure ventilation
■ drugs (for example, chlorpropamide, tolbutamide, vincristine, cyclophosphamide, haloperidol, carbamazepine, clofibrate, morphine, nicotine, barbiturates, tricyclic antidepressants, and thiazides)
■ endocrine disorders, such as adrenal insufficiency, myxedema, and anterior pituitary insufficiency
■ other conditions, such as psychosis, craniotomy (especially pituitary surgery), respiratory infection, and extreme stress and pain.

PATHOPHYSIOLOGY

Increased ADH causes excessive water reabsorption from the distal convoluted tubule and collecting ducts, leading to hyponatremia and normal to slightly increased extracellular fluid volume. (See *Understanding SIADH,* page 360.)

Neurologic system
■ Intracellular fluid shifts causing cerebral edema, which leads to increased ICP.
■ Cerebral perfusion pressure falls and cerebral blood flow decreases.

■ Ischemia leads to cellular hypoxia, which initiates vasodilation of cerebral blood vessels in an attempt to increase cerebral blood flow. Unfortunately, this causes the ICP to increase further.
■ As pressure continues to rise, compression of brain tissue and cerebral vessels further impairs cerebral blood flow.
■ With continued rise in ICP, the brain begins to shift under the extreme pressure and may herniate to an area of lesser pressure. (See *Disorders affecting management of SIADH,* pages 358 and 359.)
■ When the herniating brain tissue's blood supply is compromised, cerebral ischemia and hypoxia worsen. The herniation increases pressure in the area where the pressure was lower, thus impairing its blood supply.
■ As ICP approaches systemic blood pressure, cerebral perfusion slows even more, ceasing when ICP equals systemic blood pressure.

ASSESSMENT

The patient's medical history, including medications used, may provide a clue to the cause of SIADH. A history of cerebrovascular disease, cancer, pulmonary disease, or recent head injury is especially significant.

Clinical findings
■ Complaints of anorexia, nausea, and vomiting despite weight gain
■ Thirst and fatigue, followed by vomiting and intestinal cramping due to hyponatremia and electrolyte imbalance manifestations
■ Water retention and decreased urinary output due to hyponatremia
■ Neurologic symptoms such as lethargy, headaches, emotional and behavioral changes, restlessness, confusion, irritability, and disorientation that may progress to seizures and coma
■ Tachycardia associated with increased fluid volume
■ Sluggish deep tendon reflexes and muscle weakness.

Diagnostic test results
■ *Serum osmolarity* is less than 280 mOsm/kg of water.

DISORDERS AFFECTING MANAGEMENT OF SIADH

This chart highlights disorders that affect the management of syndrome of inappropriate antidiuretic hormone (SIADH).

DISORDER	SIGNS AND SYMPTOMS	DIAGNOSTIC TEST RESULTS
Brain herniation (complication)	◆ Drowsiness ◆ Confusion ◆ Dilation of one or both pupils ◆ Nuchal rigidity ◆ Bradycardia ◆ Changes in respiratory patterns including Cheyne-Stokes respirations or hyperventilation ◆ Decorticate or decerebrate posturing	◆ Computed tomography scan may reveal the area of herniation.
Hyponatremia (severe) (complication)	◆ Headache, nausea, or abdominal cramps ◆ Muscle twitching, tremors, or weakness ◆ Changes in level of consciousness (LOC) possibly starting as a shortened attention span, lethargy, or confusion and progressing to stupor and even coma ◆ Seizures ◆ Hypovolemia with poor skin turgor and dry, cracked mucous membranes ◆ Weak, rapid pulse ◆ Hypotension, orthostatic hypotension ◆ Possibly decreased central venous pressure, pulmonary artery pressure, and pulmonary artery wedge pressure	◆ Serum osmolality is less than 280 mOsm/kg (dilute blood). ◆ Serum sodium level is less than 135 mEq/L; if severe, less than 110 mEq/L. ◆ Urine specific gravity is elevated and urine sodium levels is above 20 mEq/L. ◆ Hematocrit and plasma protein levels are elevated.

■ *Serum sodium level* reveals hyponatremia (serum sodium less than 135 mEq/L); lower values indicate worsening condition.
■ *Urine sodium level* is elevated (more than 20 mEq/day).
■ *Serum ADH level* is elevated.
■ *Renal function tests* are normal, with no evidence of dehydration.
■ *Electrocardiography* may reveal changes suggesting hypokalemia.

COLLABORATIVE MANAGEMENT
Caring for the patient with SIADH requires a multidisciplinary approach that focuses on restricting fluids and treating the underlying cause. An endocrinologist can help manage the patient's hormone levels. A nutritionist may be consulted to devise a high-salt, high-protein diet. Social services may assist with arranging follow-up care and home care.

TREATMENT AND CARE
■ Based primarily on the patient's symptoms, begin treatment with restricted fluid intake (500 to 1,000 ml/day).
■ For some patients who continue to have symptoms, give a high-salt, high-protein diet or urea supplements to enhance fluid excretion.
■ Anticipate use of demeclocycline or lithium to help block the renal response to ADH, especially if fluid restriction is ineffective.
■ Although rare, and with severe fluid intoxication, administer 200 to 300 ml of 3% to 5% sodium chloride solution to raise the serum sodium level. A loop diuretic may also be prescribed to reduce the risk of heart failure.
■ When possible, include correction of the underlying cause of SIADH. If SIADH is due to cancer, surgery, irradiation, or chemotherapy may alleviate fluid retention.

TREATMENT AND CARE

◆ Check vital signs, LOC, and pupil size every 15 minutes.
◆ Establish and maintain a patent airway; anticipate endotracheal intubation and mechanical ventilation if necessary.
◆ Observe for cerebrospinal fluid (CSF) drainage from the patient's ears, nose, or mouth. Check pillows for CSF and look for a halo sign; test drainage for glucose with reagent strip. If the patient's nose is draining CSF, wipe it – don't let him blow it. If an ear is draining, cover it lightly with sterile gauze; don't pack it.
◆ Take seizure precautions but don't restrain the patient. Agitated behavior may be due to hypoxia or increased intracranial pressure.
◆ Speak in a calm voice and touch the patient gently. Don't make sudden, unexpected moves.
◆ Restrict total fluid intake to 1,200 to 1,500 ml/day to reduce fluid volume and intracellar swelling.

◆ Administer isotonic or hypertonic saline solution (such as 3% or 5% saline) with an infusion pump as ordered.
◆ Monitor the patient carefully during the infusion for signs of circulatory overload or worsening neurologic status. A hypertonic saline solution causes water to shift out of cells, which may lead to intravascular volume overload and serious brain damage (osmotic demyelination), especially in the pons.
◆ Accurately measure and record intake and output; obtain daily weights.
◆ Monitor for extreme changes in serum sodium levels and accompanying serum chloride levels. Also monitor other test results such as urine specific gravity and serum osmolality.
◆ Institute safety measures and seizure precautions as indicated.

■ Assess the patient's level of consciousness and ability to maintain a patent airway.
■ Monitor respiratory status closely, including respiratory rate and depth and breath sounds and oxygen saturation levels.
■ Administer supplemental oxygen as ordered. Anticipate using endotracheal intubation and mechanical ventilation if the patient can't maintain a patent airway or if he develops signs and symptoms of respiratory distress.
■ Assess vital signs, cardiac status, and hemodynamic status frequently.
■ Maintain fluid restrictions as ordered, typically 1,000 ml/24 hours. Remove liquids from the patient's bedside.
RED FLAG Meticulously monitor the patient's fluid intake, including the amount of ice chips given. When measuring ice chips as fluid intake, record the fluid as one-half of the amount of ice chips. For exam-

ple, if the patient ingests 4 oz (118 ml) of ice chips, record 2 oz (59 ml) fluid intake.
■ Administer I.V. fluids as ordered along with furosemide or mannitol I.V. to promote water excretion.
■ Obtain serial specimens to check serum and urine sodium levels, osmolarity, and urine specific gravity.
RED FLAG Monitor serum sodium levels closely to determine the rate of I.V. fluid therapy. If serum sodium levels are raised too quickly, the patient is at risk for neurologic damage (central pontine myelinosis). The goal is to raise the serum sodium level less than 12 mEq/L in 24 hours.
■ Institute measures to treat the underlying cause of the patient's condition; if medication is suspected as the cause, withhold as ordered.
■ Elevate the head of the bed approximately 10 to 20 degrees to promote venous re-

UNDERSTANDING SIADH

The flowchart below highlights the events that produce syndrome of inappropriate antidiuretic hormone (SIADH).

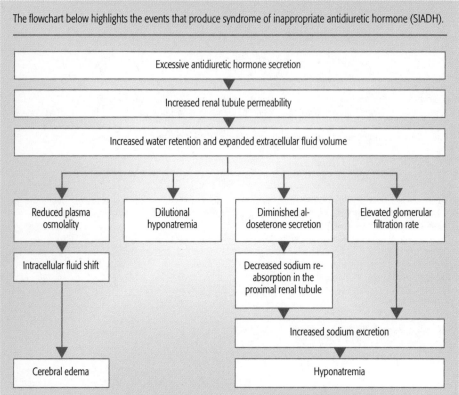

turn because decreased venous return is a stimulus for ADH release.
■ Institute seizure and safety precautions as appropriate to reduce the risk of injury.
■ Provide a calm, stress-free environment.

T-Z

Thyrotoxic crisis

Thyrotoxic crisis, also known as *thyroid storm* or *thyrotoxicosis,* is an acute manifestation of hyperthyroidism, a condition in which thyroid hormone overproduction results in a metabolic imbalance. Types of hyperthyroidism include Graves' disease (most common), toxic multinodular goiter, thyrotoxicosis factitia, functioning metastatic thyroid carcinoma, thyroid-stimulating hormone (TSH)–secreting pituitary tumor, and subacute thyroiditis.

Thyrotoxic crisis usually occurs in patients with preexisting (though commonly unrecognized) hyperthyroidism. It's a medical emergency that can lead to life-threatening cardiac, hepatic, or renal failure. Left untreated, it's invariably fatal.

ETIOLOGY
Hyperthyroidism can result from genetic and immunologic factors. In Graves' disease, thyroid-stimulating antibodies bind to and then stimulate the TSH receptors of the thyroid gland. The trigger for this autoimmune disease is unclear, although increased incidence in monozygotic twins suggests an inherited factor (probably a polygenic inheritance pattern). Graves' disease occasionally coexists with abnormal iodine metabolism and other endocrine abnormalities, such as diabetes mellitus, thyroiditis, and hyperparathyroidism. Graves' disease is also associated with production of autoantibodies, including long-acting thyroid stimulator (LATS), LATS protector, and human thyroid adenylate cyclase stimulators. A defect in suppressor-T lymphocyte function is a possible cause that allows the formation of these autoantibodies.

Thyrotoxic crisis is almost always abrupt in onset, evoked by a stressful event such as trauma, surgery, or infection. Less common causes include:
- insulin-induced hypoglycemia or diabetic ketoacidosis
- stroke
- myocardial infarction
- pulmonary embolism
- sudden discontinuation of antithyroid drug therapy
- initiation of radioactive iodine (^{131}I) therapy
- subtotal thyroidectomy with excess intake of synthetic thyroid hormone.

PATHOPHYSIOLOGY
Triiodothyronine and thyroxine (T_3 and T_4) are hormones secreted by the thyroid gland. Overproduction of T_3 and T_4 causes an increase in systemic adrenergic activity, which leads to overproduction of epinephrine. Severe hypermetabolism leads to cardiac and sympathetic nervous system decompensation. (See *Disorders affecting management of thyrotoxic crisis,* pages 362 and 363.)

Cardiopulmonary system
- Hypermetabolism causes increases in ventilation, blood volume, and cardiac output.
- Heart rate and myocardial contractility increase to compensate for the increased cardiac output, possibly leading to arrhythmias, especially atrial fibrillation.
- Heart failure and respiratory failure may occur if hypermetabolism is prolonged.

Neurologic system
- The overproduction of epinephrine leads to decompensation of the central nervous system, resulting in signs of irritability, restlessness, and tremors.

ASSESSMENT
The patient experiencing thyrotoxic crisis requires a thorough yet expedient assess-

DISORDERS AFFECTING
MANAGEMENT OF THYROTOXIC CRISIS

This chart highlights disorders that affect the management of thyrotoxic crisis.

DISORDER	SIGNS AND SYMPTOMS	DIAGNOSTIC TEST RESULTS
Atrial fibrillation (complication)	◆ Irregularly irregular pulse rhythm with normal or abnormal heart rate ◆ Radial pulse rate slower than apical pulse rate ◆ Palpable peripheral pulse with stronger contractions ◆ Evidence of decreased cardiac output, such as hypotension and light-headedness, with new-onset atrial fibrillation and a rapid ventricular rate	◆ Electrocardiography (ECG) reveals no clear P waves, irregularly irregular ventricular response and uneven baseline fibrillatory waves, and wide variation in R-R intervals resulting in loss of atrial kick. Atrial fibrillation may be preceded by premature atrial contractions. ◆ Transesophageal echocardiogram rules out the presence of thrombi in the atria.
Heart failure (complication)	*Left-sided heart failure* ◆ Dyspnea ◆ Orthopnea ◆ Paroxysmal nocturnal dyspnea ◆ Fatigue ◆ Nonproductive cough ◆ Crackles ◆ Hemoptysis ◆ Tachycardia ◆ Third and fourth heart sounds ◆ Cool, pale skin ◆ Restlessness and confusion *Right-sided heart failure* ◆ Jugular vein distention ◆ Positive hepatojugular reflux ◆ Right-upper-quadrant pain ◆ Anorexia ◆ Nausea ◆ Nocturia ◆ Weight gain ◆ Edema ◆ Ascites or anasarca	◆ Chest X-ray shows increased pulmonary vascular markings, interstitial edema, or pleural effusions and cardiomegaly. ◆ ECG may reveal hypertrophy, ischemic changes or infarction, tachycardia, and extrasystoles. ◆ Liver function test may be abnormal; blood urea nitrogen (BUN) and creatinine levels may be elevated. ◆ Prothrombin time may be prolonged. ◆ B-type natriuretic peptide immunoassay is elevated. ◆ Echocardiography may reveal left ventricular hypertrophy, dilation, and abnormal contractility. ◆ Pulmonary artery pressure, pulmonary artery wedge pressure, and left ventricular end-diastolic pressure are elevated in the presence of left-sided heart failure; right atrial or central venous pressure is elevated in right-sided heart failure. ◆ Radionuclide ventriculography may reveal ejection fraction less than 40% in diastolic dysfunction.

ment because the condition may prove fatal. The patient's history may reveal that an onset of symptoms followed a period of acute physical or emotional stress. A family history of Graves' disease is also common.

Clinical findings

- Marked tachycardia, vomiting, and stupor
- Difficulty concentrating, nervousness, irritability, and restlessness
- Vision disturbances, such as diplopia
- Angina or palpitations
- Shortness of breath, dyspnea on exertion (and possibly at rest)
- Cough
- Swollen extremities
- Fine tremors of the fingers and tongue, shaky handwriting, and clumsiness
- Emotional instability or lability and mood swings (occasional outbursts to overt psychosis)
- Flushed skin, diaphoresis
- Premature graying, increased hair loss, and fine, soft hair
- Fragile nails, possible onycholysis (the distal nail is separated from the nail bed)
- Pretibial myxedema over the dorsum of the legs or feet, which produces raised, thickened skin that may be itchy and hyperpigmented
- Plaquelike or nodular lesions
- Generalized or localized muscle atrophy and acropachy (soft-tissue swelling with underlying bone changes where new bone formation occurs)
- Infrequent blinking, characteristic stare, lid lag, exophthalmos, reddened conjunctiva and cornea, possible impaired upward gaze, convergence, and strabismus
- Asymmetrical, lobular, and enlarged thyroid gland
- Possibly enlarged liver
- Warm and moist skin with a velvety texture
- Hyperreflexia
- Paroxysmal supraventricular tachycardia and atrial fibrillation (especially in elderly patients) and, occasionally, a systolic murmur at the left sternal border
- Wide pulse pressures
- Increased bowel sounds
- In Graves' disease, an audible bruit over the thyroid gland

TREATMENT AND CARE

- Focus interventions on reducing the ventricular response rate to less than 100 beats/minute, establishing anticoagulation, and restoring and maintaining sinus rhythm.
- Administer drug therapy, such as calcium channel blockers or beta-adrenergic blockers, or expect to combine electrical cardioversion and drug therapy; administer anticoagulant therapy as ordered to prevent atrial thrombi.
- If the patient is hemodynamically unstable, perform synchronized electrical cardioversion. It's most successful if done within 48 hours after atrial fibrillation starts.
- Prepare for possible transesophageal echocardiogram before cardioversion to rule out the presence of thrombi in the atria.
- If drug therapy is used, monitor serum drug levels and observe the patient for evidence of toxicity.
- Tell the patient to report changes in pulse rate, dizziness, feeling faint, chest pain, and signs of heart failure, such as dyspnea and peripheral edema.
- Monitor the patient's peripheral and apical pulses; watch for evidence of decreased cardiac output and heart failure. If the patient isn't on a cardiac monitor, be alert for an irregular pulse and differences in the radial and apical pulse rates.

- Place the patient in Fowler's position and give supplemental oxygen.
- Weigh the patient daily, and check for peripheral edema.
- Monitor intake and output, vital signs, and mental status.
- Auscultate for third and fourth heart sounds and adventitious lung sounds such as crackles or rhonchi.
- Monitor BUN, creatinine, and serum potassium, sodium, chloride, and magnesium.
- Institute continuous cardiac monitoring to identify and treat arrhythmias promptly.
- Administer angiotensin-converting enzyme inhibitors, digoxin, diuretics, beta-adrenergic blockers, human B-type natriuretic peptides, nitrates, or morphine.
- Encourage lifestyle modifications, as appropriate.

■ High temperature, typically above 100.4° F (38° C) that begins insidiously and rises rapidly to a lethal level
■ Menstrual abnormalities

Diagnostic test results

Thyrotoxic crisis occurs only in patients with hyperthyroidism. The following laboratory test results confirm the diagnosis of hyperthyroidism.
■ *Radioimmunoassay* shows increased serum T_3 and T_4 concentrations.
■ *Thyroid scan* reveals increased uptake of 131I.
■ *Thyrotropin-releasing hormone (TRH) stimulation test* indicates hyperthyroidism if TSH level fails to rise within 30 minutes after administration of TRH.
■ Other supportive test results show increased serum protein-bound iodine and decreased serum cholesterol and total lipid levels.

COLLABORATIVE MANAGEMENT

Thyrotoxic crisis requires multidisciplinary care focused on decreasing thyroid hormone levels, restoring hemodynamic stability, regulating body temperature, and maintaining or improving ventilation, oxygenation, and cardiac function. An endocrinologist can help manage the patient's hormonal status. A pulmonologist and a respiratory therapist may be involved if the patient requires ventilatory support. A cardiac specialist may be consulted to help manage hemodynamic status and arrhythmias. A dietitian may provide diet planning. Social services may be involved to assist with financial concerns, follow-up, and long-term care planning, such as home care or referrals for community support.

TREATMENT AND CARE

■ Monitor vital signs, electrocardiogram, and cardiopulmonary status continuously.
■ Administer antithyroid drugs (propylthiouracil [PTU]) or beta-adrenergic blockers (propranolol) to block sympathetic effects.
■ Anticipate use of a corticosteroid to inhibit the conversion of T_3 and T_4 and to replace depleted cortisol.
■ Give iodide to block the release of thyroid hormones.

DRUG ALERT Don't administer aspirin to patients with thyrotoxic crisis

because it increases circulating thyroid hormones, thus exacerbating the patient's already hyperthyroid state. Acetaminophen, however, may be administered.
■ Institute cooling measures and closely monitor the patient's temperature as indicated.
■ Treat the underlying hyperthyroidism, which may include administering a single dose of 131I or partial thyroidectomy (in patients younger than age 40 with a large goiter who have experienced relapse after drug therapy).
■ Assess level of consciousness and the patient's ability to maintain a patent airway. Monitor respiratory status closely, including respiratory rate and depth, breath sounds, and oxygen saturation levels. Anticipate the need for endotracheal intubation and mechanical ventilation if the patient can't maintain a patent airway or develops signs and symptoms of respiratory distress.
■ Assess cardiac and hemodynamic status frequently, including auscultating heart sounds for changes, such as third heart sound or decreased or muffled heart sounds (which indicate heart failure), or chest pain or dyspnea (suggesting possible myocardial ischemia).
■ Monitor mean arterial pressure, central venous pressure, pulmonary artery wedge pressure, and cardiac output and note changes.

RED FLAG Mean arterial pressure is maintained at 70 mm Hg. A pressure below this level may interfere with cerebral and renal perfusion.
■ Perform continuous cardiac monitoring to evaluate for possible arrhythmias; be alert for ST-segment changes.
■ Assess core body temperature every 15 minutes for the first hour, and then every 30 minutes to 1 hour until the patient is stable.
■ Administer beta-adrenergic blockers, such as propranolol, to control tachycardia and hypertension, and be alert for possible hypotension secondary to the medication and fever.
■ Administer I.V. fluid replacement therapy as ordered while closely monitoring fluid status for overload.

DRUG ALERT If the patient exhibits signs and symptoms of overload or heart failure, cardiac glycosides and diuretics, such as furosemide, may be given. Monitor the patient's serum electrolyte levels, especially potassium levels, if the patient is receiving diuretics. Hypokalemia predisposes the patient to numerous complications, including arrhythmias and digoxin toxicity.

■ Administer antithyroid agents, such as PTU, iodide, or methimazole, as ordered. When administering PTU, monitor complete blood count results periodically to detect leukopenia, thrombocytopenia, and agranulocytosis.

DRUG ALERT *If PTU and iodide are ordered, give iodide at least 1 hour after giving PTU to enhance effectiveness. During antithyroid therapy, be alert for symptoms of hypothyroidism, such as weakness, fatigue, sensitivity to cold, weight gain, decreased level of consciousness, and bradycardia.*

■ Evaluate laboratory tests results, including thyroid hormone levels, to evaluate the effectiveness of therapy.

■ Assess for signs and symptoms of hyperglycemia, and monitor blood glucose levels closely.

RED FLAG *When thyroid hormones are excessive, glycogenolysis increases and insulin levels decrease, placing the patient at risk for hyperglycemia. Insulin therapy may be necessary.*

Traumatic brain injury

A traumatic brain injury is an insult to the brain resulting in physical, cognitive, or vocational impairment. Children ages 6 months to 2 years, those between ages 15 to 24, and elderly people are at highest risk for traumatic brain injury. Men are twice as likely as women to experience traumatic brain injury.

Mortality from head injury has declined due to the increased use of seat belts and airbags, faster emergency medical system response and transport times, and advances in treatments. The proliferation of regional trauma centers has also improved the prognosis for patients with traumatic brain injury.

ETIOLOGY

Traumatic brain injury commonly results from:

■ transportation or motor vehicle accidents (number one cause)
■ falls
■ sports-related accidents
■ assault.

PATHOPHYSIOLOGY

Traumatic brain injuries are classified as closed or open, depending on whether the cranial vault — the protective structure consisting of hair, skin, bone, meninges, and cerebrospinal fluid (CSF) — is breached. Closed trauma, the most common type of brain injury, typically results from acceleration-deceleration (also called *coup-contrecoup*). Forceful impact between the head and a stationary object causes the brain to strike the skull, injuring cranial tissues near the point of contact (coup). Residual force then causes the brain to rebound, driving it against the opposite side of the skull (contrecoup). Although the brain isn't exposed in closed trauma injuries, contusions and lacerations may occur as brain tissues slide over the rough bone of the cranial cavity. Diffuse axonal injury (or *shearing*) also occurs, damaging and severing connections between neurons.

In open trauma injuries, the cranial vault and dura are breached and brain tissues are exposed. Open trauma may result from impact (for example, in a fall or motor vehicle accident) or penetration (for example, by a knife or bullet). Open brain injuries are typically associated with skull fractures; bone fragments commonly cause hematomas and meningeal tears with consequent loss of CSF. The patient with an open trauma brain injury is also at high risk for infection.

RED FLAG *All patients with head injuries must be presumed to have spine injury until X-rays have shown otherwise.* (*See* Disorders affecting management of traumatic brain injury, *pages 366 and 367.*)

Neurologic system

■ Inflammation impairs the vascular tone of cerebral blood vessels.
■ Capillary permeability increases, disrupting the blood-brain barrier.
■ Edema leads to increased intracranial pressure (ICP), which impairs the flow of

DISORDERS AFFECTING
MANAGEMENT OF TRAUMATIC BRAIN INJURY

This chart highlights disorders that affect the management of traumatic brain injury.

DISORDER	SIGNS AND SYMPTOMS	DIAGNOSTIC TEST RESULTS
Brain herniation (complication)	◆ Drowsiness ◆ Confusion ◆ Dilation of one or both pupils ◆ Hyperventilation ◆ Nuchal rigidity ◆ Bradycardia ◆ Decorticate or decerebrate posturing ◆ Changes in respiratory patterns, including Cheyne-Stokes respirations or hyperventilation	◆ Computed tomography scan may reveal the area of herniation.
Respiratory failure (complication)	◆ Diminished chest movement ◆ Restlessness, irritability, and confusion ◆ Decreased level of consciousness (LOC) ◆ Pallor, possible cyanosis of skin, mucous membranes, lips, and nail beds ◆ Tachypnea, tachycardia (strong and rapid initially, but thready and irregular in later stages) ◆ Cold, clammy skin and frank diaphoresis are apparent, especially around the forehead and face ◆ Diminished breath sounds; possibly adventitious breath sounds ◆ Possibly cardiac arrhythmias	◆ Arterial blood gas (ABG) analysis indicates early respiratory failure when partial pressure of arterial oxygen is low (usually less than 70 mm Hg). ◆ Partial pressure of arterial carbon dioxide is greater than 45 mm Hg; bicarbonate level is normal. ◆ Serial vital capacity shows readings less than 800 ml. ◆ Electrocardiogram may demonstrate arrhythmias. ◆ Pulse oximetry reveals a decreased oxygen saturation level; oxygen levels less than 50% indicate impaired tissue oxygenation.

oxygen and nutrients to the brain as well as to other body tissues.

■ Increased ICP causes distortion of blood vessels and displacement of brain tissue, ultimately leading to herniation.

Respiratory system

■ Increased ICP disrupts nerve impulse transmissions to the diaphragm and intercostal muscles, affecting respiratory depth and rate.

■ Interruption in nerve impulse transmission to the diaphragm can lead to respiratory failure.

ASSESSMENT

Assessment findings will vary, depending on the type and location of the head injury.

Types of head injury include concussion, epidural hematoma, subdural hematoma, intracerebral hematoma, and skull fractures. (See *Types of brain injury*, pages 368 to 371.)

Clinical findings

■ History of traumatic injury (obtained from the patient, his family, eyewitnesses, or emergency personnel) to the head possibly followed by a period of unconsciousness

■ Altered level of consciousness (LOC) ranging from drowsy or easily disturbed by any form of stimulation such as noise or light to unconsciousness. (For specific signs and symptoms, see *Types of brain injury*, pages 368 to 371.)

TREATMENT AND CARE

◆ Check vital signs, LOC, and pupil size every 15 minutes.
◆ Establish and maintain a patent airway; anticipate endotracheal (ET) intubation and mechanical ventilation if necessary.
◆ Observe for cerebrospinal fluid (CSF) drainage from the patient's ears, nose, or mouth. Check pillows for a CSF leak and look for a halo sign. If the patient's nose is draining CSF, wipe it – don't let him blow it. If an ear is draining, cover it lightly with sterile gauze, don't pack it.
◆ Take seizure precautions but don't restrain the patient. Agitated behavior may be due to hypoxia or increased intracranial pressure.
◆ Speak in a calm voice and touch the patient gently. Don't make any sudden, unexpected moves.
◆ Restrict total fluid intake to 1,200 to 1,500 ml/day to reduce fluid volume and intracellular swelling.

◆ Institute oxygen therapy immediately to optimize oxygenation of pulmonary blood.
◆ Prepare for ET intubation and mechanical ventilation if necessary; anticipate the need for high-frequency or pressure ventilation to force airways open.
◆ Administer drug therapy, such as bronchodilators, to open airways; corticosteroids to reduce inflammation, continuous I.V. solutions of positive inotropic agents (which increase cardiac output) and vasopressors (which induce vasoconstriction) to maintain blood pressure; and diuretics to reduce fluid overload and edema, as ordered.
◆ Assess the patient's respiratory status at least every 2 hours, or more often as indicated. Observe for a positive response to oxygen therapy, such as improved breathing, color, and oximetry and ABG values.
◆ Maintain a normothermic environment to reduce the patient's oxygen demand.
◆ Monitor vital signs, heart rhythm, and fluid intake and output.
◆ If intubated, auscultate the lungs to check for accidental intubation of the esophagus or the mainstem bronchus. Be alert for aspiration, broken teeth, nosebleeds, and vagal reflexes causing bradycardia, arrhythmias, and hypotension. Perform suctioning, as ordered, using strict aseptic technique.
◆ Monitor oximetry and capnography values to detect important indicators of changes in the patient's condition.
◆ Check cuff pressure on the ET tube to prevent erosion from an overinflated cuff. Normal cuff pressure is about 20 mm Hg.
◆ Implement measures to prevent nasal tissue necrosis from nasotracheal tube if used.

Diagnostic test results

■ *Skull X-rays* will locate a fracture, if present, unless the fracture occurs in the cranial vault. (These fractures aren't visible or palpable.)
■ *Cerebral angiography* locates vascular disruptions from internal pressure or injuries due to cerebral contusion or skull fracture.
■ *Computed tomography scan* will disclose intracranial hemorrhage from ruptured blood vessels, ischemic or necrotic tissue, cerebral edema, areas of petechial hemorrhage, a shift in brain tissue, and subdural, epidural, and intracerebral hematomas.
■ *Magnetic resonance imaging* and a *radioisotope scan* may also disclose intracranial hemorrhage from ruptured blood vessels in a patient with a skull fracture.

COLLABORATIVE MANAGEMENT

Traumatic brain injury requires multidisciplinary care. A neurosurgeon may coordinate care if the trauma is severe enough to require surgery or invasive ICP monitoring. Physical therapy, occupational therapy, and social services may be necessary if the patient has physical or cognitive deficits from the injury and requires assistance with activities of daily living. A child with a head injury may be referred to a child life therapist for care to facilitate normal growth and development through the use of play and self-expression therapy. In cases of severe injury, the family may require spiritual support and help in considering whether the patient may be a candidate for organ donation.

(Text continues on page 370.)

TYPES OF BRAIN INJURY

TYPE	DESCRIPTION
Concussion (closed head injury)	◆ A blow to the head hard enough to make the brain hit the skull but not hard enough to cause a cerebral contusion causes temporary neural dysfunction. ◆ Recovery is usually complete within 24 to 48 hours. ◆ Repeated injuries exact a cumulative toll on the brain.
Epidural hematoma	◆ Acceleration-deceleration or coup-contrecoup injuries disrupt normal nerve functions in bruised area. ◆ Injury is directly beneath the site of impact when the brain rebounds against the skull from the force of a blow (a beating with a blunt instrument, for example), when the force of the blow drives the brain against the opposite side of the skull, or when the head is hurled forward and stopped abruptly (as in an automobile accident when a driver's head strikes the windshield). ◆ Brain continues moving and slaps against the skull (acceleration), then rebounds (deceleration). Brain may strike bony prominences inside the skull (especially the sphenoidal ridges), causing intracranial hemorrhage or hematoma that may result in tentorial herniation.
Intracerebral hematoma	◆ Subacute hematomas have better prognosis because venous bleeding tends to be slower. ◆ Traumatic or spontaneous disruption of cerebral vessels in brain parenchyma cause neurologic deficits, depending on site and amount of bleeding. ◆ Shear forces from brain movement frequently cause vessel laceration and hemorrhage into the parenchyma. ◆ Frontal and temporal lobes are common sites. Trauma is associated with few intracerebral hematomas; most caused by result of hypertension.

SIGNS AND SYMPTOMS

◆ Short-term loss of consciousness secondary to disruption of reticular activating system (RAS), possibly due to abrupt pressure changes in the areas responsible for consciousness, changes in polarity of the neurons, ischemia, or structural distortion of neurons
◆ Vomiting from localized injury and compression
◆ Anterograde and retrograde amnesia (patient can't recall events immediately after the injury or events that led up to the traumatic incident) correlating with severity of injury; all related to disruption of RAS
◆ Irritability or lethargy from localized injury and compression
◆ Behavior out of character due to focal injury
◆ Complaints of dizziness, nausea, or severe headache due to focal injury and compression

◆ Brief period of unconsciousness after injury reflecting the concussive effects of head trauma, followed by a lucid interval varying from 10 to 15 minutes to hours or, rarely, days
◆ Severe headache
◆ Progressive loss of consciousness and deterioration in neurologic signs resulting from expanding lesion and extrusion of medial portion of temporal lobe through tentorial opening
◆ Compression of brain stem by temporal lobe causing clinical manifestations of intracranial hypertension
◆ Deterioration in level of consciousness resulting from compression of brainstem reticular formation as temporal lobe herniates on its upper portion
◆ Respirations, initially deep and labored, becoming shallow and irregular as brain stem is impacted
◆ Contralateral motor deficits reflecting compression of corticospinal tracts that pass through the brainstem
◆ Ipsilateral (same-side) pupillary dilation due to compression of third cranial nerve
◆ Seizures possible from increased intracranial pressure (ICP)
◆ Continued bleeding leading to progressive neurologic degeneration, evidenced by bilateral pupillary dilation, bilateral decerebrate response, increased systemic blood pressure, decreased pulse, and profound coma with irregular respiratory patterns

◆ Unresponsive immediately or experiencing a lucid period before lapsing into a coma from increasing ICP and mass effect of hemorrhage
◆ Possible motor deficits and decorticate or decerebrate responses from compression of corticospinal tracts and brain stem

DIAGNOSTIC TEST RESULTS

◆ Computed tomography (CT) scan reveals no sign of fracture, bleeding, or other nervous system lesion.

◆ CT scan or magnetic resonance imaging (MRI) identifies abnormal masses or structural shifts within the cranium.

◆ CT scan or cerebral arteriography identifies bleeding site. CSF pressure is elevated; fluid may appear bloody or xanthochromic (yellow or straw-colored) from hemoglobin breakdown.

(continued)

TYPES OF BRAIN INJURY *(continued)*

TYPE	DESCRIPTION
Skull fracture	◆ There are four types of skull fractures, including linear, comminuted, depressed, and basilar. ◆ Fractures of the anterior and middle fossae are associated with severe head trauma and are more common than those of the posterior fossa. ◆ Blow to the head causes one or more of the types. May not be problematic unless brain is exposed or bone fragments are driven into neural tissue.
Subdural hematoma	◆ Meningeal hemorrhages, resulting from accumulation of blood in subdural space (between dura mater and arachnoid) are most common. ◆ It may be acute, subacute, and chronic; unilateral or bilateral. ◆ Usually associated with torn connecting veins in cerebral cortex; rarely from arteries. ◆ Acute hematomas are a surgical emergency.

TREATMENT AND CARE

■ Surgical treatment of traumatic brain injury may include evacuation of the hematoma or a craniotomy to elevate or remove fragments that have been driven into the brain and to extract foreign bodies and necrotic tissue, thereby reducing the risk of infection and further brain damage from fractures.

■ Observe the patient closely to detect changes in neurologic status, including LOC and pupil size, which suggest further damage or expanding hematoma.

■ Clean and debride wounds associated with skull fractures.

■ Administer medications as ordered, including diuretics (such as mannitol) and corticosteroids (such as dexamethasone) to reduce cerebral edema, analgesics (such as acetaminophen) to relieve complaints of headache, anticonvulsants (such as phenytoin) to prevent and treat seizures, and prophylactic antibiotics to prevent the onset of meningitis from CSF leakage.

DRUG ALERT Keep in mind that the use of corticosteroids may be controversial because they have been associated with poorer outcomes. Monitor doses of mannitol closely for possible accumulation of the drug because the drug can lead to renal failure and exacerbate brain edema by leaking into the brain interstitium.

■ Provide respiratory support, including mechanical ventilation and endotracheal intubation, as indicated, for respiratory failure from brain stem involvement.

■ Assess for cardiopulmonary changes.

RED FLAG Abnormal respirations could indicate a breakdown in the brain's respiratory center and, possibly, impending tentorial herniation—a neurologic emergency. Elderly patients require close monitoring because brain atrophy due to aging leads to greater space for cerebral edema. ICP may increase despite absence of signs or symptoms (in elderly patients).

SIGNS AND SYMPTOMS	DIAGNOSTIC TEST RESULTS
◆ Possibly asymptomatic, depending on underlying brain trauma ◆ Discontinuity and displacement of bone structure with severe fracture ◆ Motor sensory and cranial nerve dysfunction with associated facial fractures ◆ Persons with anterior fossa basilar skull fractures may have periorbital ecchymosis ("raccoon eyes"), anosmia (loss of smell due to first cranial nerve involvement) and pupil abnormalities (second and third cranial nerve involvement) ◆ CSF rhinorrhea (leakage through nose), CSF otorrhea (leakage from the ear), and hemotympanium (blood accumulation at the tympanic membrane) ◆ Signs of medullary dysfunction such as cardiovascular and respiratory failure (posterior fossa basilar skull fracture)	◆ CT scan and MRI reveal intracranial hemorrhage from ruptured blood vessels and swelling. ◆ Skull X-ray may reveal fracture. ◆ Lumbar puncture contraindicated by expanding lesions.
◆ Similar to epidural hematoma but significantly slower in onset because bleeding typically originates in veins	◆ CT scan, X-rays, and arteriography reveal mass and altered blood flow in the area, confirming hematoma. ◆ CT scan or MRI reveals evidence of masses and tissue shifting. ◆ CSF is yellow and has relatively low protein (chronic subdural hematoma).

■ Maintain a patent airway and monitor oxygenation saturation levels; administer supplemental oxygen as necessary.

■ Carefully observe for CSF leakage. Check sheets for a blood-tinged spot surrounded by a lighter ring (halo sign) or test fluid with a reagent strip for glucose.

RED FLAG *If the patient has CSF leakage or is unconscious, elevate the head of the bed to 30 degrees to reduce the risk of jugular compression, which can lead to increased ICP. Keep his head properly aligned.*

■ Assist with the insertion of the ICP monitoring system and continuously monitoring ICP waveforms and pressure.

■ Determine cerebral perfusion pressure (CPP) by calculation or with a cerebral blood flow monitoring system.

■ Assess hemodynamic parameters to help evaluate CPP.

■ Administer medications as ordered. If necessary, use continuous infusions of medications, such as midazolam, fentanyl, morphine, or propofol to help reduce metabolic demand and reduce the risk of increased ICP. If ICP increases, administer mannitol and furosemide, as ordered.

■ Monitor intake and output frequently to help maintain a normovolemic state.

■ Institute safety and seizure precautions if indicated.

■ Prepare the patient for a craniotomy as indicated.

■ After the patient is stabilized, clean and dress superficial scalp wounds using strict aseptic technique.

Quick-reference guide to laboratory test results

A

Acetylcholine receptor antibodies, serum
Negative

Acid mucopolysaccharides, urine
Adults: <13.3 µg glucuronic acid/mg/creatinine/24 hours

Acid phosphatase, serum
0 to 3.7 U/L (SI, 0 to 3.7 U/L)

Adrenocorticotropic hormone, plasma
<120 pg/ml (SI, <26.4 pmol/L)

Alanine aminotransferase
8 to 50 IU/L (SI, 0.14 to 0.85 µkat/L)

Aldosterone, serum
◆ Supine individuals: 3 to 16 ng/dl (SI, 80 to 440 pmol/L)
◆ Upright individuals: 7 to 30 ng/dl (SI, 190 to 832 pmol/L)

Aldosterone, urine
3 to 19 µg/24 hours (SI, 8 to 51 nmol/d)

Alkaline phosphatase, peritoneal fluid
◆ Males >18 years: 90 to 239 U/L (SI, 90 to 239 U/L)
◆ Females <45 years: 76 to 196 U/L (SI, 76 to 196 U/L); >45 years: 87 to 250 U/L (87 to 250 U/L)

Alkaline phosphatase, serum
45 to 115 U/L (SI, 45 to 115 U/L)

Alpha-fetoprotein serum
Males and nonpregnant, females: <15 ng/ml (SI, <15 mg/L)

Ammonia, peritoneal fluid
<50 ng/dl (SI, <29 µmol/L)

Amniotic fluid analysis
◆ Lecithin-sphingomyelin ratio: >2
◆ Meconium: absent (except in breech presentation)
◆ Phosphatidylglycerol: present

Amylase, peritoneal fluid
138 to 404 U/L (SI, 138 to 404 U/L)

Amylase, serum
Adults ≥18 years: 26 to 102 U/L (SI, 0.4 to 1.74 µkat/L)

Amylase, urine
1 to 17 U/hour (SI, 0.017 to 0.29 µkat/h)

Androstenedione (radioimmunoassay)
◆ Males: 75 to 205 ng/dl (SI, 2.6 to 7.2 nmol/L)
◆ Females: 85 to 275 ng/dl (SI, 3.0 to 9.6 nmol/L)

Angiotensin-converting enzyme
Adults ≥20 years: 8 to 52 U/L (SI, 0.14 to 0.88 µkat/L)

Anion gap
8 to 14 mEq/L (SI, 8 to 14 mmol/L)

Antibody screening, serum
Negative

Antidiuretic hormone, serum
1 to 5 pg/ml (SI, 1 to 5 ng/L)

Antiglobulin test, direct
Negative

Antimitochondrial antibodies, serum
Negative

Anti-smooth-muscle antibodies, serum
Negative

Antistreptolysin-O, serum
◆ Preschoolers and adults: 85 Todd units/ml
◆ School-age children: 170 Todd units/ml

Antithrombin III
80% to 120% of normal control values

Antithyroid antibodies, serum
Normal titer <1:100

Arginine test
◆ Human growth hormone levels
– Males: increase to >10 ng/ml (SI, >10 µg/L)
– Females: increase to >15 ng/ml (SI, >15 µg/L)
– Children: increase to >48 ng/ml (SI, >48 µg/L)

Arterial blood gases
- pH: 7.35 to 7.45 (SI, 7.35 to 7.45)
- Pao_2: 80 to 100 mm Hg (SI, 10.6 to 13.3 kPa)
- $Paco_2$: 35 to 45 mm Hg (SI, 4.7 to 5.3 kPa)
- O_2 CT: 15% to 23% (SI, 0.15 to 0.23)
- Sao_2: 94% to 100% (SI, 0.94 to 1.00)
- HCO_3^-: 22 to 25 mEq/L (SI, 22 to 25 mmol/L)

Arylsufatase A, urine
- Random: 16 to 42 µ/g creatinine
- 24-hour: 0.37 to 3.60 µ/day creatinine
- 1-hour test: 2 to 19 µ/1 hour (SI, 2 to 19 µ/h)
- 2-hour test: 4 to 37 µ/2 hours (SI, 4 to 37 µ/h)
- 24-hour test: 170 to 2,000 µ/24 hours (SI, 2.89 to 34.0 µkat/L)

Aspartate aminotransferase
12 to 31 U/L (SI, 0.21 to 0.53 µkat/L)

Aspergillosis antibody, serum
Normal titer < 1:8

Atrial natriuretic factor, plasma
20 to 77 pg/ml

B

Bacterial meningitis antigen
Negative

Bence Jones protein, urine
Negative

Beta-hydroxybutyrate
<0.4 mmol/L (SI, 0.4 mmol/L)

Bilirubin, amniotic fluid
- Early: <0.075 mg/dl (SI, <1.3 µmol/L)
- Term: <0.025 mg/dl (SI, <0.41 µmol/L)

Bilirubin, serum
- Adults
- Direct: <0.5 mg/dl (SI, <6.8 µmol/L)
- Indirect: 1.1 mg/dl (SI, 19 µmol/L)
- Neonates
- Total: 1 to 12 mg/dl (SI, 34 to 205 µmol/L)

Bilirubin, urine
Negative

Blastomycosis antibody, serum
Normal titer < 1:8

Bleeding time
- Template: 3 to 6 minutes (SI, 3 to 6 m)
- Ivy: 3 to 6 minutes (SI, 3 to 6 m)
- Duke: 1 to 3 minutes (SI, 1 to 3 m)

Blood urea nitrogen
8 to 20 mg/dl (SI, 2.9 to 7.5 mmol/L)

B-lymphocyte count
270 to 640/µl

C

Calcitonin, plasma
- Baseline
- Males: < 16 pg/ml (SI, < 16 ng/L)
- Females: < 8 pg/ml (SI, < 8 ng/L)

Calcium, serum
- Adults: 8.2 to 10.2 mg/dl (SI, 2.05 to 2.54 mmol/L)
- Children: 8.6 to 11.2 mg/dl (SI, 2.15 to 2.79 mmol/L)
- Ionized: 4.65 to 5.28 mg/dl (SI, 1.1 to 1.25 mmol/L)

Calcium, urine
100 to 300 mg/24 hours (SI, 2.50 to 7.50 mmol/d)

Candida antibodies, serum
Negative

Capillary fragility
Petechiae per 5 cm:	Score:
11 to 20	2 +
21 to 50	3 +
over 50	4 +

Carbon dioxide, total, blood
22 to 26 mEq/L (SI, 22 to 26 mmol/L)

Carcinoembryonic antigen, serum
<5 ng/ml (SI, <5 mg/L)

Catecholamines, plasma
- Supine
- Epinephrine: undetectable to 110 pg/ml (SI, undetectable to 600 pmol/L)
- Norepinephrine: 70 to 750 pg/ml (SI, 413 to 4,432 pmol/L)
- Standing
- epinephrine: undetectable to 140 pg/ml (SI, undetectable to 764 pmol/L)
- norepinephrine: 200 to 1,700 pg/ml (SI, 1,182 to 10,047 pmol/L)

Catecholamines, urine
◆ Epinephrine: 0 to 20 µg/24 hours (SI, 0 to 109 nmol/24 h)
◆ Norepinephrine: 15 to 80 µg/24 hours (SI, 89 to 473 nmol/24 h)
◆ Dopamine: 65 to 400 µg/24 hours (SI, 425 to 2,610 nmol/24 h)

Cerebrospinal fluid
◆ Pressure: 50 to 180 mm H_2O
◆ Appearance: clear, colorless
◆ Gram stain: no organisms

Ceruloplasmin, serum
22.9 to 43.1 mg/dl (SI, 0.22 to 0.43 g/L)

Chloride, cerebrospinal fluid
118 to 130 mEq/L (SI, 118 to 130 mmol/L)

Chloride, serum
100 to 108 mEq/L (SI, 100 to 108 mmol/L)

Chloride, urine
◆ Adults: 110 to 250 mmol/24 hours (SI, 110 to 250 mmol/d)
◆ Children: 15 to 40 mmol/24 hours (SI, 15 to 40 mmol/d)
◆ Infants: 2 to 10 mmol/24 hours (SI, 2 to 10 mmol/d)

Cholinesterase (pseudocholinesterase)
204 to 532 IU/dl (SI, 2.04 to 5.32 kU/L)

Coccidioidomycosis antibody, serum
Normal titer <1:2

Cold agglutinins, serum
Normal titer <1:64

Complement, serum
◆ Total
− 40 to 90 U/ml (SI, 0.4 to 0.9 g/L)
◆ C3
− Males: 80 to 180 mg/dl (SI, 0.8 to 1.8 g/L)
− Females: 76 to 120 mg/dl (SI, 0.76 to 1.2 g/L)
◆ C4
− Males: 15 to 60 mg/dl (SI, 0.15 to 0.6 g/L)
− Females: 15 to 52 mg/dl (SI, 0.15 to 0.52 g/L)

Copper, urine
3 to 35 µg/24 hours (SI, 0.05 to 0.55 µmol/d)

Cortisol, free, urine
<50 µg/24 hours (SI, <138 nmol/d)

Cortisol, plasma
◆ Morning: 7 to 25 mcg/dl (SI, 0.2 to 0.7 µmol/L)
◆ Afternoon: 2 to 14 mcg/dl (SI, 0.06 to 0.39 µmol/L)

C-reactive protein, serum
<0.8 mg/dl (SI, <8 mg/L)

Creatine kinase
Total
− Males: 55 to 170 U/L (SI, 0.94 to 2.89 µkat/L)
− Females: 30 to 135 U/L (SI, 0.51 to 2.3 µkat/L)

Creatinine clearance
◆ Males: 94 to 140 ml/min/1.73 m² (SI, 0.91 to 1.35 ml/s/m²)
◆ Females: 72 to 110 ml/min/1.73 m² (SI, 0.69 to 1.06 ml/s/m²)

Creatinine, serum
◆ Males: 0.8 to 1.2 mg/dl (SI, 62 to 115 µmol/L)
◆ Females: 0.6 to 0.9 mg/dl (SI, 53 to 97 µmol/L)

Creatinine, urine
◆ Males: 14 to 26 mg/kg body weight/24 hours (SI, 124 to 230 µmol/kg body weight/d)
◆ Females: 11 to 20 mg/kg body weight/24 hours (SI, 97 to 177 µmol/kg body weight/d)

Cryoglobulins, serum
Negative

Cyclic adenosine monophosphate, urine
◆ 0.3 to 3.6 mg/day (SI, 100 to 723 µmol/d)
or
◆ 0.29 to 2.1 mg/g creatinine (SI, 100 to 723 µmol/mol creatinine)

Cytomegalovirus antibodies, serum
Negative

D

D-xylose absorption
◆ Blood
− Adults: 25 to 40 mg/dl in 2 hours
− Children: >30 mg/dl in 1 hour
◆ Urine
− Adults: >3.5 g excreted in 5 hours (age 65 of older, >5 g in 24 hours)
− Children: 16% to 33% excreted in 5 hours

E

Epstein-Barr virus antibodies
Negative

Erythrocyte sedimentation rate
- Males: 0 to 10 mm/hour (SI, 0 to 10 mm/h)
- Females: 0 to 20 mm/hour (SI, 0 to 20 mm/h)

Esophageal acidity
pH >5.0

Estrogens, serum
- Females
- Menstruating: 26 to 149 pg/ml (SI, 90 to 550 pmol/L)
- Postmenopausal: 0 to 34 pg/ml (SI, 0 to 125 pmol/L)
- Males
- 12 to 34 pg/ml (SI, 40 to 125 pmol/L)
- Children
- <6 years: 3 to 10 pg/ml (SI, 10 to 36 pmol/L)

Euglobulin lysis time
2 to 4 hours (SI, 2 to 4 h)

F

Factor assay, one-stage
50% to 150% of normal activity (SI, 0.50 to 1.50)

Febrile agglutination, serum
- Salmonella antibody: <1:80
- Brucellosis antibody: <1:80
- Tularemia antibody: <1:40
- Rickettsial antibody: <1:40

Ferritin, serum
- Males
- 20 to 300 ng/ml (SI, 20 to 300 µg/L)
- Females
- 20 to 120 ng/ml (SI, 20 to 120 µg/L)
- Infants
- 1 month: 200 to 600 ng/ml (SI, 200 to 600 µg/L)
- 2 to 5 months: 50 to 200 ng/ml (SI, 50 to 200 µg/L)
- 6 months to 15 years: 7 to 140 ng/ml (SI, 7 to 140 µg/L)
- Neonates
- 25 to 200 ng/ml (SI, 25 to 200 µg/L)

Fibrinogen, plasma
200 to 400 mg/dl (SI, 2 to 4 g/L)

Fibrin split products
- Screening assay: <10 µg/ml (SI, <10 mg/L)
- Quantitative assay: <3 µg/ml (SI, <3 mg/L)

Fluorescent treponemal antibody absorption, serum
Negative

Folic acid, serum
1.8 to 20 ng/ml (SI, 4 to 45.3 nmol/L)

Follicle-stimulating hormone, serum
- Menstruating females
- Follicular phase: 5 to 20 mIU/ml (SI, 5 to 20 IU/L)
- Ovulatory phase: 15 to 30 mIU/ml (SI, 15 to 30 IU/L)
- Luteal phase: 5 to 15 mIU/ml (SI, 5 to 15 IU/L)
- Menopausal females
- 5 to 100 mIU/ml (SI, 50 to 100 IU/L)
- Males
- 5 to 20 mIU/ml (5 to 20 IU/L)

Free thyroxine, serum
0.9 to 2.3 ng/dl (SI, 10 to 30 nmol/L)

Free triiodothyronine
0.2 to 0.6 ng/dl (SI, 0.003 to 0.009 nmol/L)

G

Galactose 1-phosphate uridyl transferase
- Qualitative: negative
- Quantitative: 18.5 to 28.5 U/g of hemoglobin

Gamma-glutamyl transferase
- Males ≥16 years: 6 to 38 U/L (SI, 0.10 to 0.63 µkat/L)
- Females 16 to 45 years: 4 to 27 U/L (SI, 0.08 to 0.46 µkat/L); >45 years: 6 to 38 U/L (SI, 0.10 to 0.63 µkat/L)
- Children: 3 to 30 U/L (SI, 0.05 to 0.51 µkat)

Gastric acid stimulation
- Males: 18 to 28 mEq/hour
- Females: 11 to 21 mEq/hour

Gastric secretion, basal
- Males: 1 to 5 mEq/hour
- Females: 0.2 to 3.3 mEq/hour

Gastrin, serum
50 to 150 pg/ml (SI, 50 to 150 ng/L)

Globulin, peritoneal fluid
30% to 45% of total protein

Glucose, amniotic fluid
<45 mg/dl (SI, <2.3 mmol/L)

Glucose, cerebrospinal fluid
50 to 80 mg/dl (SI, 2.8 to 4.4 mmol/L)

Glucose, peritoneal fluid
70 to 100 mg/dl (SI, 3.5 to 5 mmol/L)

Glucose, plasma, fasting
70 to 100 mg/dl (SI, 3.9 to 6.1 mmol/L)

Glucose-6-phosphate dehydrogenase
4.3 to 11.8 U/g (SI, 0.28 to 0.76 mU/mol) of hemoglobin

Glucose tolerance, oral
Peak at 160 to 180 mg/dl (SI, 8.8 to 9.9 mmol/L) 30 to 60 minutes after challenge dose

Growth hormone suppression
Undetectable to 3 ng/ml (SI, undetectable to 3 µg/L) after 30 minutes to 2 hours

H

Ham test
Negative

Haptoglobin, serum
40 to 180 mg/dl (SI, 0.4 to 1.8 g/L)

Heinz bodies
Negative

Hematocrit
- Males
  - 42% to 52% (SI, 0.42 to 0.52)
- Females
  - 36% to 48% (SI, 0.36 to 0.48)
- Children
  - 10 years: 36% to 40% (SI, 0.36 to 0.40)
- Infants
  - 3 months: 30% to 36% (SI, 0.30 to 0.36)
  - 1 year: 29% to 41% (SI, 0.29 to 0.41)
- Neonates
  - At birth: 55% to 68% (SI, 0.55 to 0.68)
  - 1 week: 47% to 65% (SI, 0.47 to 0.65)
  - 1 month: 37% to 49% (SI, 0.37 to 0.49)

Hemoglobin (Hb) electrophoresis
- Hb A: 95% (SI, 0.95)
- Hb A$_2$: 1.5% to 3% (SI, 0.015 to 0.03)
- Hb F: <2% (SI, <0.02)

Hemoglobin, unstable
- Heat stability: negative
- Isopropanol: stable

Hemoglobin, urine
Negative

Hemosiderin, urine
Negative

Hepatitis B surface antigen, serum
Negative

Herpes simplex antibodies, serum
Negative

Heterophil agglutination, serum
Normal titer <1:56

Hexosaminidase A and B, serum
Total: 5 to 12.9 U/L (hexosaminidase A constitutes 55% to 76% of total)

Histoplasmosis antibody, serum
Normal titer <1:8

Homovanillic acid, urine
<10 mg/24 hours (SI, <55 µmol/d)

Human chorionic gonadotropin, serum
<4 IU/L

Human chorionic gonadotropin, urine
Pregnant women
- First trimester: 500,000 IU/24 hours
- Second trimester: 10,000 to 25,000 IU/24 hours
- Third trimester: 5,000 to 15,000 IU/24 hours

Human growth hormone, serum
- Males: undetectable to 5 ng/ml (SI, undetectable to 5 µg/L)
- Females: undetectable to 10 ng/ml (SI, undetectable to 10 µg/L)
- Children: undetectable to 16 ng/ml (SI, undetectable to 16 µg/L)

Human immunodeficiency virus antibody, serum
Negative

Human placental lactogen, serum
- Males and nonpregnant females: <0.5 µg/ml
- Pregnant females at term: 9 to 11 µg/ml

17-hydroxycorticosteroids, urine
- Males
  - 4.5 to 12 mg/24 hours (SI, 12.4 to 33.1 µmol/d)
- Females
  - 2.5 to 10 mg/24 hours (SI, 6.9 to 27.6 µmol/d)
- Children
  - 8 to 12 years: <4.5 mg/24 hours (SI, < 12.4 µmol/d)
  - <8 years: <1.5 mg/24 hours (SI, <4.14 µmol/d)

5-hydroxyindoleacetic acid, urine
2 to 7 mg/24 hours (SI, 10.4 to 36.6 µmol/d)

Hydroxyproline, total, urine
1 to 9 mg/24 hours (SI, 1.0 to 3.4 IU/d)

I J

Immune complex, serum
Negative

Immunoglobulins (Ig), serum
- IgG: 800 to 1,800 mg/dl (SI, 8 to 18 g/L)
- IgA: 100 to 400 mg/dl (SI, 1 to 4 g/L)
- IgM: 55 to 150 mg/dl (SI, 0.55 to 1.5 g/L)

Insulin, serum
0 to 35 µU/ml (SI, 144 to 243 pmol/L)

Insulin tolerance test
10- to 20-ng/dl (SI, 10- to 20-µg/L) increase over baseline levels of human growth hormone and adrenocorticotropic hormone

Iron, serum
- Males: 65 to 175 mcg/dl (SI, 11.6 to 31.3 µmol/L)
- Females: 50 to 170 mcg/dl (SI, 9 to 30.4 µmol/L)

Iron, total binding capacity, serum
300 to 360 µg/dl (SI, 54 to 64 µmol/L)

K

17-ketogenic steroids, urine
- Males: 4 to 14 mg/24 hours (SI, 13 to 49 µmol/d)
- Females: 2 to 12 mg/24 hours (SI, 7 to 42 µmol/d)
- Children
- Infants to 11 years: 0.1 to 4 mg/24 hours (SI, 0.3 to 14 µmol/d)
- 11 to 14 years: 2 to 9 mg/24 hours (SI, 7 to 31 µmol/d)

Ketones, urine
Negative

17-ketosteroids, urine
- Males: 10 to 25 mg/24 hours (SI, 35 to 87 µmol/d)
- Females: 4 to 6 mg/24 hours (SI, 4 to 21 µmol/d)
- Children
- Infants to 10 years: <3 mg/24 hours (SI, < 10 µmol/d)
- 10 to 14 years: 1 to 6 mg/24 hours (SI, 2 to 21 µmol/d)

L

Lactate dehydrogenase (LD)
- Total: 71 to 207 IU/L (SI, 1.2 to 3.52 µkat/L)
- LD_1: 14% to 26% (SI, 0.14 to 0.26)
- LD_2: 29% to 39% (SI, 0.29 to 0.39)
- LD_3: 20% to 26% (SI, 0.20 to 0.26)
- LD_4: 8% to 16% (SI, 0.08 to 0.16)
- LD_5: 6% to 16% (SI, 0.06 to 0.16)

Lactic acid, blood
0.5 to 2.2 mEq/L (SI, 0.5 to 2.2 mmol/L)

Leucine aminopeptidase
- Males: 80 to 200 U/ml (SI, 80 to 200 kU/L)
- Females: 75 to 185 U/ml (SI, 75 to 185 kU/L)

Leukoagglutinins
Negative

Lipase, serum
10 to 73 U/L (SI, 0.17 to 1.24 µkat/L)

Lipids, fecal
Constitute <20% of excreted solids; <7 g excreted in 24 hours

Lipoproteins, serum
- High-density lipoprotein cholesterol
- Males: 37 to 70 mg/dl (SI, 0.96 to 1.8 mmol/L)
- Females: 40 to 85 mg/dl (SI, 1.03 to 2.2 mmol/L)
- Low-density lipoprotein cholesterol:
- In individuals who don't have coronary artery disease: <130 mg/dl (SI, <3.36 mmol/L)

Long-acting thyroid stimulator, serum
Negative

Lupus erythematosus cell preparation
Negative

Luteinizing hormone, serum
- Menstruating women
- Follicular phase: 5 to 15 mIU/ml (SI, 5 to 15 IU/L)
- Ovulatory phase: 30 to 60 mIU/ml (SI, 30 to 60 IU/L)
- Luteal phase: 5 to 15 mIU/ml (SI, 5 to 15 IU/L)
- Postmenopausal women
- 50 to 100 mIU/ml (SI, 50 to 100 IU/L)
- Males
- 5 to 20 mIU/ml (SI, 5 to 20 IU/L)
- Children
- 4 to 20 mIU/ml (SI, 4 to 20 IU/L)

Lyme disease serology
Nonreactive

Lysozyme, urine
0 to 3 mg/24 hours

M

Magnesium, serum
1.3 to 2.1 mg/dl (SI, 0.65 to 1.05 mmol/L)

Magnesium, urine
6 to 10 mEq/24 hours (SI, 3 to 5 mmol/d)

Manganese, serum
0.4 to 1.4 µg/ml

Melanin, urine
Negative

Myoglobin, urine
Negative

N

5'-nucleotidase
2 to 17 U/L (SI, 0.034 to 0.29 µkat/L)

O

Occult blood, fecal
<2.5 ml

Oxalate, urine
≤40 mg/24 hours (SI, ≤456 µmol/d)

P Q

Parathyroid hormone, serum
◆ Intact: 10 to 50 pg/ml (SI, 1.1 to 5.3 pmol/L)
◆ N-terminal fraction: 8 to 24 pg/ml (SI, 0.8 to 2.5 pmol/L)
◆ C-terminal fraction: 0 to 340 pg/ml (SI, 0 to 35.8 pmol/L)

Partial thromboplastin time
21 to 35 seconds (SI, 21 to 35 s)

Pericardial fluid
◆ Amount: 10 to 50 ml
◆ Appearance: clear, straw-colored
◆ White blood cell count: <1,000/µl (SI, <1.0 × 10⁹/L)
◆ Glucose: approximately whole blood level

Peritoneal fluid
◆ Amount: <50 ml
◆ Appearance: clear, straw-colored

Phenylalanine, serum
<2 mg/dl (SI, <121 µmol/L)

Phosphates, serum
◆ Adults: 2.7 to 4.5 mEq/L (SI, 0.87 to 1.45 mmol/L)
◆ Children: 4.5 to 6.7 mEq/L (SI, 1.45 to 1.78 mmol/L)

Phosphates, urine
<1,000 mg/24 hours

Phospholipids, plasma
180 to 320 mg/dl (SI, 1.80 to 3.20 g/L)

Plasma renin activity
◆ Normal sodium diet: 1.1 to 4.1 ng/ml/hour (SI, 0.30 to 1.14 ng LS)
◆ Restricted sodium diet: 6.2 to 12.4 ng/ml/hour (SI, 1.72 to 3.44 ng LS)

Phosphate, tubular reabsorption, urine and plasma
80% reabsorption

Plasminogen, plasma
80% to 130%

Platelet aggregation
3 to 5 minutes (SI, 3 to 5 m)

Platelet count
◆ Adults: 140,000 to 400,000/µl (SI, 140 to 400 × 10⁹/L)
◆ Children: 150,000 to 450,000/µl (SI, 150 to 450 × 10⁹/L)

Potassium, serum
3.5 to 5 mEq/L (SI, 3.5 to 5 mmol/L)

Potassium, urine
◆ Adults: 25 to 125 mmol/24 hours (SI, 25 to 125 mmol/d)
◆ Children: 22 to 57 mmol/24 hours (SI, 22 to 57 mmol/d)

Pregnanediol, urine
◆ Nonpregnant females
– 0.5 to 1.5 mg/24 hours (during the follicular phase of the menstrual cycle)
◆ Pregnant females
– First trimester: 10 to 30 mg/24 hours
– Second trimester: 35 to 70 mg/24 hours
– Third trimester: 70 to 100 mg/24 hours
◆ Postmenopausal females
– 0.2 to 1 mg/24 hours
◆ Males
– 0 to 1 mg/24 hours

Pregnanetriol, urine
◆ Males ≥ 16 years: 0.4 to 2.5 mg/24 hours (SI, 1.2 to 7.5 µmol/d)
◆ Females ≥ 16 years: 0 to 1.8 mg/ hours (SI, 0.3 to 5.3 µmol/d)

Progesterone, plasma
◆ Menstruating females
– Follicular phase: <150 ng/dl (SI, <5 nmol/L)
– Luteal phase: 300 to 1,200 ng/dl (SI, 10 to 40 nmol/L)
◆ Pregnant women
– First trimester: 1,500 to 5,000 ng/dl (SI, 50 to 160 nmol/L)
– Second and third trimesters: 8,000 to 20,000 ng/dl (SI, 250 to 650 nmol/L)

Prolactin, serum
Undetectable to 23 ng/ml (SI, undetectable to 23 µg/L)

Prostate-specific antigen
◆ 40 to 50 years: 2 to 2.8 ng/ml (SI, 2 to 2.8 µg/L)
◆ 51 to 60 years: 2.9 to 3.8 ng/ml (SI, 2.9 to 3.8 µg/L)
◆ 61 to 70 years: 4 to 5.3 ng/ml (SI, 4 to 5.3 µg/L)
◆ ≥71 years: 5.6 to 7.2 ng/ml (SI, 5.6 to 7.2 µg/L)

Protein, cerebrospinal fluid
15 to 50 mg/dl (SI, 0.15 to 0.5 g/L)

Protein C, plasma
70% to 140% (SI, 0.70 to 1.40)

Protein, total, peritoneal fluid
0.3 to 4.1 g/dl (SI, 3 to 41 g/L)

Protein, urine
50 to 80 mg/24 hours (SI, 50 to 80 mg/d)

Prothrombin time
10 to 14 seconds (10 to 14 s)

Pulmonary artery pressures
◆ Right atrial: 1 to 6 mm Hg
◆ Left atrial: approximately 10 mm Hg
◆ Systolic: 20 to 30 mm Hg
◆ Systolic right ventricular: 20 to 30 mm Hg
◆ Diastolic: 10 to 15 mm Hg
◆ End-diastolic right ventricular: <5 mm Hg
◆ Mean: <20 mm Hg
◆ Pulmonary artery wedge pressure: 6 to 12 mm Hg

Pyruvate kinase
◆ Ultraviolet: 9 to 22 U/g of hemoglobin
◆ Low substrate assay: 1.7 to 6.8 U/g of hemoglobin

Pyruvic acid, blood
0.08 to 0.16 mEq/L (SI, 0.08 to 0.16 mmol/L)

R

Red blood cell count
◆ Males: 4.2 to 5.4 × 106/mm³ (SI, 4.2 to 5.4 × 10^{12}/L)
◆ Females: 3.6 to 5.0 × 106/mm³ (SI, 3.6 to 5 × 10^{12}/L)
◆ Neonates: 4.4 to 5.8 million/µl (SI, 4.4 to 5.8 × 10^{12}/L)
◆ 2 months: 3 to 3.8 million/µl (SI, 3 to 3.8 × 10^{12}/L)
(increasing slowly)
◆ Children: 4.6 to 4.8 million/µl (SI, 4.6 to 4.8 × 10^{12}/L)

Red blood cell survival time
25 to 35 days

Red blood cells, urine
0 to 3 per high-power field

Red cell indices
◆ Mean corpuscular volume: 84 to 99 µm3 (SI, 84 to 99 fL)
◆ Mean corpuscular hemoglobin: 26 to 32 pg/cell (SI, 0.40 to 0.53 fmol/cell)
◆ Mean corpuscular hemoglobin concentration: 30 to 36 g/dl (SI, 300 to 360 g/L)

Respiratory syncytial virus antibodies, serum
Negative

Reticulocyte count
◆ Adults: 0.5% to 2.5% (SI, 0.005 to 0.025)
◆ Infants (at birth): 2% to 6% (SI, 0.02 to 0.06), decreasing to adult levels in 1 to 2 weeks

Rheumatoid factor, serum
Negative or titer <1:20

Ribonucleoprotein antibodies
Negative

Rubella antibodies, serum
Titer of 1:8 or less indicates little or no immunity; titer more than 1:10 indicates adequate protection against rubella

S

Semen analysis
◆ Volume: 0.7 to 6.5 ml
◆ pH: 7.3 to 7.9
◆ Liquefaction: within 20 minutes
◆ Sperm count: 20 to 150 million/ml

Sickle cell test
Negative

Sjögren's antibodies
Negative

Sodium chloride, urine
110 to 250 mEq/L (SI, 100 to 250 mmol/d)

Sodium, serum
135 to 145 mEq/L (SI, 135 to 145 mmol/L)

Sodium, urine
◆ Adults: 40 to 220 mEq/L/24 hours (SI, 40 to 220 mmol/d)
◆ Children: 41 to 115 mEq/L/24 hours (SI, 41 to 115 mmol/d)

Sporotrichosis antibody, serum
Normal titers <1:40

T

Terminal deoxynucleotidyl transferase, serum
◆ Bone marrow: <2%
◆ Blood: undetectable

Testosterone, plasma or serum
◆ Males: 300 to 1,200 ng/dl (SI, 10.4 to 41.6 nmol/L)
◆ Females: 20 to 80 ng/dl (SI, 0.7 to 2.8 nmol/L)

Thrombin time, plasma
10 to 15 seconds (10 to 15 s)

Thyroid-stimulating hormone, neonatal
◆ ≤2 days: 25 to 30 µIU/ml (SI, 25 to 30 mU/L)
◆ >2 days: <25 µIU/ml (SI, <25 mU/L)

Thyroid-stimulating hormone, serum
Undetectable to 15 µIU/ml (SI, undetectable to 15 mU/L)

Thyroid-stimulating immunoglobulin, serum
Negative

Thyroxine, total, serum
5 to 13.5 µg/dl (SI, 60 to 165 nmol/L)

T-lymphocyte count
1,500 to 3,000/µl

Transferrin, serum
200 to 400 mg/dl (SI, 2 to 4 g/L)

Triglycerides, serum
◆ Males: 44 to 180 mg/dl (SI, 0.44 to 2.01 mmol/L)
◆ Females: 11 to 190 mg/dl (SI, 0.11 to 2.21 mmol/L)

Triiodothyronine, serum
80 to 200 ng/dl (SI, 1.2 to 3 nmol/L)

U

Uric acid, serum
◆ Males: 3.4 to 7 mg/dl (SI, 202 to 416 µmol/L)
◆ Females: 2.3 to 6 mg/dl (SI, 143 to 357 µmol/L)

Uric acid, urine
250 to 750 mg/24 hours (SI, 1.48 to 4.43 mmol/d)

Urinalysis, routine
◆ Color: straw to dark yellow
◆ Appearance: clear
◆ Specific gravity: 1.005 to 1.035
◆ pH: 4.5 to 8.0
◆ Epithelial cells: 0 to 5 per high-power field
◆ Casts: none, except 1 to 2 hyaline casts per low-power field
◆ Crystals: present

Urine osmolality
◆ 24-hour urine: 300 to 900 mOsm/kg
◆ Random urine: 50 to 1,400 mOsm/kg

Urobilinogen, fecal
50 to 300 mg/24 hours (SI, 100 to 400 EU/100 g)

Urobilinogen, urine
◆ 0.1 to 0.8 EU/2 hours (SI 0.1 to 0.8 EU/2 h)
or
◆ 0.5 to 4.0 EU/24 hours (SI, 0.5 to 4.0 EU/d)

Uroporphyrinogen I synthase
≥7 nmol/second/L

V

Vanillylmandelic acid, urine
1.4 to 6.5 mg/24 hours (SI, 7 to 33 µmol/day)

Venereal Disease Research Laboratory test, cerebrospinal fluid
Negative

Venereal Disease Research Laboratory test, serum
Negative

Vitamin A, serum
30 to 80 µg/dl (SI, 1.05 to 2.8 µmol/L)

Vitamin B_2, serum
3 to 15 µg/dl

Vitamin B_{12}, serum
200 to 900 pg/ml (SI, 148 to 664 pmol/L)

Vitamin C, plasma
0.2 to 2 mg/dl (SI, 11 to 114 µmol/L)

Vitamin C, urine
30 mg/24 hours

Vitamin D_3, serum
10 to 60 ng/ml (SI, 25 to 150 nmol/L)

W X Y

White blood cell count, blood
4,000 to 10,000/µl (SI, 4 to 10 × 10⁹/L)

White blood cell count, peritoneal fluid
<300/µl (SI, <300 × 10⁹/L)

White blood cell count, urine
0 to 4 per high-power field

White blood cell differential, blood
◆ Adults
- Neutrophils: 54% to 75% (SI, 0.54 to 0.75)
- Lymphocytes: 25% to 40% (SI, 0.25 to 0.40)
- Monocytes: 2% to 8% (SI, 0.02 to 0.08)
- Eosinophils: 1% to 4% (SI, 0.01 to 0.04)
- Basophils: 0 to 1% (SI, 0 to 0.01)

Z

Zinc, serum
70 to 120 µg/dl (SI, 10.7 to 18.4 µmol/L)

Blood factors and products

ABO COMPATIBILITY
- Cross-matching method of typing blood that identifies two antigens on red blood cells (RBCs): A and B
  - Type A blood has A antigens and anti-B antibodies (may receive type A and O blood)
  - Type B blood has B antigens and anti-A antibodies (may receive type B and O blood)
  - Type O blood has no antigens and anti-A and anti-B antibodies (universal donor; may receive type O blood)
  - Type AB blood has both A and B antigens and no antibodies (universal recipient)
- Ideally, transfusions should use the patient's own blood type.

RH FACTOR
- Rh-positive blood possesses the Rh antigen.
- Rh-negative blood doesn't possess the Rh antigen.
- If an Rh-negative patient is exposed to Rh-positive blood, an injection of Rh immune globulin can be given within 72 hours of exposure.

HUMAN LEUKOCYTE ANTIGEN (HLA)
- Located on the surface of circulating platelets, white blood cells (WBCs), and most tissue cells.
- Responsible for febrile reactions during blood transfusions.
- Administration of HLA-matched platelets before administration of blood with platelets from several donors decreases the risk of an antigen-antibody reaction.

TYPES OF BLOOD PRODUCTS
Whole blood
- Used when the patient has lost more than 25% total blood volume.
- Used to treat hemorrhage, trauma, or major burns.
- Should be avoided if fluid overload is a concern.

Packed RBCs
- Prepared by removing about 90% of the plasma surrounding the cells and adding an anticoagulant preservative.
- Helps to restore or maintain the oxygen-carrying capacity of the blood in patients with anemia or to correct blood losses during or after surgery.
- Removal of about 70% of leukocytes reduces the risk of febrile, nonhemolytic reactions.

Granulocytes (WBCs)
- Rarely used.
- May be given to treat gram-negative sepsis or progressive soft-tissue infection that's unresponsive to an antimicrobial.

Fresh frozen plasma
- Prepared by separating plasma from RBCs and freezing it within 6 hours of collection.
- Contains plasma proteins, water, fibrinogen, some clotting factors, electrolytes, sugar, vitamins, minerals, hormones, and antibodies.
- Used to treat hemorrhage, expand plasma volume, correct undetermined coagulation factor deficiencies, replace specific clotting factors, and correct factor deficiencies resulting from liver disease.

Cryoprecipitate (factor VIII)
- Consists of insoluble portion of plasma recovered from fresh frozen plasma.
- Used to treat von Willebrand's disease, hypofibrinogenemia, factor VIII deficiency (antihemophilic factor), hemophilia A, and disseminated intravascular coagulation.

Albumin
- Extracted from plasma; contains globulin and other proteins.
- Used for patients with acute liver failure, burns, or trauma; those who have had surgery; and neonates with hemolytic disease when crystalloids prove ineffective.
- Increases plasma oncotic pressure, coaxing fluid from the interstitial space across normal capillary membranes and into the intravascular space.
- Also used to treat hypoproteinemia with or without edema.

Platelets
- Used for patients who have platelet dysfunction or thrombocytopenia; those who have had multiple transfusions of stored blood; acute leukemia; or bone marrow abnormalities.
- May cause febrile or mild allergic reactions.

Internet resources

AIDS
National AIDS Hotline
www.ashastd.org/nah

CDC National Prevention Information
Network
www.cdcnpin.org

Association of Nurses in AIDS Care
www.anacnet.org

Alcoholism
Al-Anon/Alateen Family Group
Headquarters
www.al-anon-alateen.org

Alcoholics Anonymous world Services
www.alcoholics-anonymous.org

Alzheimer's disease
The Alzheimer's Association
www.alz.org

Alzheimer's Disease Education & Referral
Center
www.alzheimers.org

Arthritis
Arthritis Foundation
www.arthritis.org

National Institute of Arthritis and
Musculoskeletal and Skin Diseases
www.nih.gov/niams

Asthma
Asthma & Allergy Foundation of America
www.aafa.org

American Academy of Allergy, Asthma &
Immunology
www.aaaai.org

American Lung Association
www.lungusa.com

Cancer
American Cancer Society
www.cancer.org

Skin Cancer Foundation
www.skincancer.org

Cancer Information Service
www.cis.nci.nih.gov

Cancer Care
www.cancercare.org

Association of Cancer Online Resources
www.acor.org

National Alliance of Breast Cancer
Organizations
www.nabco.org

The Susan G. Komen Breast Cancer
Foundations
www.komen.org

Y-Me National Breast Cancer Organization
www.y-me.org

Us Too! International
www.ustoo.com

Dermatology
American Academy of Dermatology
www.aad.org

Diabetes
American Diabetes Association
www.diabetes.org

Juvenile Diabetes Foundation
www.jdf.org

American Association of Diabetes Educators
www.aadenet.org

The Neuropathy Association
www.neuropathy.org

Epilepsy
Epilepsy Foundation of America
www.efa.org

Genetic disorders
Cystic Fibrosis Foundation
www.cff.org

National Marfan Foundation
www.marfan.org

National Tay-Sachs and Allied Diseases
Association
www.ntsad.org

Gastrointestinal disorders
Crohn's and Colitis Foundation of America
www.ccfa.org

National Institute of Diabetes and Digestive
and Kidney Diseases
www.niddk.nih.gov

Headache
American Council for Headache Education
www.achenet.org

National Headache Foundation
www.headaches.org

New England Center for Headache
www.headachenech.com

Heart disease
American Heart Association
www.americanheart.org

Hemophilia
National Hemophilia Foundation
www.hemophilia.org

Hepatitis
American Liver Foundation
www.liverfoundation.org

Hepatitis Foundation International
www.hepfi.org

Hepatitis B Foundation
www.hepb.org

Infectious diseases
Centers for Disease Control and Prevention
www.cdc.gov

Lupus
Lupus Foundation of American
www.lupus.org

Lyme disease
Lyme Disease Foundation
www.lyme.org

Mental retardation
Association for Retarded Citizens
www.thearc.org

Miscellaneous
National Library of Medicine
www.nlm.nih.gov

American Academy of Family Physicians
www.aafp.org

National Heart, Lung & Blood Institute
www.nhlbi.nih.gov

United Ostomy Association
www.uoa.org

Wound, Ostomy & Continence Nurse
Society
www.wocn.org

American Academy of Otolaryngology —
Head and Neck Surgery
www.entnet.org

American Rhinologic Society
www.american-rhinologic.org

American Lung Association
www.lungusa.org

Multiple sclerosis
National Multiple Sclerosis Society
www.nmss.org

Myasthenia gravis
Myasthenia Gravis Foundation
www.myasthenia.org

Neurofibromatosis
National Neurofibromatosis Foundation
www.nf.org

Orthopedics
American Society for Surgery of the Hand
www.assh.org

American Academy of Orthopaedic Surgeons
www.aaos.org

National Osteoporosis Foundation
www.nof.org

Pain
American Chronic Pain Association
www.theacpa.org

Parkinson's disease
National Parkinson Foundation
www.parkinson.org

American Parkinson Disease Foundation
www.apdaparkinson.com

Pediatrics
American Academy of Pediatrics
www.aap.org

Psychiatric & mental Illness
Depression and Bipolar Support Alliance
www.dbsalliance.org

National Foundation for Depressive Illness
www.depression.org

National Mental Health Association
www.nmha.org

Renal
National Kidney Foundation
www.kidney.org

Reye's syndrome
National Reye's Syndrome Foundation
www.reyessyndrome.org

Sickle cell anemia
Sickle Cell Disease Association of America
www.sicklecelldisease.org

Stroke
National Stroke Association
www.stroke.org

National Institute of Neurological Disorders
and Stroke
www.ninds.nih.gov

Thyroid
Thyroid Foundation of America
www.tsh.com

Selected references

Berry, B., and Pinard, A. "Assessing Tissue Oxygenation," *Critical Care Nurse* 22(3):22-40, June 2002.

Braunwald, E., et al. *Harrison's Principles of Internal Medicine,* 16th ed. New York: McGraw-Hill Book Co., 2005.

Cheung, R.T., and Hachinski V. "Cardiac Effects of Stroke: Current Treatment Options," *Cardiovascular Medicine* 6(3):199-207, June 2004.

Eliopoulos, C. *Gerontological Nursing,* 6th ed. Philadelphia: Lippincott Williams & Wilkins, 2005.

Habif, T.P. *Clinical Dermatology,* 4th ed. St.Louis: Mosby–Year Book, Inc., 2003.

Hickey, J. *The Clinical Practice of Neurological and Neurosurgical Nursing,* 5th ed. Philadelphia: Lippincott Williams & Wilkins, 2003.

Ignatavicius, D.D., and Workman, M.L. *Medical-Surgical Nursing: Critical Thinking for Collaborative Care,* 5th ed. Philadelphia: W.B. Saunders Co., 2005.

Nursing2004 Herbal Medicine Handbook, 2nd ed. Philadelphia: Lippincott Williams & Wilkins, 2004.

Okada, Y., and Ohtomo, K. "Abdominal Computed Tomography Manifestation of Multiple-Organ-System Disorders," *Radiologist* 10(6):309-22, November 2003.

Paran, D., et al. "Pulmonary Disease in Systemic Lupus Erythematosus and the Antiphospholpid Syndrome," *Autoimmune Review* 3(1):70-75, January 2004.

Porth, C.M. *Pathophysiology Concepts of Altered Health States,* 7th ed. Philadelphia: Lippincott Williams & Wilkins, 2005.

Professional Guide to Diseases, 8th ed. Philadelphia: Lippincott Williams & Wilkins, 2005.

Professional Guide to Pathophysiology. Philadelphia: Lippincott Williams & Wilkins. 2003.

Woods, S., et al. *Cardiac Nursing,* 5th ed. Philadelphia: Lippincott Williams & Wilkins, 2005.

Index

i refers to an illustration; t refers to a table.

i refers to an illustration; t refers to a table.

i refers to an illustration; t refers to a table.

---

i refers to an illustration; t refers to a table.

i refers to an illustration; t refers to a table.

i refers to an illustration; t refers to a table.

i refers to an illustration; t refers to a table.

i refers to an illustration; t refers to a table.

---

i refers to an illustration; t refers to a table.

i refers to an illustration; t refers to a table.

i refers to an illustration; t refers to a table.

i refers to an illustration; t refers to a table.

i refers to an illustration; t refers to a table.

i refers to an illustration; t refers to a table.